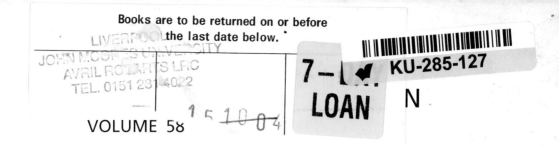

The changing face of HIV and AIDS

Scientific Editors

Robin A Weiss

Michael W Adler

Sarah L Rowland-Jones

Series Editors
L K Borysiewicz PhD FRCP
M J Walport PhD FRCP

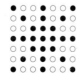

OXFORD
UNIVERSITY PRESS

PUBLISHED FOR THE BRITISH COUNCIL BY
OXFORD UNIVERSITY PRESS

OXFORD UNIVERSITY PRESS
Great Clarendon Street, Oxford OX2 6DP, UK

British Library Cataloguing in Publication Data
A catalogue record for this book is available from the British Library
ISBN 0–19–922486–2
ISSN 0007–1420

Subscription information *British Medical Bulletin* is published quarterly on behalf of The British Council. Subscription rates for 2001 are £160/$275 for four volumes, each of one issue. Prices include distribution and is distributed by surface mail within Europe, by air freight and second class post within the USA*, and by various methods of air-speeded delivery to all other countries. Subscription orders, single issue orders and enquiries for 2001 should be sent to:

Oxford University Press, Great Clarendon Street, Oxford OX2 6DP, UK
(Tel +44 (0)1865 267907; Fax +44(0)1865 267485; E-mail: jnl.orders@oup.co.uk

*Periodicals postage paid at Rahway, NJ. US Postmaster: Send address changes to *British Medical Bulletin*, c/o Mercury Airfreight International Ltd, 365 Blair Road, Avenel, NJ 07001, USA.

Back numbers of titles published 1996–2000 (see inside back cover) are available from The Royal Society of Medicine Press Limited, 1 Wimpole St, London W1G 0AE, UK. (Tel. +44 (0)20 7290 2921; Fax +44 (0)20 7290 2929); www.rsm.ac.uk/pub/bmb/htm).

Pre-1996 back numbers: Contact Jill Kettley, Subscriptions Manager, Harcourt Brace, Foots Cray, Sidcup, Kent DA14 5HP (Tel +44 (0)20 8308 5700; Fax +44 (0)20 8309 0807).

This journal is indexed, abstracted and/or published online in the following media: Adonis, Biosis, BRS Colleague (full text), Chemical Abstracts, Colleague (Online), Current Contents/ Clinical Medicine, Current Contents/Life Sciences, Elsevier BIOBASE/Current Awareness in Biological Sciences, EMBASE/Excerpta Medica, Index Medicus/Medline, Medical Documentation Service, Reference Update, Research Alert, Science Citation Index, Scisearch, SIIC-Database Argentina, UMI (Microfilms)

Editorial services and typesetting by BA & GM Haddock, Ford, Midlothian, Scotland
Printed in Great Britain by Bell & Bain Ltd, Glasgow, Scotland.

The changing face of HIV and AIDS

Scientific Editors: *Robin A Weiss, Michael W Adler and Sarah L Rowland-Jones*

http://www.bmb.oupjournals.org

Acknowledgements

The planning committee for this issue of the *British Medical Bulletin* was chaired by Professor Robin Weiss and also included Professor Michael Adler and Professor Sarah Rowland-Jones.

The British Council and Oxford University Press are most grateful to them for their help and advice and for their valuable work as Scientific Editors in completing this issue.

Preface

It is now 20 years since acquired immune deficiency syndrome (AIDS) was first recognised as a novel disease. Since then, it has burgeoned from a few sentinel cases among 'high risk' groups to become a world-wide pandemic. Some 22 million people have died as a result of AIDS and over 37 million women, men and children are currently infected with the human immunodeficiency virus (HIV). The epidemic has left behind a cumulative total of over 13 million orphans. Traditional family structures and extended families are breaking down under the strain of HIV. Population growth and death rates are increasingly affected. Life expectancies in countries with adult prevalences of over 10% (*e.g.* Botswana, Kenya, Zimbabwe, South Africa, Zambia, Rwanda) are expected to see an average reduction of 17 years by 2010–2015. Young, highly productive adults die at the peak of their output which has considerable impact on a country's economy.

HIV actually constitutes two distinct types of lentivirus, HIV-1 and HIV-2, which have a slightly different genetic make-up and different origins. HIV-1 is further classified into three major groups, M, N and O. Group M, which represents the global spread of HIV, comprises numerous subtypes or clades, A to H, that have blossomed in different geographic regions. Both HIV-1 and HIV-2 are new infections to humankind. HIV-1 is thought to have crossed host species to humans from chimpanzees, whereas HIV-2 clearly comes from sooty mangabey monkeys. Both types of HIV cause AIDS with essentially the same symptoms of disease, but a higher proportion of those infected with HIV-2 appear to survive as long-term non-progressors.

There has been rapid progress in our medical and scientific understanding of AIDS and HIV. Within 2 years of noting AIDS as a distinctive syndrome in 1981, HIV-1 was identified, and within a year of learning how to propagate the virus, experimental serological research had been developed into reliable and robust diagnostic tests for blood screening. By late 1985, all industrialised countries had instituted universal screening of blood and tissue donors. The first anti-HIV drug started clinical trials in 1986 and, since 1996, combination anti-retroviral therapy has resulted in a 67% fall in AIDS mortality among those HIV-infected persons who had access to treatment. On the other hand, progress in translating immunological and virological research into a safe, efficacious vaccine has not yet matched the progress in treatment.

HIV/AIDS has emerged to become the overwhelming health issue confronting the world today. Daunting medical, social and economic problems remain in designing, delivering and implementing preventive measures to curb the HIV pandemic. In the following pages, leading investigators of HIV and AIDS present authoritative overviews on the nature of HIV, its epidemiology and pathogenesis, on the medical and social impact of intervention, treatment and prevention. We are grateful to them all for presenting an up-to-date and balanced account of the changing face of HIV and AIDS.

Robin A Weiss
Michael W Adler
Sarah L Rowland-Jones

Introduction

Peter Piot

Executive Director, UNAIDS, Geneva, Switzerland

In June 2001, the world not only marked the twentieth anniversary of the first report of AIDS, but also held its highest level meeting ever on the subject: a special session of the United Nations General Assembly.

Twenty years of the epidemic have taught us that HIV is a formidable enemy both biologically and socio-politically. HIV is perhaps the most complex problem facing humanity today – without doubt it is the most devastating disease humankind has ever faced. A cumulative total of 60 million people have been infected, 22 million of whom have died.

Recent months have seen a new level of energy from scientific and policy communities in insisting that the world is ready to vastly increase the scale of the AIDS response as well as deal with its complexity.

The General Assembly Special Session on HIV/AIDS set new ground-rules for national accountability. Every member state of the United Nations signed on to a Declaration that commits them to a comprehensive AIDS response. The agreed Declaration of Commitment endorsed specific targets against which progress in responding to the epidemic can be measured – for example in relation to young people, where the goal is a 25% reduction in prevalence in the most affected countries by 2005 and 25% globally by 2010.

But even the full and immediate implementation of these commitments will not see the end of the epidemic. At best it will represent 'the end of the beginning'.

In order to make significant progress in meeting any of the targets set by the General Assembly, there needs to be an order-of-magnitude boost in spending on the AIDS response in non-industrialised countries. The General Assembly joined other bodies such as the Organisation of African Unity and the G8 in declaring support for a new Global AIDS and Health Fund. By July, $1.4 billion had already been pledged to the Fund, which was called for by United Nations' Secretary General Kofi Annan only in April 2001.

The fund will be an important new source of resources, but it cannot be the only one. Continued intergovernmental assistance through bilateral channels, national budget allocations, funds liberated through further debt relief or cancellation, social insurance, and private sector efforts will all be needed.

The detailed calculations by UNAIDS and its collaborators on the resource needs of low-and middle-income countries show that by 2005,

Correspondence to:
Dr Peter Piot, Executive
Director, UNAIDS,
20 avenue Appia, 1211
Geneva 27, Switzerland

$9.2 billion ought to be spent on AIDS annually: $4.8 billion on prevention and $4.4 billion on care[1].

This level of spending would provide 6 billion condoms, treatment for 22 million sexually transmitted infections, and voluntary counselling and testing for 9 million people. An additional 35 million women would receive testing at prenatal clinics and 900,000 would receive antiretrovirals to prevent mother-to-child transmission. Special prevention programs would reach almost 6 million sex workers, 28 million men who have sex with men and 3 million injecting drug users.

The past year has seen a convergence of science, economics and policy on the question of resources. Demanding billions for the response to AIDS in the non-industrialised world has moved from being a naïve plea to a political imperative.

At the same time, access to a wider range of HIV care has moved from the realm of the impossible to the possible. For many years, the price of drugs seemed to be an impassable barrier. But today, preferential prices for non-industrialised countries for AIDS drugs have been widely accepted within both the pharmaceutical industry and by policy makers, with benchmark prices for non-industrialised countries falling to 5% or less of those paid in wealthy countries.

A radically new context is emerging in which the prospects for major global advances in both HIV care and prevention have markedly improved. Progress depends on linking prevention and care, as both work best when they work together. Successful prevention and care build a common constituency for action.

In the North, where most people with HIV have been able to access the new combinations of HIV antiretrovirals, mortality dropped sharply in 1996 and 1997 and has since plateaued. Attention has been focused on the complex medical problem of adjusting drug combinations to stay one step ahead of a mutating drug-resistant virus, but meanwhile, progress on prevention fell behind.

In nearly every high-income country, the past few years have seen the epidemic move into poorer and more marginalised parts of the community. Indigenous, migrant and heterosexual populations are comprising a growing proportion of a more complex epidemic. Among gay men, once the champions of behaviour change, unsafe sex is on the rise – from London to San Francisco, Sydney to Vancouver – and rising HIV infections are the result.

Meanwhile, in the South, the slogan 'prevention is the only cure' began to sound morally bankrupt in the face of growing numbers of infections and the limited level of national and global resources available to address the epidemic. For as long as the South is denied access to the treatments that have transformed AIDS in wealthy countries, it is denied not only hope, but also any incentive for people to go for HIV testing.

Antiretrovirals are no magic bullet, and unless extending access is managed carefully their benefits in lives prolonged will last for only a few years. But there is a key opportunity for the South to gain the benefits of sustainably enhanced care while avoiding the divorce between prevention and care that threatens to undermine the response in the North.

AIDS is a large-scale humanitarian emergency, but it is a long-term emergency. We are only just beginning to realise that, globally, the epidemic is still in its early stages. The natural dynamic of AIDS is to show up first among the most exposed populations, but only after decades will the final shape of the epidemic become evident.

The thought that the AIDS epidemic is only beginning is a daunting one – but it ought also be a hopeful one. The fact is that the future course of the epidemic can be changed. Investment now will prevent tens of millions of new infections as well as extend the lives of millions already living with HIV. It also justifies according special priority to young people – changing behaviours and expectations early will result in a life-time of benefit both in HIV prevention and in helping to overcome HIV-related stigma.

For the first time in the history of this epidemic we have the opportunity to turn the tide on a truly large scale – the scale that matches the extent of the epidemic. We know what we need to do to slow new infections, and provide care for those who are ill. The only question, 20 years after that first report of the disease called AIDS, is whether we have the will to do it. History will be our judge.

Reference

1   Schwartländer B, Stover J, Walker N *et al*. Resource needs for HIV/AIDS. *Science* 2001; **292**: 2434–6

The global epidemiology of HIV/AIDS

Linda Morison

MRC Tropical Epidemiology Group, Infectious Disease Epidemiology Unit, Department of Infectious and Tropical Diseases, London School of Hygiene and Tropical Medicine, London, UK

In this paper, the ways in which HIV is transmitted and factors facilitating transmission are described, although we still do not fully understand why the HIV epidemic has spread so heterogeneously across the globe. Estimates of HIV prevalence vary in quality but give some idea of trends in different countries and regions. Of all regions in the world, sub-Saharan Africa is the hardest hit by HIV, containing around 70% of people living with HIV/AIDS. There are, however, recent signs of hope in Africa due to a slight reduction in the number of new HIV cases in the year 2000. Most countries in Asia have not seen explosive epidemics in the general population up to now but patterns of injecting drug use (IDU) and sex work are conducive to the spread of HIV so there is no room for complacency. Unpredictable epidemics among IDU in the former Soviet Union have the potential to spread into the general population. Some countries in Central America and the Caribbean have growing HIV epidemics with adult prevalences second only to sub-Saharan Africa. Reductions in morbidity and mortality through the use of highly active antiretroviral therapy are at present limited to high-income and some Latin American countries. Both the cost of these therapies and the poor health care delivery systems in many affected countries need to be addressed before antiretrovirals can benefit the majority of people living with HIV/AIDS.

Correspondence to:
Dr Linda Morison, MRC Tropical Epidemiology Group, Infectious Disease Epidemiology Unit, Department of Infectious and Tropical Diseases, London School of Hygiene and Tropical Medicine, Keppel Street, London WC1E 7HT, UK

In 1981, the Centers for Disease Control and Prevention reported unusual clusters of *Pneumocystis carinii* pneumonia and Kaposi's sarcoma in gay men in parts of the US[1]. These were the first reported cases of Acquired Immune Deficiency Syndrome (AIDS). Twenty years later, the global HIV/AIDS epidemic has killed an estimated 21.8 million people and another 36.1 million are living with HIV infection[2]. Around 95% of these people live in non-industrialised countries with few financial resources to deal with the HIV/AIDS epidemic and where hard won social and economic development is most vulnerable to the heavy burden that HIV/AIDS puts upon it. Over 90% of people living with HIV/AIDS do not know they are infected and even if they did antiretroviral therapies (ART) are not at present an option for them. Most people living with HIV/AIDS are in the economically productive age-group supporting children and elderly relatives and most will receive minimal care when they finally develop AIDS-related illness. From many aspects the global HIV/AIDS epidemic is an enormous tragedy for humankind.

HIV transmission

The estimated 57.9 million people who have been infected with HIV since the pandemic began have, with a few exceptions, caught the virus by one of three modes of transmission: sexual, parenteral and mother-to-child. HIV-1 is the virus type responsible for the global pandemic. HIV-2 is less easily transmitted than HIV-1 and is confined mainly to West Africa[3]. There is at present no convincing evidence to suggest that different HIV-1 subtypes have different transmission probabilities[4].

Sexual transmission of HIV

Sexual transmission is by far the most common mode of transmission globally. Obviously the probability of a person being infected *via* sexual intercourse depends on the likelihood of unprotected sex with an infected partner, so sexual behaviour patterns and the background prevalence of HIV are of major importance. Interventions to change sexual behaviour (mainly partner reduction) and to promote condom use are, therefore, a vital component of any HIV control programme and have been shown to be effective in individual studies and at the national level[5,6].

The chance that a person becomes infected with HIV during one particular sexual contact varies greatly and depends on many factors[7]. Male to female penile-vaginal transmission appears to be 2–3 times more efficient than female to male transmission[8,9] and there is some evidence that first sexual intercourse for females may be associated with particularly high transmission probabilities[10,11]. Receptive anal intercourse appears to be more risky than receptive vaginal intercourse with obvious implications for spread amongst men who have sex with men (MSM)[12]. Cases of infection by oral sex have been reported but this mode of transmission is believed to be much less risky than penile-vaginal or penile-anal sex[7].

Sexual transmission of HIV also depends greatly on the infectiousness of the infected partner. Higher viral loads in the later stages of the disease are associated with increased probability of transmission but infectiousness has also been shown to be higher around the time of seroconversion[13,14]. ART, which reduces infectiousness, therefore has implications for transmission of HIV as well as affecting the morbidity and mortality of those living with HIV/AIDS[15,16].

Sexual transmission of HIV is enhanced by the presence of another sexually transmitted infection (STI), especially an ulcerative one such as chancroid, syphilis or herpes simplex virus 2 (HSV2)[17,18]. STI control programmes are, therefore, an important component of HIV prevention programmes and have been shown to be effective in reducing incidence of HIV in the early stages of an HIV epidemic where a substantial proportion of STIs are treatable[19]. However, there is some doubt about their effectiveness for HIV control in areas where the HIV epidemic is mature and transmission probabilities are dominated by viral load and infections which are difficult to treat in non-industrialised countries, such as HSV2 and bacterial vaginosis[20,21].

The evidence for a partially protective effect of male circumcision is now compelling[22,23] and studies examining the acceptability and feasibility of promoting male circumcision for HIV prevention are underway[24]. Other factors which may increase the transmission probability of HIV include the insertion of herbs or other substances into the vagina by some women in sub-Saharan Africa to facilitate dry and tight sex[25] and use of some types of contraception[7]. Recent reviews[26,27] suggest that forced or coercive sex may also be associated with increased transmission probabilities for women.

Parenteral transmission of HIV

Parenteral transmission of HIV occurs most commonly among IDU when needles are shared. Prevention of transmission between IDU can be achieved by community outreach and needle exchange programmes[5] although political reluctance to work with IDU can be difficult to overcome. Parenteral transmission can also occur by the transfusion of infected blood, so screening blood and/or reducing the unnecessary use of transfusions are necessary to minimise transmission by this route. Contaminated needles for injections and needlestick injuries among health professionals are another source of infection. Contaminated blood products (such as Factor VIII) and infected organs or semen have also been shown to transmit infection.

Mother-to-child transmission of HIV

Since the beginning of the epidemic, an estimated 5.1 million children world-wide have been infected with HIV. Mother-to-child transmission (MTCT) is believed to be responsible for more than 90% of these infections[28]. Around two-thirds of MTCT occurs *in utero* and at delivery and one-third occurs during breast feeding. Long regimens of ART have been shown to be highly effective in preventing MTCT but shorter, less complex and cheaper regimens have also been shown to reduce MTCT by half in infants who are not breast fed[29]. Implementing this intervention on a large scale in non-industrialised countries is complicated by the lack of safe alternatives to breast feeding, the issue of HIV testing and costs of the drug, service delivery and HIV tests.

Core groups

Within countries, there are sub-populations who are particularly vulnerable to HIV infection, such as sex workers and their clients, MSM and IDU. The HIV virus is often found predominantly within these subpopulations (sometimes called core-groups) at the beginning of an epidemic when prevalence is extremely low in the general population[30,31]. HIV prevention activities have been found to be particularly effective when focused on these vulnerable groups at the early stages of an epidemic[5,31,32]. If not controlled while it is predominantly within these groups, HIV can spread into the general population *via*, for example, wives or girlfriends of men who use sex workers or sexual partners of IDU. Subpopulations at a particularly high risk of HIV tend to be situated in urban areas so when HIV starts to spread into the general population, urban areas are usually affected before rural areas.

Social, cultural, economic and political context

The fact that HIV raises the culturally sensitive issues of sexuality, gender inequality, commercial sex, MSM and IDU has often led to denial of the problem and reluctance to address it, which obviously exacerbates the problem. Gender inequality means that women are often not in a position to negotiate safe sex and are put at risk of infection by husbands and partners. The development of female controlled methods of HIV prevention, such as the female condom and microbicides, are therefore particularly urgent. Migration, which separates people from their families, can result in higher levels of commercial and casual sex. The very low level of financial resources available to most affected countries make decisions about the priority of HIV control extremely difficult and also limits the general level of health services available. These are just a few examples of how the social, cultural, economic and political context have a major impact on HIV epidemics.

The relative importance of factors driving HIV epidemics

In addition to the factors mentioned above, the susceptibility of an individual to HIV infection may depend on genetic factors, although it is not widely believed at present that this is a major factor driving the different HIV epidemics. A study of sexual behaviour and factors affecting transmission probabilities in four cities in sub-Saharan Africa[33] suggests that male circumcision, prevalence of HSV2 and high levels of sexual debut at an early age for females are important in driving the HIV epidemics in sub-Saharan Africa. An analysis of more macro social and economic factors thought to affect HIV in 72 non-industrialised countries found that indicators of poverty, income inequality, gender inequality, poor economic growth, high levels of immigration and high levels of militarisation explained between a half and a third of the variation in HIV prevalences between countries[34]. However, we are a long way from fully understanding how and why the enormous variations in the HIV epidemic seen around the world have developed.

Estimating the magnitude of the epidemic

Where HIV has spread into the general population, ongoing HIV surveillance in women attending antenatal care can give a good indication of trends within a population. In addition, community-based surveys give estimates of prevalence, and sometimes incidence, in the general population and aid interpretation of antenatal surveillance data. STI clinic attendees are often included in HIV surveillance to give an idea of prevalence in high risk groups. However, access to many high risk groups for surveillance is difficult, so estimates in countries where HIV is still mainly restricted to these groups are usually less reliable. There is great variation between countries in the effort to gather data on HIV. Some countries have carried out widespread surveillance since the 1980s, whilst in others coverage is patchy or barely existent. UNAIDS takes estimates available from published studies and combines them with unpublished data, which is collected as part of AIDS control programmes in many countries, to produce national estimates of prevalence and deaths. Obviously, these estimates are only as good as the data on which they are based but they are the most comprehensive available. UNAIDS reports for the year 2000[2,35] will be drawn on heavily in the following sections describing regional trends around the world.

Global trends in the HIV pandemic

Sub-Saharan Africa

Sub-Saharan Africa has been devastated by the HIV/AIDS epidemic. While only 10% of the world's population lives in sub-Saharan Africa,

Table 1 Regional HIV/AIDS statistics and features at the end of 2000

Region	Epidemic started	Adults and children living with HIV/AIDS	Adult prevalence rate[a]	% of HIV positive adults who are women	Main mode of transmission[b] for adults living with HIV/AIDS
Sub-Saharan Africa	Late 1970s, early 1980s	25.3 million	8.8%	55%	Hetero
North Africa and Middle East	Late 1980s	400,000	0.2%	40%	Hetero, IDU
South & South-East Asia	Late 1980s	5.8 million	0.56%	35%	Hetero, IDU
East Asia & Pacific	Late 1980s	640,000	0.07%	13%	IDU, Hetero, MSM
Latin America	Late 1970s, early 1980s	1.4 million	0.5%	25%	MSM, IDU, Hetero
Caribbean	Late 1970s, early 1980s	390,000	2.3%	35%	Hetero, MSM
Eastern Europe & Central Asia	Early 1990s	700,000	0.35%	25%	IDU
Western Europe	Late 1970s, early 1980s	540,000	0.24%	25%	MSM, IDU
North America	Late 1970s early 1980s	920,000	0.6%	20%	MSM, IDU, Hetero
Australia & New Zealand	Late 1970s, early 1980s	15,000	0.13%	10%	MSM
Total		**36.1 million**	**1.1%**	**47%**	

[a]The proportion of adults (15–49 years of age) living with HIV/AIDS in 2000.
[b]Hetero, heterosexual transmission; IDU, transmission through injecting drug use; MSM, sexual transmission among men who have sex with men. Source UNAIDS[2].

an estimated 70% of all HIV infected adults and children are found there (Table 1). Heterosexual sexual transmission is predominant and sub-Saharan Africa is the only region where more women than men are infected. Patterns of sexual behaviour whereby young women have sex with older men, in combination with high susceptibility to infection in very young women, has resulted in extremely high infection rates in young women in some parts of Africa[11]. The inaccessibility of antiretroviral treatment in this region means that the vast majority of HIV infected people die around 8–10 years after infection, with tuberculosis being the most common AIDS-related illness. In the year 2000, 2.4 million adults and children were estimated to have died from AIDS in sub-Saharan Africa.

The first area to experience high prevalences of HIV was East Africa with countries in this area now experiencing adult prevalence rates of around 8–10%. Rates in two of these countries, Kenya and Somalia, appear to be still rising. West Africa has been relatively less affected by HIV with adult prevalence rates in most countries still estimated as less than 3%. However, there are worrying signs in two of the largest countries in West Africa with prevalences of 11% in Côte D'Ivoire and 5% in Nigeria. The most shocking statistics are from southern Africa where adult HIV prevalences have risen rapidly in the last few years to around 20%, with a staggering 35% prevalence in Botswana. South Africa is now the country with the highest number of people with HIV/AIDS in the world. However, there is some good news. After a strong HIV prevention programme in Uganda, adult prevalence has decreased from 14% in the early 1990s to around 8% in 2000. Also while the number of children and adults living with HIV/AIDS in sub-Saharan Africa increased during 2000, the increase (3.8 million) was slightly less than in 1999 (4.0 million). However, if rates start rising rapidly in some of the more populous countries, such as Nigeria, this trend could easily be reversed.

HIV/AIDS epidemics in North Africa and the Middle-East

HIV data from this region are very sparse. Best estimates are that around 400,000 adults and children were living with HIV in this region at the end of the year 2000 (Table 1). While adult HIV prevalence is at present low (an estimated 0.2%), recent data from Algeria and Sudan give warning signs that HIV may be spreading into the general population.

South and South-East Asia

Despite an overall estimated adult prevalence rate of only 0.56% (Table 1), this region contains around 16% of the total number of people in the world living with HIV/AIDS. There are enormous variations in how the HIV epidemic has spread within this region. National estimates put the prevalence at around 0.7% or less for all countries except Cambodia (4%), Myanmar (2%) and Thailand (2%). Thailand has a well-documented epidemic which showed rapid rises in HIV prevalence in the late 1980s which were reversed through a vigorous campaign to promote condom use, especially for contact with sex workers[6,32]. There are hopeful signs that a similar approach by Cambodia may be limiting the spread of HIV into the general population there.

India is one of the most populous countries in the world and with a relatively low overall adult HIV prevalence of 0.7% already has the second highest number of people living with AIDS in the world. There is wide variation within India. By 1998, Maharashtra and Andhra Pradesh states had antenatal prevalences of 2% or more while others had prevalences close to zero[36]. National and some state governments have implemented prevention programmes to try and limit HIV infection in IDU and sex workers. They have also launched mass publicity campaigns to reduce risky sexual behaviour, especially among young men, in an effort to avert large scale infection in the general population. The success of these campaigns remains to be seen, as does the pattern of HIV prevalence in other South and South-East Asian countries which have similar patterns of risk factors but very low current HIV prevalence in the general population.

East Asia and the Pacific

Estimated adult HIV prevalence is extremely low (< 0.07%) in this region except for Papua New Guinea where it is still relatively low (0.22%). There is, however, no room for complacency because patterns of IDU and sex work in this region show a potential for the spread of HIV and mobility between and within countries is high. The most populous country in the world, China, has recently seen worrying levels of HIV among IDU and then in sex workers close to the borders of Myanmar, Thailand and Laos[37]. An upsurge in STI rates in China after almost eradicating them in the 1960s also signals a worrying potential for HIV spread[38].

Latin America and the Caribbean

In Latin America, the highest rates of HIV prevalence are seen in the central American countries of Belize (2%), Guatemala (1.4%), Honduras (1.9%) and Panama (1.54%) and on the Caribbean coast in Guyana (3%) and Suriname (1.3%). Transmission within these countries is predominantly through heterosexual intercourse and in many of these countries HIV is spreading rapidly. In other Latin American countries, HIV transmission tends to be among MSM and IDU and prevalence rates in the general population have remained relatively low. In Brazil, the epidemic is characterised by heterosexual sexual transmission as well as transmission among MSM and IDU. Brazil (along with Argentina and Mexico) is attempting to provide antiretroviral treatment and high standards of care for people living with HIV/AIDS. The reduction in mortality due to the impact of these treatments results in higher numbers of people living with HIV/AIDS in these countries which masks the success of vigorous campaigns to prevent new infections.

The Caribbean has been badly affected by the HIV/AIDS epidemic with an overall adult prevalence rate of 2.1% at the end of 2000 (Table 1), second worst in the world after sub-Saharan Africa. The most badly affected countries are Haiti with an adult prevalence rate of 5.2%, the Bahamas (4.1%) and the Dominican Republic (2.8%). In these countries, transmission is predominantly heterosexual and rates are particularly high amongst young women (as in sub-Saharan Africa). High HIV rates have also been seen among IDU and MSM in these regions.

Eastern Europe and Central Asia

HIV/AIDS was rare in this region until the mid-1990s but since then HIV prevalence has risen exponentially, although still mainly restricted to IDU. At the end of 1999, Ukraine, Belarus, Moldova and the Russian Federation were the most badly affected countries. The epidemics occurring in different populations of IDU throughout the region make the overall epidemic highly unstable and there are worrying signs of a potential for spread. Economic instability may be exacerbating drug use and sex work and there are signs that HIV may have entered the general population in Ukraine. A rapid rise in syphilis in many parts of this region during the 1990s indicated a potential for sexual HIV spread, although there are some indications that this may have peaked around 1997[39,40]. More optimistically, many countries in this region are improving sentinel surveillance and implementing political and legal reforms which will facilitate HIV prevention efforts.

Western Europe, North America and Australasia

HIV infection in these regions is confined largely to IDU and MSM. High prevalences of HIV among IDU reflect a reluctance to implement community outreach and needle exchange programmes in many countries in these regions. MSM were hit very hard by the epidemic in the early 1980s but mobilised themselves against the disease very effectively and rates of new infections dropped after the mid-1980s. However, there are fears of complacency in the latest generation of MSM, who have not seen peers die of AIDS and who have access to highly active antiretroviral treatment (HAART)[41].

There have been slow and steady rises in heterosexual transmission of HIV in these regions and it has become the predominant mode of transmission in some western European countries[42,43], although prevalences are still very low. Examination of HIV infections by ethnic group in the US and UK show that many ethnic minorities are at a disproportionately high risk of HIV infection and have not benefited as much from HAART as the rest of the population.

The most striking feature of the HIV/AIDS epidemics in these regions is the marked reductions in AIDS-related illness and death seen as a result of the introduction of HAART in the mid-1990s. However, rates have now levelled out, possibly due to treatment intolerance, poor compliance, drug resistance and late diagnosis of HIV/AIDS. HAART has also substantially reduced mother-to-child transmission of HIV with most perinatal infections in these regions now occurring in women who have not sought antenatal care and/or not been diagnosed as HIV positive.

Conclusions

Although our understanding of the factors affecting the spread of HIV has increased greatly, we still do not fully understand why different parts of the globe have experienced such different HIV epidemics. Data on HIV prevalence in different countries are compiled by UNAIDS. They vary greatly in quality but gives us some idea of the magnitude of the problem and trends. Sub-Saharan Africa has been hardest hit by the HIV pandemic with extremely high prevalences currently being observed in southern Africa. There are, however, signs of hope due to a slight reduction in the number of new cases in 2000. Most countries in Asia have not seen explosive epidemics up to now, but patterns of IDU and sex work are conducive to the spread of HIV so there is no room for complacency. Unpredictable epidemics among IDU in the former Soviet Union have the potential to spread into the general population. Some countries in central America and the Caribbean have growing epidemics with prevalences second only to sub-Saharan Africa. HAART has reduced mortality and morbidity due to AIDS in high-income countries and in some countries in Latin America but it is still inaccessible to the vast majority of the world's infected population. Negotiations are taking place to provide more affordable ART to non-industrialised countries, especially for MTCT; however, the ability of the health systems to deliver ART effectively in many of these countries needs also to be addressed.

Acknowledgement

Linda Morison is funded by the UK Medical Research Council.

References

1   CDC. Kaposi's sarcoma and pneumocystis pneumonia among homosexual men – New York and California. *Morb Mortal Wkly Rep* 1981; **30**: 305–8

2   UNAIDS. *AIDS Epidemic Update: December 2000*. Geneva: UNAIDS/WHO, 2000

3   De Cock K, Adjorlo G, Ekpini E *et al*. Epidemiology and transmission of HIV-2 – why there is not an HIV-2 pandemic. *JAMA* 1993; **270**: 2083–6

4   Hu DJ, Buvé A, Baggs J, van der Groen G, Dondero TJ. What role does HIV-1 subtype play in transmission and pathogenesis? An epidemiological perspective. *AIDS* 1999; **13**: 873–81

5   Merson MH, Dayton JM, O'Reilly K. Effectiveness of HIV prevention interventions in developing countries. *AIDS* 2000; **24 (Suppl 2)**: s68–84

6   Robinson NJ, Silarug N, Surasiengsunk S, Auvert B, Hanenberg R. Two million HIV infections prevented in Thailand: estimate of the impact of increased condom use. XI *International AIDS Conference, Vancouver*, July 1996 [Abstract Mo. C904]

7   Mastro TD, de Vincenzi I. Probabilities of HIV-1 transmission. *AIDS* 1996; **10 (Suppl A)**: s75–82

8   de Vincenzi I. Longitudinal study of human immunodeficiency virus transmission by heterosexual partners. *N Engl J Med* 1994; **331**: 341–6

9   Nicolosi A, Correa Leite ML, Musicco M, Arici C, Gavazzeni G, Lazzarin A. The efficiency of male-to-female and female-to-male sexual transmission of the human immunodeficiency virus: a study of 730 stable couple. Italian Study Group of HIV Heterosexual Transmission. *Epidemiology* 1994; **5**: 570–5

10 Bouvet E, de Vincenzi I, Ancelle R, Vachon F. Defloration as a risk factor for heterosexual HIV transmission. *Lancet* 1989; **1**: 615

11 Glynn JR, Carael M, Buve A *et al*. Why do young women have a much higher prevalence of HIV than young men? A study in Kisumu, Kenya and Ndola, Zambia. *XIII International AIDS Conference* Durban, July 9–14 2000 [abstract MoPpC1097]

12 Caceres CF, van Griensen GJP. Male homosexual transmission of HIV-1. *AIDS* 1994; **8**: 1051–61

13 Vernazza PL, Eron JJ, Fiscus SA, Cohen MS. Sexual transmission of HIV: infectiousness and prevention. *AIDS* 1999; **13**: 155–66

14 Leynaert B, Downs AM, de Vincenzi for the European Study Group on Heterosexual Transmission of HIV. Heterosexual transmission of human immunodeficiency virus. *Am J Epidemiol* 1998; **148**: 88–96

15 Vernazza PL, Troiani L, Flepp MJ *et al*. Potent antiretroviral treatment of HIV-infection results in suppression of the seminal shedding of HIV, The Swiss HIV cohort study. *AIDS* 2000; **14**: 117–21

16 Wood E, Braitstein P, Montaner JSG *et al*. Extent to which low-level use of antiretroviral treatment could curb the AIDS epidemic in sub-Saharan Africa. *Lancet* 2000; **355**: 2095–100

17 Fleming DT, Wasserheit JN. From epidemiological synergy to public health policy and practice: the contribution of other sexually transmitted diseases to sexual transmission of HIV infection. *Sex Transm Infect* 1999; **75**: 3–17

18 Hayes RJ, Schulz KF, Plummer FA. The cofactor effect of genital ulcers on the per-exposure risk of HIV transmission in sub-Saharan Africa. *J Trop Med Hyg* 1995; **98**: 1–8

19 Grosskurth H, Mosha F, Todd J *et al*. Impact of improved treatment of sexually transmitted diseases on HIV infection in rural Tanzania: randomised controlled trial. *Lancet* 1995: **346**: 530–6

20 Wawer MJ, Sewankambo N, Serwadda D *et al*. Control of sexually transmitted diseases for AIDS prevention in Uganda: a randomised community trial. *Lancet* 1999: **353**: 525–35

21 Grosskurth H, Gray R, Hayes R, Mabey D, Wawer M. Control of sexually transmitted diseases for HIV-1 prevention: understanding the implications of the Mwanza and Rakai trials. *Lancet* 2000; **355**: 1981–7

22 Quigley MA, Weiss HA, Hayes RJ. Male circumcision as a measure to control HIV infection and other sexually transmitted diseases. *Curr Opin Infect Dis* 2001; **14**: 71-5

23 Weiss HA, Quigley MA, Hayes RJ. Male circumcision and risk of HIV infection in sub-Saharan Africa: a systematic review and meta-analysis. *AIDS* 2000; **14**: 2361–70

24 Bailey R, Muga R, Poulussen R. Trial intervention introducing male circumcision to reduce HIV/STD infections in Nyanza province, Kenya: baseline results. *XIII International AIDS Conference Durban*, July 9–14 2000 [abstract MoOrC196]

25 Brown JE, Brown RC. Traditional intravaginal practices and the heterosexual transmission of disease: a review. *Sex Transm Dis* 2000; **27**(4): 183–7

26 Garcia-Moreno C, Watts C. Violence against women: its importance for HIV/AIDS. *AIDS* 2000; **14** (**Suppl 3**): s253–65

27 Maman S, Campbell J, Sweat MD, Gielen AC. The intersections of HIV and violence: directions for future research and interventions. *Soc Sci Med* 2000; **50**: 459–78

28 UNAIDS. Preventing mother-to-child transmission: technical experts recommend use of antiretroviral regimens beyond pilot projects [Press release]. Geneva: UNAIDS, 2000

29 UNAIDS. *Mother-to Child Transmission. Summary Booklet of Best Practices*. Geneva: UNAIDS, 2000

30 Plummer FA, Nagelkerke NJ, Moses S, Ndinya-Achola JO, Bwayo J, Ngugi E. The importance of core groups in the epidemiology and control of HIV-1 infection. *AIDS* 1991; **5** (**Suppl 1**): s169–76

31 Mills S. Back to behaviour: prevention priorities in countries with low HIV prevalence. *AIDS* 2000; **14** (**Suppl 3**): s267–73

32 Hanenberg RS, Rojanapithayakorn W, Kunasoi P, Sokal DC. Impact of Thailand's HIV control programmed as indicated by the decline of sexually transmitted diseases. *Lancet* 1994; **344**: 243–5

33 Buvé A for the Study Group on Heterogeneity of HIV Epidemics in African Cities. HIV/AIDS in Africa: why so severe, why so heterogeneous? *7th Conference on Retroviruses and Opportunistic Infections*. San Francisco, CA, USA. February 2000 [Abstract S28]

34 Over M. The evidence of societal variables on urban rates of HIV infection in developing countries: an exploratory analysis. In: Ainsworth M, Fransen L, Over M. (eds) *Confronting AIDS: Evidence from the Developing World. Selected Background Papers for the World Bank Policy Research Report Confronting AIDS: Public Priorities in a Global Epidemic*. New York: World Bank, 1998

35 UNAIDS. *Report on the Global HIV/AIDS Epidemic*. Geneva: UNAIDS, 2000

36 NACO HIV/AIDS HIV prevalence among antenatal women in India 1998. *The Indian Scenario*. [http://www.naco.nic.in/vsnaco/indianscene/indscen.htm]

37 MAP. The status and trends of the HIV/AIDS/STD epidemics in Asia and the Pacific. *Fifth International Congress on AIDS in Asia and the Pacific*. Kuala Lumpur, October 1999

38 MAP. The status and trends of the HIV/AIDS epidemics in the world. *XIII International AIDS conference*. Durban, South Africa, July 2000

39 Dehne KL, Pokrovskiy V, Kobyshcha, Schwartländer B. Update on the epidemics of HIV and other sexually transmitted infections in the newly independent states of the former Soviet Union. *AIDS* 2000; **14** (**Suppl 3**): s75–84

40 Riedner G, Dehne KL, Gromyko A. Recent declines in reported syphilis rates in eastern Europe and central Asia: are the epidemics over? *Sex Transm Infect* 2000; **76**: 363–5

41 Stall RD, Hays RB, Waldo CR, Ekstrand M, McFarland W. The gay '90s: a review of research in the 1990s on sexual behaviour and HIV risk among men who have sex with men. *AIDS* 2000; **14** (**Suppl 3**): s101–14

42 European Centre for the Epidemiological Monitoring of AIDS. *HIV/AIDS Surveillance in Europe: Half Yearly Report*. Sainte Maurice: WHO/UNAIDS-EC, 1999

43 CDSC. AIDS and HIV infection in the United Kingdom: monthly report. *Commun Dis Rep Wkly* 2000; **9**: 415

Evolutionary and immunological implications of contemporary HIV-1 variation

Bette Korber[*,†], **Brian Gaschen**[*], **Karina Yusim**[*,†], **Rama Thakallapally**[*], **Can Kesmir**[†,‡] and **Vincent Detours**[*,†]

Division of Theoretical Biology and Biophysics, Los Alamos National Laboratory, Los Alamos, New Mexico, USA
†*The Santa Fe Institute, Santa Fe, New Mexico, USA*
‡*Center for Biological Sequence Analysis, Department of Biotechnology, Technical University of Denmark, Denmark*

Evolutionary modelling studies indicate less than a century has passed since the most recent common ancestor of the HIV-1 pandemic strains and, in that time frame, an extraordinarily diverse viral population has developed. HIV-1 employs a multitude of schemes to generate variants: accumulation of base substitutions, insertions and deletions, addition and loss of glycosylation sites in the envelope protein, and recombination. A comparison between HIV and influenza virus illustrates the extraordinary scale of HIV variation, and underscores the importance of exploring innovative HIV vaccine strategies. Deeper understanding of the implications of variation for both antibody and T-cell responses may help in the effort to rationally design vaccines that stimulate broad cross-reactivity. The impact of HIV-1 variation on host immune response is reviewed in this context.

The natural variability of HIV-1 provides a framework for understanding the complex biology of the virus. As we strive to understand immune evasion and drug resistance, our fundamental knowledge of mutational processes and selection is expanded. Phylogenetic analysis of variable forms of HIV can provide a glimpse into the evolutionary and epidemiological history of the virus. Recent studies have exploited advances both in sequencing technology and in modelling methods. Interpretation of global data sets through the application of improved analysis strategies enables researchers to trace the roots of HIV in terms of primate lentiviral evolution, to estimate divergence rates and the timing of the most recent common ancestor of the epidemic strains, and to model demographic trends in the epidemic. Simultaneously, new experimental methods in immunology[1] have rapidly expanded our understanding of the host's response to the virus and the consequences of immune pressure. Scientists are now poised to conduct large scale population studies combining viral sequencing, host genetics, and immunology.

HIV-1's great diversity is seeded by the lack of a proof-reading mechanism in RNA viral polymerase reverse transcriptase, and the

Correspondence to:
Dr Bette Korber, Division of Theoretical Biology and Biophysics, Los Alamos National, Laboratory, Los Alamos, New Mexico 98545, USA

British Medical Bulletin 2001;**58**: 19–42

consequential high error rate (0.2–2 mutations per genome per cycle)[2]; but that is not the full story. For example, HTLV-I, like HIV-1, infects CD4+ T-cells and goes though a reverse transcription step, but is far less variable; this may be attributed to differences in the dynamics of the two viruses[3]. A high replication rate accompanied by rapid viral turn-over[4], as well as pressure for change coupled with tolerance of change must be part of the story. Beyond base-substitution, HIV is subject to recombination and relatively large insertions and deletions (indels), which rapidly generate radically divergent forms.

An HIV infection starts out with a homogeneous viral population[5,6]; over the course of a typical infection, viruses which have mutated to alter more than 10% of their DNA bases in the envelope gene arise[6–8]. The concept of a viral quasispecies was originally introduced to model within-host viral populations and assumes that the frequency of viral forms in the population will be dictated by their relative fitness; the quasispecies is the realization of the distribution of forms within the sequence space[9]. However, the term quasispecies has come to be used more loosely in the HIV literature to simply refer to the set of viruses found in an infected individual. Under circumstances of selective pressure, such as therapy[10] or immune pressure[11–13], the frequency of forms in the viral population can shift. An 'archive' of earlier forms of the virus is retained in proviral DNA and these forms on occasion can re-emerge[6,7,14], presumably under changing circumstances in the host or through recombination. Combination therapy is effective despite within-host variation because multiple mutations required for resistance to three or more drugs are difficult to achieve unless selected for sequentially[15]. The correlation between long asymptomatic periods and the breadth of the T-cell immune response[16], and the association of HLA-homozygosity with accelerated progression to AIDS[17], may be manifestations of this same phenomenon, as simultaneous evasion of multiple immune responses may be difficult for the virus to achieve.

While immune escape clearly can drive positive selection in specific HIV epitopes[11,13,18,19], neutral mutations and genetic drift can also contribute to the overall diversity of the virus[20,21]. One strategy used to try to understand the relative importance of positive selection through immune evasion in HIV evolution is to quantify the force of positive selection within a given gene through analyzing the ratio of synonymous to non-synonymous substitutions[22,23]. Interpretation of average values is complicated because positive selection can be limited to narrow immunogenic domains within proteins, and average values of these ratios for full genes can be misleading. Many forces concurrently influence the evolutionary pattern *in vivo*, such as counterbalancing influences of retention of protein structure and function. Hence, there has been a recent interest in estimating these parameters for each site[21,24–26]. It will be important to establish how mutations which arise in the context of immune evasion within a single host can influence HIV diversity in populations. Such information will help define what is required at a molecular level for stimulating broadly cross-reactive immune responses.

HIV-1 subtypes are distinct lineages of the virus that are defined on the basis of genetic distances and phylogenetic clustering and are labelled A–K (Fig. 1f). It remains unclear whether these genetically defined subtypes will provide a useful way to consider global or regional variation for vaccine design. Neutralizing antibody serotypes do not correlate well with genetically defined subtypes[27,28]; the antigenic domains that define reactive sites are generally cross-reactive with a subset of viruses, and both cross-reactive and non-reactive viral forms can be found within the same subtype and within different subtypes. Cytotoxic T-cell (CTL) epitopes show a spectrum of cross-reactive responses to epitopes derived from proteins of different subtypes than the stimulation strain[29–34].

In this paper, we will consider the impact of variation in several ways. The first section concerns what can be learned from viral genetic diversity and phylogenetics about the history of the epidemic and rate of evolution. The second section is a summary of the extent of HIV variation as it is known today. The third briefly reviews the influence of variation on design and selection of the annual influenza vaccine (Fig. 2), and contrasts influenza and contemporary HIV-1 variation (Fig. 1). The influenza vaccine is often suggested to be a model system for HIV; however, the variability issues facing those involved with influenza vaccine design, while scientifically challenging and complex, are fundamentally distinct from the issues that need to be faced for an HIV vaccine. Finally, in the last section, the relationship between subtypes and known CTL epitopes is discussed, and the potential impact of variation on epitope processing is modelled.

The origins of contemporary HIV-1 diversity

Primate lentiviruses

Lentiviruses have been found in many African primate species[35], and the phylogenetic relationships between the viruses have been used to study the primate origins of HIVs[36]. HIV-2, the distant cousin of HIV-1 that also causes AIDS in humans, is most closely related to simian immunodeficiency viruses (SIVs) found in sooty mangabeys[37,38], while HIV-1 is most closely related to viruses that have been isolated from chimpanzees[36,39,40]. HIV-1 has three distantly related groups: (i) the main group (M), the group of viruses that cause the global pandemic; (ii) O, a form that is found with a low prevalence in west central Africa and has also been found in Europe[41,42]; and (iii) N, a very rare form found in Africa[43]. There are only a small number of viral sequences available from chimpanzees, and they are very diverse[36]; more information is needed before the precise relationships between chimpanzee viruses and HIV-1 M, N, and O groups can be elucidated.

Modelling the history of the HIV epidemic through phylogenetics

The earliest human sample found to contain HIV-1 was taken in 1959, and found among stored samples from the city now known as Kinshasa in the Democratic Republic of the Congo[44]. Phylogenetic analysis was used to validate the sample; it behaved like an older sequence would be expected to behave in terms of its position in the tree, branching closer to the root than modern sequences[44]. So the epidemic had its origins sometime prior to 1959. The lack of hard data prior to 1959 makes this a nebulous period, but important in the human history of HIV. Assuming the evolutionary behaviour of the virus is consistent, one can extrapolate into this pre-1959 period by estimating the rate of diversification using modern isolates with known dates of sampling. This allows a projection based on genetic distances and time, that can be used to estimate the most recent common ancestor of a given viral lineage[14,45,46]. Current estimates point to an origin of the HIV-1 M group near 1930, with error bars that span roughly a decade or so, depending on the method used[14,45]. These methods depend upon models of evolution that have inherent assumptions that are imperfectly met by real data[47,48]. Despite this, the method used in Korber et al[14] was validated through accurately estimating the timing of two control time points: the 1959 sample, and the beginning of the epidemic in Thailand. Salemi et al[45] used a strategy that excluded the most variable positions, and used a hepatitis sequence set as their control.

These analyses provide information about the rate of evolution, and also the rate of expansion of the epidemic. Dating the most recent ancestral sequence of the pandemic strains does not, however, decisively show when the first M group ancestral virus infected a human. There could have been an ancestral virus in chimpanzee with multiple subsequent cross-over events between species, or a period of time during which the virus was carried in humans prior to the expansion of the M group. If the evolution of the HIV-1 M group took place in humans, then the time of the most recent common ancestor of the M group would be an upper bound on the cross-species transmission event that ultimately gave rise to the epidemic.

Coalescent theory provides a way to extend the boundaries of what can be learned through phylogenetic studies, and model the demographic history of an epidemic through the phylogenetic branching pattern in a tree[49–52]. But to move beyond the phylogenetic tree into modelling estimations of past epidemic growth, additional assumptions are required. Current coalescent methods are based on the assumptions that: (i) the variance in the reproductive rate of the virus is constant in time (the reproductive rate is related to the number of new infections that arise from a single infection); (ii) the available sequences are sampled randomly; and (iii) the population is panmictic, *i.e.* the virus is circulating within a population that is not subdividing into isolated lineages and that there is no immigration of new forms into the population. Allowing for these assumptions, again imperfectly met by real data (although clearly some data sets are in better accordance with the assumptions than others), one can model the expansion of the effective population size through the history of the epidemic lineages represented in a tree. Coalescent theory has been applied to the study of HIV at many levels: within a person[50], comparisons of subtypes[49,51], and to the evolution of the M group virus in the Democratic Republic of the Congo (DRC)[52]. The DRC set is the most diverse set of HIV-1 M group sequences currently available from any nation, and is considered to be from a region of Africa which harboured the virus for much of its history in humans[53]. Analysis of this set of central African viruses suggested a period of slow expansion early in the epidemic, with more rapid expansion in recent decades[52], consistent with the timing estimates that suggest the virus was in the human population for many decades prior to AIDS being detected and defined[14,45].

The extent of contemporary HIV-1 diversity

HIV subtypes

HIV-1 genetic subtypes have a certain arbitrariness in terms of their definition, and biologists can (and do) reasonably argue for different nomenclature schemes. Nonetheless, a standard nomenclature system is important, as it provides a common language for referring to related lineages and captures a fundamental feature of the virus: the gene and protein sequences within a subtype are more closely related to one another than to the HIV genes and proteins from other subtypes. The associations and groupings of the subtypes can be statistically validated through phylogenetic analysis (Fig. 1f)[54–56]. For the sake of uniformity in the field and to facilitate communication, a team of experts recently assembled to update the nomenclature system[57,58]. The genetically distinct subtypes are labelled A–K (with no subtype E or I). Circulating recombinant forms (CRFs) describe viral genomes that contain clearly

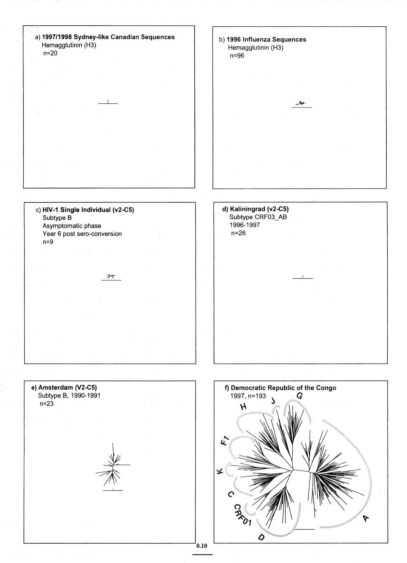

Fig. 1 A comparison of evolutionary distances of HIV-1 envelope sequences encoding V2-C5 and influenza HA1 domain of the HA gene through phylogenetic analysis. All panels show maximum likelihood trees using a REV model allowing for rate variation at different sites, following the strategy described in Korber *et al*[14]. The scale bar is the same in a–f for comparisons. (a) Tree based on 20 HA1 domain sequences of A/Sydney-like viruses circulating in Canada during the first half of the 1997–1998 flu season (Osiowy CK, unpublished observations. Accession numbers: AF087700-AF087708 and AF096306-AF096316). (b) Tree based on 96 HA1 domain sequences of human influenza H3N2 viruses. The tree contains all sequences from the Influenza Sequence Database, Los Alamos National Laboratory[131], with an isolation year of 1996. (c) Tree based on 9 V2-C5 sequences from a single asymptomatic individual collected at one time point 73 months post-seroconversion – this was a subtype B infection, and is typical of intrapatient diversity[7]. (d) Tree based on HIV-1 subtype CRF03_AB V2-C5 sequences from 26 individuals from Kaliningrad, representing a unique situation where a recombinant form of the virus spread explosively through a population of i.v. drug users, and all viruses were very closely related to a single common ancestor[65]. These samples were collected during 1997–1998, within a year of the introduction of the strain into the population. (e) Tree based on HIV-1 V2-C5 env sequences from a subtype B epidemic, sampled from 23 individuals residing in Amsterdam in 1990–1991[117]. (f) Tree based on HIV-1 V2-C5 sequences sampled in 1997 from 193 individuals residing in the Democratic Republic of the Congo (DRC), a remarkably diverse set[53].

delineated sections derived from different subtypes, that share a common ancestor, and that are the basis of multiple infections. CRFs are thus epidemic strains, which, like subtypes, are of global importance. There are currently 11 defined CRFs, and more are in the pipeline. Some of the CRFs infect great numbers of people: CRF01(AE) in Asia (originally identified in Thailand and called subtype E[59,60]), CRF02(AG), with a prototype isolate IbNg, found throughout western and central Africa[61–63], a newly defined subtype B and C CRF common in China[64], and a subtype A and B recombinant form found in Russia[65]. Given the exquisite specificity of immune receptors, the genetic relatedness of subtypes and CRFs viruses will certainly have some immunological consequences, but the implications for vaccine design are unclear.

More extensive sampling in regions of sub-Saharan Africa with great viral diversity has resulted in ever greater indications of the potential complexity of HIV diversity. In regions where multiple subtypes are co-circulating with a high prevalence, intersubtype recombination is common[61] and recombination between recombinants has also been observed. The large number of novel recombinants found suggests that multiple infections of HIV are not uncommon. Several new isolated examples of strains that are not clearly related to any defined subtype, and that are not obviously recombinants, have also been found. The subtypes themselves are growing ever more diverse with time. The combination of these factors results in a massive pressure on the current nomenclature system, and probably will eventually result in a breakdown of our current HIV classification scheme.

Measures of diversity

There are many ways to compare and contrast the extent of diversity found in HIV-1, and the individual proteins show different levels and patterns of variation. One very basic measure is a tally of sites that are preserved throughout all of the M group, of sites that tolerate insertions and deletions, and of sites that are variable because of nucleotide substitutions. In an alignment of the 132 nearly full-length M group sequences publicly available in the HIV database alignment[66], spanning a region from the start of *gag* to the end of *env*, there are a total of 7667 bases in HXB2. HXB2 is a sequence derived from the first HIV-1 isolate[67] and is a standard reference strain. Roughly 13% (992) of the positions in HXB2 have deletions in one or more of the other 131 HIV-M group sequences, leaving 6675 positions in HXB2 that do not contain any deletions in the alignment. Of these 6675 alignable positions, 2301 bases (30% of the total 7667 bases) are invariant, and 4374 (57%) of the positions have substitutions.

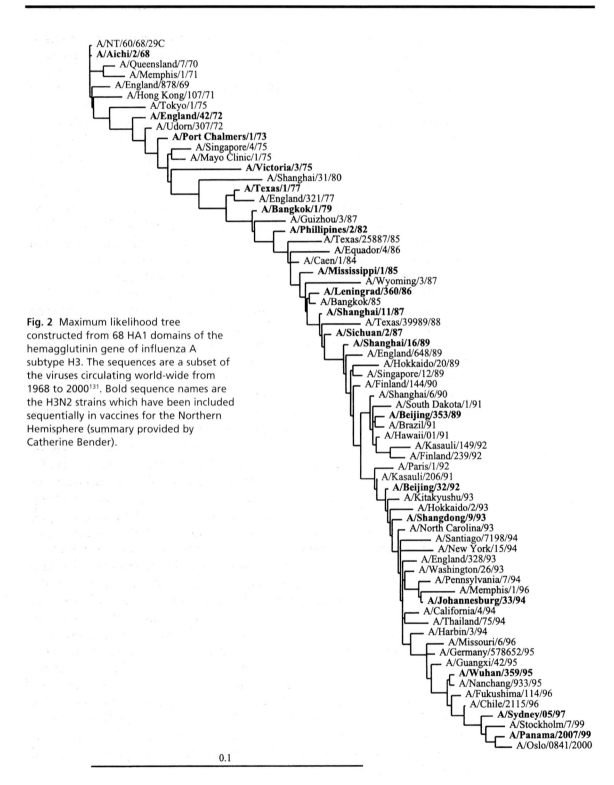

Fig. 2 Maximum likelihood tree constructed from 68 HA1 domains of the hemagglutinin gene of influenza A subtype H3. The sequences are a subset of the viruses circulating world-wide from 1968 to 2000[131]. Bold sequence names are the H3N2 strains which have been included sequentially in vaccines for the Northern Hemisphere (summary provided by Catherine Bender).

Another way to consider variation is distinctive lengths and glycosylation patterns found in envelope proteins. Among the current database collection (December, 2000) of 566 full-length gp120 protein sequences, protein lengths vary from 484 to 543 amino acids because of the insertions and deletions found in hypervariable regions. The hypervariable regions are typically excluded from phylogenetic analysis, as insertions and deletions do not follow the evolutionary base substitution models used to determine phylogenetic relationships. Thus the branch lengths in the *env*-based trees are a profound underestimate of the true diversity of the protein, because they capture only one aspect of the variation. Many of the hypervariable sites and insertions and deletions involve glycosylation sequons (the amino acids NX[S or T], sites where N-linked glycosylation occurs). The number of N-linked glycosylation sites in gp120 ranges from 18–33, with a median value of 25. Glycosylation can reduce accessibility to neutralizing antibody epitopes[68].

Considering relative HIV variation by protein can also be informative. Using the full-length genome alignment, so a fair comparison between genes can be made, one can model the relative rate of variation between all sites in an alignment using maximum likelihood phylogenies, and then build more accurate phylogenies by including site-specific rate variation[69]. A gamma distribution was used to assign one of seven evolutionary rates to each site in the nearly full-length HIV-1 M group alignment (the 6675 positions with no insertions or deletions described above). The sites that were evolving most slowly were assigned to category 1, and the fastest were assigned to category 7; in this model, category 7 was estimated to be evolving 20 times faster than category 1. For simplicity, just four HIV-1 genes are shown in Figure 3, representative of the spectrum of evolutionary rates found in HIV-1: gp120, the most rapidly evolving protein; tat; and the gag genes encoding p17, and p24. Gag p24, like pol, is highly conserved. We also used the program SNAP[24] to measure the non-synonymous substitution rate for genes included in the full-length genome alignment. In this case, we were not trying to calculate the ratio of non-synonymous to synonymous substitution within genes, but the relative rates of non-synonymous substitution between genes in the 132 full-length sequences. Tat in particular has overlapping coding regions in different frames, and its synonymous substitution rates are low and strongly biased by this. But, as the full-length genome alignment was used to examine the different coding regions, the non-synonymous rates for the different genes can be compared directly. The highest rate of non-synonymous substitutions (dn) was found in Tat, lowest in gp24 (dn values: Tat, 0.170 ± 0.022; gp120, 0.130 ± 0.015; p17, 0.104 ± 0.180; and p24, 0.039 ± 0.010). The high rate of substitution found in Tat is particularly important in the light of recent interest in Tat as a early and potent CTL target[13].

Influenza vaccines: responding to change

Influenza diversity and vaccine design

Influenza A viruses infect many mammalian and avian hosts, including duck, swine, human, geese, quail, whale, seal, and chicken. The viral genome has eight segments and is categorized by the serological and genetic characteristics of its two surface glycoproteins, the neuraminidase gene (NA) and the hemagglutinin gene (HA)[70]. To date, 15 subtypes of the HA gene and 9 subtypes of the NA gene have been isolated from mammalian and avian hosts; all 15 HA genes occur naturally within the

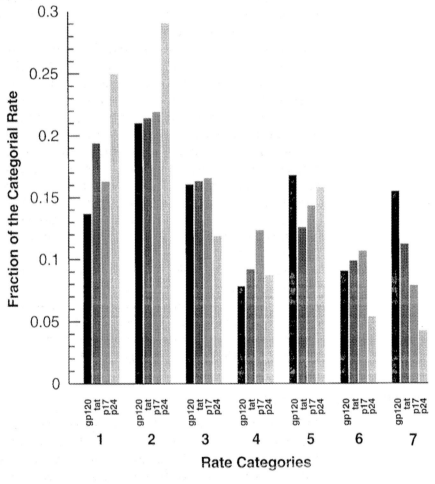

Fig. 3 Histogram showing frequency of mutation rate categories assigned to different sites in HIV-1 proteins coding regions, with category one being the slowest evolving sites, category seven the fastest. The rates were calculated based on a full genome maximum likelihood tree, excluding recombinant sequences, using a gamma distribution, and the frequency of assigned rates within gp120, tat, p17 and p24 are shown.

avian population[71]. Two kinds of viral evolution have been observed in human hosts over the last century, which have been termed antigenic drift and antigenic shift. Antigenic drift is the gradual change in the nucleotide sequence which is due to point mutations accumulating over time. Normally, changes made in the influenza vaccine are made in response to the antigenic drift of the virus. Antigenic shift, on the other hand, is an abrupt change in the serological and genetic properties of the virus due to the introduction of new HA or NA subtypes into previously unexposed populations. Since 1900, four HA genes (H1, H3, H5 and H9) and two NA (N1 and N2) have been isolated from human hosts[72–75]. Currently, two influenza A subtypes are found co-circulating in the human population, H3N2, a result of an antigenic shift in 1968, and H1N1, a result of a re-introduction of an H1N1 strain in 1977 similar to H1N1 strains circulating around 1950[76,77].

Because of the annual cost and the threat of particularly dangerous world-wide influenza pandemics, the World Health Organization (WHO) global influenza network was established in 1948. The network comprises over 110 laboratories in 80 countries, and four WHO Collaborative Laboratories[78]. Both unusual and representative samples of influenza virus are sent by the national laboratories year-round to a Collaborative Laboratory where antigenic and molecular analyses are performed. New viruses are antigenically screened for cross-reactivity with the current vaccine strains by the HA inhibition assay (HI), using antiserum stimulated by the vaccine. Members of the WHO network meet to recommend strains for inclusion in the vaccine for the coming year, currently two influenza A strains (H3N2 and H1N1) and one B strain. Recommendations are made based on the antigenic and molecular analyses of recent isolates, epidemiological data, and post-vaccination serological studies in humans[79]. In the years spanning 1968–2001, the H3N2 component of the influenza vaccine was changed a total of 17 times (Fig. 2), in one case necessitated by antigenic drift of as little as 3 amino acids substitutions in the 307 amino acid HA1 component of HA (A/Shanghai/16/89 to A/Beijing/353/89).

Influenza and HIV compared

Although influenza, like HIV, is a rapidly evolving virus, a comparison of HIV and influenza A evolution reveals very different patterns. HIV evolution is characterized by a radial spread outward from an ancestral node, while influenza is characterized by bottlenecks and global drift from year to year. Within a single 9 month flu season, little variation was typically found between geographically distinct influenza isolates after the emergence of the epidemic strain. HIV, on the other hand, shows increasing genetic diversity within a population through time. A phylogenetic tree of HA sequences sampled world-wide in 1996 (Fig. 1b) shows much less diversity than a sampling of subtype B HIV-1 envelope sequences from a single city, Amsterdam in 1990–1991 (Fig. 1e). In stark contrast, a sampling of HIV sequences from the Democratic Republic of the Congo in 1997 shows extraordinary diversity, with virtually all HIV subtypes co-circulating in one geographic region (Fig. 1f). The diversity of influenza sequences world-wide in any given year appears to be roughly comparable to the diversity of HIV sequences found within a single infected individual at one time point (Fig. 1c). Thus, while influenza does have a relatively fast rate of mutation when measured over decades (Fig. 2), the vaccine for any given year is targeted towards a relatively homogeneous viral population. Small numbers of changes in the viral amino acid sequence at antigenic sites require a change in the vaccine strain to induce an immunologically appropriate response for currently circulating strains. Thus the diversity which an HIV-1 vaccine must counter through stimulating a broadly reactive immune response is far greater than the diversity countered by the influenza vaccine. If current evolutionary trends continue, the situation will only become worse from an HIV vaccine design standpoint. This is daunting when considered in the context of the small number of amino acid substitutions that result in a loss of antigenic cross-reactivity sufficient to diminish influenza vaccine efficacy (Fig. 2). Thus innovative approaches may be critical for success with HIV-1 vaccines.

Immunological responses to a rapidly evolving pathogen

Strategies for eliciting cross-reactive B-cell responses

Three broadly cross-reactive neutralizing HIV-1 Env-directed monoclonal antibodies have been found (2F5, IgG1b12, and 2G12)[80,81]. These bind to conserved parts of Env essential for viral entry, so are promising as vaccine targets. The epitopes tend to be poorly revealed, best exposed during key transitional periods, and the antibodies have high affinity for the native trimer suggesting that they were raised in response to the oligomer on the virion surface rather than dissociated subunits[82]. This contrasts with the most exposed regions on Env gp120, the V3 and C5; antibodies directed at these sites tend to have weak cross-reactive neutralizing ability[83]. This could explain the limited neutralizing antibody responses elicited by gp120 vaccines[84,85]. Novel strategies for designing HIV Env in open conformations, intended to expose conserved critical regions, are being explored, with the hope that such reagents may elicit cross-reactive neutralizing responses[81]. Examples of such strategies include: (i) disulphide linked gp120–gp41 that mimics a native oligomeric conformation of Env[82]; (ii) glycosylation-deficient forms of Env that leave neutralizing epitopes exposed and increase their antigenicity[68]; (iii) Env linked to other immunogenic proteins[86]; (iv) locking Env into a conformation adopted part way through the fusion process[87,88]; and (v) deleting variable loops to expose key epitopes[89].

CTL responses in HIV vaccines

Several lines of evidence support the notion that CTL contribute to the control of natural infections. HIV CTL have been found in a significant fraction of HIV-1 seronegative high-risk sexual partners of HIV-1 positive individuals[90,91]. In particular, HIV-specific gamma-interferon secreting cells were detected in cervical mucosa and vaginal washes of exposed seronegative women[92,93], suggesting protective immune responses may occur in women chronically exposed to HIV-1, in whom HIV infection cannot be detected virologically or clinically. Broadly cross-reactive CTL were found in highly-exposed seronegative sex-workers in two regions in Africa[94], suggesting that broadly cross-reactive CTLs provide protection. Strong CTL responses and T-helper responses are also associated with long-term survival and non-progression in HIV-1 human[95,96] and SIV macaque infections[97]. Some human HLA types, including HLA B51[98], are associated with slow disease progression; HLA B51 presents epitopes located in highly conserved regions of HIV-1[99]. Finally, CTL escape mutations have been noted to arise in conjunction with progression to AIDS[100].

CTL cross-reactivity and implications for vaccine design

Various degrees of CTL cross-subtype reactivity have been documented, including examples of complete cross-reactivity, diminished cross-subtype responses, as well as cases where the response is completely abrogated[30–34,94,101,102]. Different target proteins can yield different experimental results in terms of CTL responses to proteins[103]. CTL experiments often probe the immune response with a single variant, and may favour the detection of responses to conserved epitopes – in other words, a CTL response could be experimentally silent if the probe was sufficiently different from the infecting and stimulating strain in a CTL epitope, and such differences are more likely to occur in highly variable regions. CTL specific for early expressed proteins like Tat may be particularly important for controlling viral replication[13,104], but there are few defined HIV-1 Tat specific CTL responses[105]. Tat responses may be hard to detect[106] due to the variability of the Tat protein (see above) and the potential for rapid escape[13]. It is not clear what the practical implications of viral variation will be for CTL-stimulating vaccines, and how the complexity of host genetics and HLA alleles will factor-in, but people are beginning to attempt to address these issues[107–109].

Defining an optimum vaccine to stimulate protective CTL responses against the breadth of circulating viruses in a complex host population is a challenging problem, but DNA vaccines allow great flexibility[110,111], and so have great potential for rational design. The biology, however, can be complex. For example, even in the most parallel of infections, identical twins infected with the same batch of factor VIII, profound differences in immune escape and immunodominant CTL responses were observed[19]. This is a humbling result. If it is characteristic of host-viral interactions, then rational design of a vaccine based on discerning common patterns of response in diverse individuals will be very difficult. One very basic vaccine approach that may be broad enough to over-ride such issues is simply the inclusion of multiple whole HIV-1 protein coding regions to maximize the potential breadth of the response[112,113]. Another strategy is to concatenate DNA encoding epitopes tailored to maximize potential responses for a population with a particular HLA distribution into a single contiguous DNA-vaccine[107]. Alternatively, one could use the HIV-1 immunology database to define conserved epitope-rich domains[105,108], or to experimentally identify maximally reactive peptide regions[109] – such approaches are not exclusive, and can show significant overlap (Fig. 4). Yet another strategy, not directly addressing cross-reactivity but rather potency (which may in turn enhance cross-reactive potential), explores optimization of vaccination with immuno-modulatory agents in addition to HIV antigens that both strengthen and tailor the nature of the immune response[114–116].

Consensus sequences are more central than modern sequences

Consensus, or most recent common ancestor sequences, might provide a better reference strains than modern viral sequences for designing peptides for immunological testing, and for vaccine preparations. A consensus is 'central', and thus more similar to circulating strains than they are to each other, and can remain relatively stable over time[117]. To provide a sense of the magnitude of the overall differences within and between subtypes, and of the virtues of consensus sequences, diversity was estimated through tallying the number of amino acid substitutions in pairwise comparisons of subtype A and subtype B protein sequence alignments from the year 2000 HIV Sequence Database[66]. Subtypes A and B were selected because numerous well-characterized sequences were available (17 subtype A and 95 B Env sequences; 12 A and 37 B Tat sequences; and 7 A and 35 B Gag sequences are included in the following summary). Positions with insertions and deletions were excluded.

Comparisons of actual sequences to their subtype consensus

Median percentage of amino acid differences are 10% (range 7–14%) in Env, 9% (4–14%) in Tat, and 5% in Gag (1–10%).

Pairwise comparisons of within subtype protein sequences

Median percentage of amino acid differences are 17% (4–30%) in Env, 15% (3–30%) in Tat, and 8% (2-15%) in Gag. (Note that sequences within a subtype are generally much more distant from one another than they are from the consensus of their subtype.)

Inter-subtype comparisons between A and B subtype sequences

Median number of amino acid changes is 25% (20–36%) in Env, 35% (27–42%) in Tat, and 17% (15–22%) in Gag.

Variable regions in all HIV proteins are not evenly distributed, but clustered with patterns that probably reflect conservation of functional domains, regions that tolerate change, and regions that are subject to immune pressure. Still, 11% amino acid substitution roughly translates to an average of about one change per epitope. A detailed summary of the number of substitutions found for actual experimentally defined epitopes between and within subtypes can be found in Korber *et al*[118].

Epitope processing and variation

Viral proteins are not recognized by CTL in their native form, but are cleaved into peptides in the cytosol of infected cells[119,120], transported to the endoplasmic reticulum[120,121], and loaded into a groove on class I HLA molecules[120,122]. Peptide-loaded class I molecules are then expressed on the surface of infected cells, accessible to antigen-specific receptors of CTLs. The class I peptide binding groove accommodates peptides of length 8–11 amino acids, and peptide binding to a particular class I molecule depends most critically upon amino acids known as anchor residues[122].

Virus variability may influence any step in epitope processing[123]. Immune escape driven by mutations in epitope flanking regions has been documented *in vivo*[124,125], showing that escape through processing abrogation can be of immunological significance. Protein cleavage is usually carried out by the proteasome[119] and can be sequence-dependent[119,126]; thus, viral variation might alter cleavage points, and positions with potential to serve as epitope boundaries may differ among viral strains. There are also alternatives to proteasomal cleavage pathways[127], and proteasomal cleavage products can require additional trimming by cytosolic proteases for epitope generation[128]. After cleavage and trimming, the transporter associated with antigen processing (TAP) translocates peptides into the endoplasmic reticulum for loading onto HLA class I molecules[121]. TAP affinity for peptides also can contribute to epitope selection[129].

Epitope clustering and the potential importance of processing

As noted before, there are regions in proteins in which experimentally defined CTL epitopes cluster (Fig. 4), and the biology underlying this non-uniform distribution is not yet understood. One possible contributing factor is the presence of conserved proteasomal cleavage sites at the boundaries of the epitope rich regions. We explored this possibility through use of an artificial neural network program that predicts C-terminal epitope boundaries (http://www.cbs.dtu.dk/services/NetChop/)[130]. This program correctly predicts 65% of cleavage sites and 85% of non-cleavage sites, using a training set of human peptides eluted from class I proteins, and a window of 19 residues surrounding the putative cleavage site as a basis for the prediction[130]. A value is assigned to each position in a protein, such that higher values indicate sites that are most likely to be cleaved, and to be the C-terminus of an epitope. Predicted cleavage sites for HXB2 (Fig. 4) often coincided with, or are within one or two amino acids of, experimentally-defined C-terminal amino acids of epitope or epitope rich regions. Sites with the highest cleavage site prediction scores vary between HIV-1 sequences and subtypes (Fig. 4).

Detailed examples of the influence of variation on cleavage site predictions are shown in Figure 5. The predicted cleavage scores for positions in the B subtype HXB2 p17 protein sequence are highly correlated with predicted cleavage scores for same position in the B subtype consensus sequence ($R^2 = 0.95$). But for the more variable Nef protein, the correlation between cleavage scores breaks down somewhat ($R^2 = 0.63$), even for these two very closely related sequences. For both p17 and Nef, HXB2 and consensus sequences from other subtypes have very different predicted C-terminal cleavage site scores at most positions. This suggests that cleavage may be subtype-specific and processing might be important. It is worth noting that this effect might go undetected in many of the cross-reactivity experiments that have been conducted to date, as often the optimal peptide is defined, the sequence variants within the optimal peptide are synthesized and tested for recognition, but processing is not tested.

Epitope clustering was apparent from the first compilation of experimentally defined HIV-1 CTL epitopes in the 1995 HIV Immunology Database[105], and has become increasingly evident with each new release of the HIV Immunology Database. This, we believe, might have broad practical implications. One could preferentially exclude from vaccines regions that do not encode known epitopes, and focus instead on

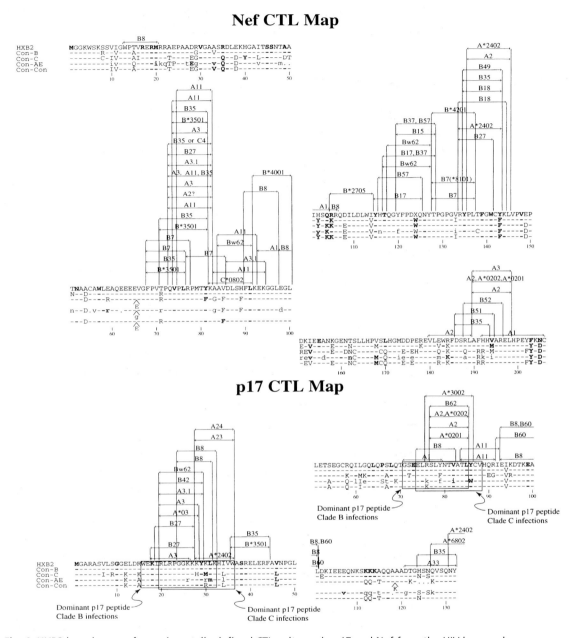

Fig. 4 HXB2 based maps of experimentally-defined CTL epitopes in p17 and Nef from the HIV immunology compendium (http://hiv-web.lanl.gov/). p17 and Nef have very distinctive epitope clustering patterns. The clustering patterns coincide with peptides that were found to serve as a stimulating antigen for CTL from many individuals (although the frequency depended on the HLA types in the population); the maximally reactive peptides are shown in grey[109]. HLA presenting molecules are shown above delineated epitopes from the database. Alignments show amino acid variation between the HXB2 reference strain and consensus sequences of different subtypes; subtype C and CRF01 were selected as they are important vaccine candidates. Predicted C-terminal proteasome cleavage sites are marked as bold letters, and differ between subtypes. Note that subtype consensus sequences are more closely related to each other than would be modern circulating strains.

epitope dense regions. Such constructs may produce safer vaccines than coding regions of full proteins, while preserving essentially full immunological potential for CTL. Shorter gene regions might also allow

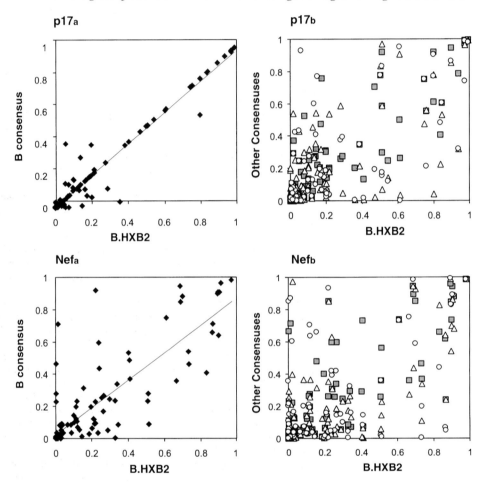

Fig. 5 Distinctions between proteasomal cleavage sites within and between subtypes. This scatter diagram shows the correlation between the predicted probability of a site being a proteasome cleavage site based on a program developed by Can Kesmir *et al* (www.cbs.dtu.dk/services/NetChop/). The HXB2 sequence (x-axis) is compared to the subtype B, C, and AE consensus sequences as well as consensus of subtype consensus sequences (y-axis). The consensus sequences were aligned to HXB2 (see Fig. 4). Each point on the graph corresponds to an amino acid position and has two co-ordinates: cleavage prediction for this position in HXB2 and the cleavage prediction for the appropriate consensus sequence. Points representing the B consensus sequence cleavage prediction as ordinate are denoted by filled diamonds; C consensus, empty triangles; CRF01_AE consensus sequence, empty circles; the main group consensus, grey rectangles. p17a and Nefa: cleavage predictions for B consensus versus B.HXB2 in p17 and Nef, respectively. R^2 values for best fit lines are 0.95 for p17 and for 0.63 for Nef. p17b and Nefb: cleavage predictions for other consensus sequences versus HXB2 in p17 and Nef, respectively. R^2 values are 0.52 for p17 and 0.55 in Nef for the C consensus; 0.54 in p17 and 0.38 in Nef for the CRF01_AE consensus; and 0.77 for p17 and 0.62 for Nef for the M group consensus.

for inclusion of a cocktail of variants. Furthermore, epitope dense regions may make possible natural processing of epitopes that polyepitope vaccines could not. Thus it may be worth considering incorporating clustering information in vaccine design strategies.

References

1   Kaul R, Rowland-Jones S. Methods of detection of HIV-specific CTL and their role in protection against HIV infection. In: Korber BTM, Moore JP, Brander BFHC, Walker BD, Koup R. (eds) *HIV Molecular Immunology Database*, part IV. Los Alamos, NM: Theoretical Biology and Biophysics, Los Alamos National Laboratory, 1999 (http://hiv-web.lanl.gov)

2   Drake JW. Rates of spontaneous mutation among RNA viruses. *Proc Natl Acad Sci USA* 1993; **90**: 4171–5

3   Wodarz D, Bangham C. Evolutionary dynamics of HTLV-I. *Mol Evol* 2000; **50**: 448–55

4   Perelson AS, Essunger P, Cao Y *et al*. Decay characteristics of HIV-1-infected compartments during combination therapy. *Nature* 1997; **387**: 188–91

5   Zhang LQ, MacKenzie P, Cleland A, Holmes EC, Leigh-Brown AJ, Simmonds P. Selection for specific sequences in the external envelope protein of human immunodeficiency virus type 1 upon primary infection. *J Virol* 1993; **67**: 3345–3356

6   Wolinsky S, Korber B, Neumann A *et al*. Adaptive evolution of human immunodeficiency virus type 1 during the natural course of infection. *Science* 1996; **277**: 537–42

7   Shankarappa R, Margolick J, Gange S *et al*. Consistent viral evolutionary changes associated with the progression of human immunodeficiency virus type 1 infection. *J Virol* 1999; **73**: 10489–502

8   Lukashov VV, Kuiken CL, Goudsmit J. Intrahost human immunodeficiency virus type 1 evolution is related to length of the immunocompetent period. *J Virol* 1995; **69**: 6911–6

9   Eigen M. On the nature of virus quasispecies. *Trends Microbiol* 1996; **4**: 216–8

10 Condra JH. Resistance to HIV protease inhibitors. *Haemophilia* 1998; **4**: 610–5

11 Price DA, Goulder PJ, Klenerman P *et al*. Positive selection of HIV-1 cytotoxic T lymphocyte escape variants during primary infection. *Proc Natl Acad Sci USA* 1997; **94**: 1890–5

12 Poignard P, Sabbe R, Picchio GR *et al*. Neutralizing antibodies have limited effects on the control of established HIV-1 infection *in vivo*. *Immunity* 1999; **10**: 431–8

13 Allen TM, O'Connor DH, Jing P *et al*. Tat-specific cytotoxic T lymphocytes select for SIV escape variants during resolution of primary viraemia. *Nature* 2000; **407**: 386–90

14 Korber B, Muldoon M, Theiler J *et al*. Timing the ancestor of the HIV-1 pandemic strains. *Science* 2000; **288**: 1789–96

15 Colgrove R. A combinatorial ledge: reverse transcriptase fidelity, total body viral burden, and the implications of multiple-drug HIV therapy for the evolution of antiviral resistance. *Antiviral Res* 1999; **41**: 45–56

16 Lubaki NM, Ray SC, Dhruva B, Quinn TC, Siliciano RF, Bollinger RC. Characterization of a polyclonal cytolytic T lymphocyte response to human immunodeficiency virus in persons without clinical progression. *J Infect Dis* 1997; **6**: 1360–7

17 Tang J, Costello C, Keet IP *et al*. HLA class I homozygosity accelerates disease progression in human. *AIDS Res Hum Retroviruses* 1999; **15**: 317–24

18 Borrow P, Lewicki H, Wei X *et al*. Anti-viral pressure exerted by HIV-1-specific cytotoxic T lymphocytes (CTLs) during primary infection demonstrated by rapid selection of CTL escape virus. *Nat Med* 1997; **3**: 205–11

19 Goulder P, Sewell A, Lalloo D *et al*. Patterns of immunodominance in HIV-1-specific cytotoxic T lymphocyte responses in two human histocompatibility leukocyte antigens (HLA)-identical siblings with HLA-A*0201 are influenced by epitope mutation. *J Exp Med* 1997; **8**: 1423–33

20 Sala M, Wain-Hobson S. Are RNA viruses adapting or merely changing? *Mol Evol* 2000; **51**: 12–20

21 Yang Z, Nielsen R, Goldman N, Pedersen AM. Codon-substitution models for heterogeneous selection pressure at amino acid sites. *Genetics* 2000; **155**: 431–49

22 Gojobori T, Yamaguchi Y, Ikeo K, Mizokami M. Evolution of pathogenic viruses with special reference to the rates of synonymous and non-synonymous substitutions. *Jpn J Genet* 2000; **69**: 481–8

23 Simmonds P, Balfe P, Ludlam CA, Holmes EC, Leigh-Brown AJ. Analysis of sequence diversity in hypervariable regions of the external glycoprotein of human immunodeficiency virus type 1. *J Virol* 1990; **64**: 5840–50

24 Korber B. HIV signature and sequence variation analysis. In: Rodrigo AG, Learn GH. (eds) *Computational Analysis of HIV Molecular Sequences*. Dordrecht, The Netherlands: Kluwer, 2000

25 Yamaguchi-Kabata Y, Gojobori T. Re-evaluation of amino acid variability of the human immunodeficiency virus type 1 gp120 envelope glycoprotein and prediction of new discontinuous epitopes. *J Virol* 2000; **74**: 4335–50

26 Zanotto PM, Kallas EG, de Souza RF, Holmes EC. Genealogical evidence for positive selection in the nef gene of HIV-1. *Genetics* 1999; **153**: 1077–89

27 Moore JP, Cao Y, Leu J, Qin L, Korber B, Ho DD. Inter- and intra-subtype neutralization of human immunodeficiency virus type 1: the genetic subtypes do not correspond to neutralization serotypes but partially correspond to gp120 antigenic serotypes. *J Virol* 1995; **70**: 427–444

28 Nyambi PN, Nkengasong J, Lewi P *et al.* Multivariate analysis of human immunodeficiency virus type 1 neutralization data. *J Virol* 1996; **70**: 6235–43

29 Menendez-Arias L, Mas A, Domingo E. Cytotoxic T-lymphocyte responses to HIV-1 reverse transcriptase. *Viral Immunol* 1998; **11**: 167–81

30 Dorrell L, Dong T, Ogg GS *et al.* Distinct recognition of non-clade B human immunodeficiency virus type 1 epitopes by cytotoxic T lymphocytes generated from donors infected in Africa. *J Virol* 1999; **73**: 1708–14

31 Cao H, Kanki P, Sankale JL *et al.* CTL cross-reactivity among different HIV-1 clades: implications for vaccine development. *J Virol* 1997; **71**: 8615–23

32 Durali D, Morvan J, Letourneur F *et al.* Cross-reactions between the cytotoxic T-lymphocyte responses of human immunodeficiency virus-infected African and European patients. *J Virol* 1998; **72**: 3547–53

33 Rowland-Jones SL, Dong T, Fowke KR *et al.* Cytotoxic T cell responses to multiple conserved HIV epitopes in HIV-resistant prostitutes in Nairobi. *J Clin Invest* 1988; **102**: 1758–65

34 Buseyne F, Chaix ML, Fleury B *et al.* Cross-clade-specific cytotoxic T lymphocytes in HIV-1-infected children. *Virology* 1998; **250**: 316–24

35 Beer BE, Bailes E, Sharp PM, Hirsch VM. Diversity and evolution of primate lentiviruses. In: Kuiken CL, B. Foley B, B. Hahn B *et al.* (eds) *AIDS and Human Retroviruses HIV Sequence Database*, part III. Los Alamos, NM: Theoretical Biology and Biophysics, Los Alamos National Laboratory, 1999 (http://hiv-web.lanl.gov)

36 Hahn B, Shaw G, De Cock K, Sharp P. AIDS as a zoonosis: scientific and public health implications. *Science* 2000; **287**: 607–14

37 Chen Z, Telfier P, Gettie A *et al.* Genetic characterization of new West African simian immunodeficiency virus SIVsm: geographic clustering of household-derived SIV strains with human immunodeficiency virus type 2 subtypes and genetically diverse viruses from a single feral sooty mangabey troop. *J Virol* 1996; **70**: 3617–27

38 Chen A, Luckay A, Sodora DL *et al.* Human immunodeficiency virus type 2 (HIV-2) seroprevalence and characterization of a distinct HIV-2 genetic subtype from the natural range of simian immunodeficiency virus-infected sooty mangabeys. *J Virol* 1997; **71**: 3953–60

39 Peeters M, Honore C, Huet T *et al.* Isolation and partial characterization of an HIV-related virus occurring naturally in chimpanzees in Gabon. *AIDS* 1989; **10**: 625–30

40 Gao F, Bailes E, Robertson DL *et al.* Origin of HIV-1 in the chimpanzee Pan troglodytes. *Nature* 1999; **397**: 436–41

41 Mauclere P, Loussert-Ajaka I, Damond F *et al.* Serological and virological characterization of HIV-1 group O infection in Cameroon. *AIDS* 1997; **11**: 445–53

42 Peeters M, Gueye A, M'Boup S *et al.* Geographical distribution of HIV-1 group O viruses in Africa. *AIDS* 1997; **11**: 493–8

43 Simon F, Mauclere P, Roques P *et al.* Identification of a new human immunodeficiency virus type 1 distinct from group M and group O. *Nat Med* 1998; **4**: 1032–7

44 Zhu T, Korber BT, Nahmias AJ, Hooper E, Sharp PM, Ho DD. An African HIV-1 sequence from 1959 and implications for the origin of the epidemic. *Nature* 1998; **391**: 594–6

45 Salemi M, Strimmer K, Hall WW *et al.* Dating the common ancestor of SIVcpz and HIV-1 group M and the origin of HIV-1 subtypes by using a new method to uncover clock-like molecular evolution. *FASEB J Express* 2000; On line, Dec 8: Article 10.1096/fj.00–0449fje

46 Sharp PM, Bailes E, Gao F, Beer BE, Hirsch VM, Hahn BH. Origins and evolution of AIDS viruses: estimating the time-scale. *Biochem Soc Trans* 2000; **28**: 275–82

47 Hillis DM, Mable BK, Moritz C. Application of molecular systematics: the state of the field and a look to the future. In: Hillis DM, Moritz C, Mable BK. (eds) *Molecular Systematics*, 2nd edn. Sunderland, MA: Sinauer, 1996; 515–43

48 Korber B, Theiler J, Wolinsky S. Limitations of a molecular clock applied to considerations of the origins of HIV-1. *Science* 1998; **280**: 1868–71

49 Grassly NC, Harvey PH, Holmes EC. Population dynamics of HIV-1 inferred from gene sequences. *Genetics* 1999; **151**: 427–38

50 Rodrigo AG, Shpaer EG, Delwart EL *et al.* Coalescent estimates of HIV-1 generation time *in vivo*. *Proc Natl Acad Sci USA* 1999; **96**: 2187–91

51 Pybus OG, Rambaut A, Harvey PH. An integrated framework for the inference of viral population history from reconstructed genealogies. *Genetics* 2000; **155**: 1429–37

52 Yusim K, Peeters M, Pybus OG, Bhattacharya T, Delaporte E, Mulanga C *et al.* Using HIV-1 sequences to infer historical features of the AIDS epidemic and HIV evolution. *Philos Trans R Soc Lond B Biol Sci* 2001; **356**: 855–65

53 Vidal N, Peeters M, Mulanga-Kabeya C, Nzilambi N, Robertson D, Ilunga W *et al.* Unprecedented degree of human immunodeficiency virus type 1 (HIV-1) group M genetic diversity in the Democratic Republic of Congo suggests that the HIV-1 pandemic originated in Central Africa. *J Virol* 2000; **74**: 10498–507

54 Louwagie J, McCutchan FE, Peeters M *et al.* Phylogenetic analysis of gag genes from 70 international HIV-1 isolates provides evidence for multiple genotypes. *AIDS* 1993; 7: 769–80

55 Gao F, Robertson DL, Carruthers CD *et al.* A comprehensive panel of near-full-length clones and reference sequences for non-subtype B isolates of human immunodeficiency virus type 1. *J Virol* 1998; **72**: 5680–98

56 The European Commission and the Joint United Nations Programme on HIV/AIDS. HIV-1 subtypes: implications for epidemiology, pathogenicity, vaccines and diagnostics. *AIDS* 1997; **11**: 17–36

57 Robertson D, Anderson J, Bradac J *et al.* HIV-1 nomenclature proposal. In: Kuiken CL, Foley B, Hahn B *et al.* (eds) *AIDS and Human Retroviruses HIV Sequence Database*, part III. Los Alamos, NM: Theoretical Biology and Biophysics, Los Alamos National Laboratory, 1999 (http://hiv-web.lanl.gov)

58 Robertson D, Anderson J, Bradac J *et al.* HIV-1 nomenclature proposal. *Science* 2000; **288**: 55–6

59 Gao F, Robertson DL, Morrison SG *et al.* The heterosexual human immunodeficiency virus type 1 epidemic in Thailand is caused by an intersubtype (A/E) recombinant of African origin. *J Virol* 1996; 70: 7013–29

60 Carr JK, Salminen MO, Koch C *et al.* Full-length sequence and mosaic structure of a human immunodeficiency virus type 1 isolate from Thailand. *J Virol* 1996; 70: 5935–43

61 McCutchan FE, Carr JK, Bajani M *et al.* Subtype G and multiple forms of A/G intersubtype recombinant human immunodeficiency virus type 1 in Nigeria. *Virology* 1999; **254**: 226–34

62 Cornelissen M, van Den Burg R, Zorgdrager F, Goudsmit J. Spread of distinct human immunodeficiency virus type 1 AG recombinant lineages in Africa. *J Gen Virol* 2000; **81**: 515–23

63 Carr JK, Laukkanen T, Salminen MO *et al.* Characterization of subtype A HIV-1 from Africa by full genome sequencing. *AIDS* 1999; **13**: 1819–26

64 Su L, Graf M, Zhang Y *et al.* Characterization of a virtually full-length human immunodeficiency virus type 1 genome of a prevalent intersubtype (C/B') recombinant strain in China. *J Virol* 2000; **74**: 11367–76

65 Liitsola K, Tashkinova I, Laukkanen T *et al.* HIV-1 genetic subtype A/B recombinant strain causing an explosive epidemic in injecting drug users in Kaliningrad. *AIDS* 1998; **12**: 1907–19

66 Kuiken C. HIV-1 sequence alignments. In: Kuiken CL, Foley B, Hahn B *et al.* (eds) *AIDS and Human Retroviruses HIV Sequence Database*, part I. Los Alamos, NM: Theoretical Biology and Biophysics, Los Alamos National Laboratory, 1999 (http://hiv-web.lanl.gov)

67 Hahn BH, Shaw GM, Arya SK, Popovic M, Gallo RC, Wong-Staal F. Molecular cloning and characterization of the HTLV-III virus associated with AIDS. *Nature* 1984; **312**: 166–9

68 Reitter J, Means R, Desrosiers R. A role for carbohydrates in immune evasion in AIDS. *Nat Med* 1998; **4**: 679–84

69 Yang Z. Maximum likelihood phylogenetic estimation from DNA sequences with variable rates over sites: approximate methods. *J Mol Evol* 1994; **39**: 306–14

70 Lamb RA. Genes and proteins of the influenza viruses. In: Krug RM. (ed) *The Influenza Viruses*. New York: Plenum, 1989; 1–87

71 Alexander DJ. A review of avian influenza in different bird species. *Vet Microbiol* 2000; **74**: 3–13

72 Smith FI, Palese P. Variation in influenza virus genes. In: Krug RM. (ed) *The Influenza Viruses*. New York: Plenum, 1989; 319–59

73 Subbarao K, Klimov A, Katz J *et al.* Characterization of an avian influenza A (H5N1) virus isolated from a child with a fatal respiratory illness [see comments]. *Science* 1998; **279**: 393–6

74 Guo Y, Li J, Cheng X *et al.* Discovery of men infected by avian influenza A (H9N2) virus. *Chin J Exp Cline Virol* 1999; **13**: 105–8

75 Peiris M, Yuen KY, Leung CW *et al.* Human infection with influenza H9N2 [letter]. *Lancet* 1999; **354**: 916–7

76 Nakajima K, Desselberger U, Palese P. Recent human influenza A (H1N1) viruses are closely related genetically to strains isolated in 1950. *Nature* 1978; **274**: 334–9

77 Kendal AP, Noble GR, Skehel JJ, Dowdle WR. Antigenic similarity of influenza A (H1N1) viruses from epidemics in 1977–1978 to 'Scandinavian' strains isolated in epidemics of 1950–1951. *Virology* 1978; **89**: 632–6

78 Stamboulian D, Bonvehi PE, Nacinovich FM, Cox N. Influenza. *Infect Dis Cline North Am* 2000; **14**: 141–66

79 Hay A, Gust I, Hampson A *et al.* Update: influenza activity – United States and worldwide, 1999–2000 season, and composition of the 2000–01 influenza vaccine. *MMWR* 2000; **78**: 1913–8

80 D'Souza MP, Livnat D, Bradac JA, Bridges SH. Evaluation of monoclonal antibodies to human immunodeficiency virus type 1 primary isolates by neutralization assays: performance criteria for selecting candidate antibodies for clinical trials. *Infect Dis* 1997; **175**: 1056–62

81 Parren PW, Moore JP, Burton DR, Sattentau QJ. The neutralizing antibody response to HIV-1: viral evasion and escape from humoral immunity. *AIDS* 1999; **13** (**Suppl A**): S137–62

82 Binley J, Sanders R, Clas B *et al.* A recombinant human immunodeficiency virus type I envelope glycoprotein complex stabilized by an intermolecular disulfide bond between the gp120 and gp41 subunits is an antigenic mimic of the trimeric virion-associated structure. *J Virol* 2000; **74**: 627–43

83 Nyambi P, Mbah H, Burda S, Gorny M, Nadas A, Zolla-Pazner S. Conserved and exposed epitopes on intact, native, primary human immunodeficiency virus type I virions of group M. *J Virol* 2000; **74**: 7096–107

84 Connor R, Korber BTM, Cao Y *et al.* Immunological and virological analyses of persons infected by human immunodeficiency virus type 1 while participating in trials of recombinant gp120 subunit vaccines. *J Virol* 1998; **72**: 1552–76

85 Locher CP, Grant RM, Collisson EA *et al.* Antibody and cellular immune responses in breakthrough infection subjects after HIV type 1 glycoprotein 120 vaccination. *AIDS Res Hum Retroviruses* 1999; **15**: 1685–9

86 Collado M, Rodriguez D, Rodriguez J, Vazquez I, Gonzalo R, Esteban M. Chimeras between the human immunodeficiency virus (HIV-1) Env and vaccinia virus immunogenic proteins p14 and p39 generate in mice broadly reactive antibodies and specific activation of CD8+ T cell responses to Env. *Vaccine* 2000; **18**: 3123–33

87 LaCasse R, Follis K, Trahey M, Scarborough JD, Littman DR, Nunberg J. Fusion-competent vaccines: broad neutralization of primary isolates of HIV. *Science* 1999; **283**: 357–62

88 Salzwedel K, Smith ED, Dey B, Berger EA. Sequential CD4-coreceptor interactions in human immunodeficiency virus type 1 Env function: soluble CD4 activates Env for coreceptor-dependent fusion and reveals blocking activities of antibodies against cryptic conserved epitopes on gp120. *J Virol* 2000; **74**: 326–33

89 Stamatatos L, Cheng-Mayer C. An envelope modification that renders a primary, neutralization-resistant clade B human immunodeficiency virus type 1 isolate highly susceptible to neutralization by sera from other clades. *J Virol* 2000; **72**: 7840–5

90 Bernard NF, Yannakis CM, Lee JS, Tsoukas CM. Human immunodeficiency virus (HIV)-specific cytotoxic T lymphocyte activity in HIV-exposed seronegative persons. *J Infect Dis* 1999; **179**: 538–47

91 Goh WC, Markee J, Akridge RE *et al*. Protection against human immunodeficiency virus type 1 infection in persons with repeated exposure: evidence for T cell immunity in the absence of inherited CCR5 coreceptor defects. J Infect Dis 1999; **179**: 548–57

92 Biasin M, Caputo SL, Speciale L *et al*. Mucosal and systemic immune activation is present in human immunodeficiency virus-exposed seronegative women. *J Infect Dis* 2000; **182**: 1365–74

93 Kaul R, Plummer F, Kimani J *et al*. HIV-1-specific mucosal CD8+ lymphocyte responses in the cervix of HIV-1-resistant prostitutes in Nairobi. *J Immunol* 2000; **164**: 1602–11

94 Rowland-Jones SL, Dong T, Dorrell L *et al*. Broadly cross-reactive HIV-specific cytotoxic T-lymphocytes in highly-exposed persistently seronegative donors. *Immunol Lett* 1999; **66**: 914

95 Greenough TC, Brettler DB, Kirchhoff F *et al*. Long-term non-progressive infection with human immunodeficiency virus type 1 in a hemophilia cohort. *J Infect Dis* 1999; **180**: 1790–802

96 Rosenberg E, Walker B. HIV type 1-specific helper T cells: a critical host defense. *AIDS Res Hum Retroviruses* 1998; **14** (**Suppl 2**): S143–7

97 Evans D, Knapp L, Jing P *et al*. Rapid and slow progressors differ by a single MHC class I haplotype in a family of MHC-defined rhesus macaques infected with SIV. *Immunol Lett* 1999; **613**: 53–9

98 Kaslow RA, Carrington M, Apple R *et al*. Influence of combinations of MHC genes on the course of HIV-1 infection. *Nat Med* 1996; **2**: 405

99 Tomiyama H, Sakaguchi T, Miwa K *et al*. Identification of multiple HIV-1 CTL epitopes presented by HLA-B*5101 molecules. *Hum Immunol* 1999; **60**: 177–86

100 Goulder P, Phillips RE, Colbert RA *et al*. Late escape from an immunodominant cytotoxic T-lymphocyte response associated with progression to AIDS. *Nat Med* 1997; **3**: 212–6

101 Paranjape RS, Gadkari DA, Lubaki M, Quinn TC, Bollinger RC. Crossreactive HIV-1-specific CTL in recent seroconverters from Pune, India. *Indian J Med Res* 2000; **108**: 35–41

102 Gotch F. Cross-clade T cell recognition of HIV-1. *Curr Opin Immunol* 2000; **10**: 388–92

103 Jin X, Roberts CG, Nixon DF *et al*. Longitudinal and cross-sectional analysis of cytotoxic T lymphocyte responses and their relationship to vertical human immunodeficiency virus transmission. *J Infect Dis* 1998; **178**:1317–26

104 van Baalen CA, Pontesilli O, Huisman RC *et al*. Human immunodeficiency virus type 1 Rev- and Tat-specific cytotoxic T lymphocyte frequencies inversely correlate with rapid progression to AIDS. *J Gen Virol* 1997; **78**: 1913–8

105 Korber B. CTL epitopes. In: Korber BTM, Moore JP, Brander BFHC, Walker BD, Koup R. (eds) *HIV Molecular Immunology Database*, part 1. Los Alamos, NM: Theoretical Biology and Biophysics, Los Alamos National Laboratory, 1999 (http://hiv-web.lanl.gov)

106 Legrand E, Pellegrin I, Neau D *et al*. Course of specific T lymphocyte cytotoxicity, plasma and cellular viral loads, and neutralizing antibody titers in 17 recently seroconverted HIV type 1-infected patients. *AIDS Res Hum Retroviruses* 1997; **13**: 1383–94

107 Hanke T, McMichael A. Pre-clinical development of a multi-CTL epitope-based DNA prime MVA boost vaccine for AIDS. *Immunol Lett* 1999; **66**: 177–81

108 Ferrari G, Kostyu DD, Cox J *et al*. Identification of highly conserved and broadly cross-reactive HIV type 1 cytotoxic T lymphocyte epitopes as candidate immunogens for inclusion in *Mycobacterium bovis* BCG-vectored HIV vaccines. *AIDS Res Hum Retroviruses* 2000; **16**: 1433–43

109 Goulder PJ, Brander C, Annamalai K *et al*. Differential narrow focusing of immunodominant human immunodeficiency virus gag-specific cytotoxic T-lymphocyte responses in infected African and Caucasoid adults and children. *J Virol* 2000; **74**: 5679-90

110 Fomsgaard A. HIV-1 DNA vaccines. *Immunol Lett* 1999; **65**: 127–31

111 Wagner R, Shao Y, Wolf H. Correlates of protection, antigen delivery and molecular epidemiology: basics for designing an HIV vaccine. *Vaccine* 1999; **17**: 1706–10

112 Evans TG, Keefer MC, Weinhold KJ *et al*. A canarypox vaccine expressing multiple human immunodeficiency virus type 1 genes given alone or with rgp120 elicits broad and durable CD8+ cytotoxic T lymphocyte responses in seronegative volunteers. *J Infect Dis* 1999; **180**: 290–8

113 Akahata W, Ido E, Shimada T *et al*. DNA vaccination of macaques by a full genome HIV-1 plasmid which produces non-infectious virus particles. *Virology* 2000; **275**: 116–24

114 Hamajima K, Fukushima J, Bukawa H *et al*. Strong augment effect of IL-12 expression plasmid on the induction of HIV-specific cytotoxic T lymphocyte activity by a peptide vaccine candidate. *Cline Immunol Immunopathol* 1997; **83**: 179–84

115 Xin KQ, Hamajima K, Sasaki S *et al*. IL-15 expression plasmid enhances cell-mediated immunity induced by an HIV-1 DNA vaccine. *Vaccine* 1999; **17**: 858–66

116 Barouch DH, Craiu A, Kuroda MJ *et al*. Augmentation of immune responses to HIV-1 and simian immunodeficiency virus DNA vaccines by IL-2/Ig plasmid administration in rhesus monkeys. *Proc Natl Acad Sci USA* 2000; **97**: 4192–7

117 Lukashov VV, Goudsmit J. Evolution of the human immunodeficiency virus type 1 subtype-specific V3 domain is confined to a sequence space with a fixed distance to the subtype consensus. *J Virol* 1997; **71**: 6332–8

118 Korber B, Foley B, Gaschen B, Kuiken C. Epidemiological and immunological implications of the global variability of HIV-1. In: Pantaleo G, Walker B (eds) *Retroviral Immunology: Immune Response and Restoration*. Totowa, NJ: Humana, 2001; In press

119 Orlowski M, Wilk S. Catalytic activities of the 20 S proteasome, a multicatalytic proteinase complex. *Arch Biochem Biophys* 2000; **383**: 1–16

120 Pamer E, Cresswell P. Mechanisms of MHC class I-restricted antigen processing. *Annu Rev Immunol* 1998; **16**: 323–58

121 Abele R, Tampe R. Function of the transport complex TAP in cellular immune recognition. *Biochim Biophys Acta* 1999; **1461**: 405–19

122 Rammensee H, Bachmann J, Stevanovic S. Norwell, MA: *MHC Ligands and Peptide Motifs*. Chapman & Hall, Kluwer Academic, 1999

123 Paradela A, Alvarez T, Garcia-Peydro M *et al*. Limited diversity of peptides related to an alloreactive T cell epitope in the HLA-B27-bound peptide repertoire results from restrictions at multiple steps along the processing-loading pathway. *J Immunol* 2000; **164**: 329–37

124 Beekman N, van Veelen P, van Hall T *et al*. Abrogation of CTL epitope processing by single amino acid substitution flanking the C-terminal proteasome cleavage site. *J Immunol* 2000; **164**: 1898–905

125 Chassin D, Andrieu M, Cohen W *et al*. Dendritic cells transfected with the nef genes of HIV-1 primary isolates specifically activate cytotoxic T lymphocytes from seropositive subjects. *Eur J Immunol* 1999; **29**: 196–202

126 Niedermann G, Geier E, Lucchiari Hartz M, Hitziger N, Ramsperger A, Eichmann K. The specificity of proteasomes: impact on MHC class I processing and presentation of antigens. *Immunol Rev* 1999; **172**: 29–48

127 Geier E, Pfeifer G, Wilm M *et al*. A giant protease with potential to substitute for some functions of the proteasome. *Science* 1999; **283**: 978–81

128 Stoltze L, Schirle M, Schwarz G *et al*. Two new proteases in the MHC class I processing pathway. *Nat Immunol* 2000; **1**: 413–8

129 Daniel S, Brusic V, Caillat Zucman S *et al*. Relationship between peptide selectivities of human transporters associated with antigen processing and HLA class I molecules. *J Immunol* 1998; **161**: 617–24

130 Kesmir C, Nussbaum A, Schild H, Detours V, Brunak S. Program available on the web: <http://www.cbs.dtu.dk/services/NetChop>. Manuscript submitted, 2001

131 Macken C, and The Influenza Sequence Database Staff. *Influenza Sequence Database*. 2000 <http://www.flu.lanl.gov>

HIV-1 receptors and cell tropism

Paul R Clapham* and **Áine McKnight†**

**Center for AIDS Research, Program in Molecular Medicine, Department of Molecular Genetics and Microbiology, University of Massachusetts Medical School, Worcester, Massachusetts, USA
†The Wohl Virion Center, Department of Immunology and Molecular Pathology, The Windeyer Institute for Medical Sciences, University College, London, UK*

HIV virus particles interact with several receptors on cell surfaces. Two receptors, CD4 and a co-receptor act sequentially to trigger fusion of viral and cellular membranes and confer virus entry into cells. For HIV-1, the chemokine receptor CCR5 is the predominant co-receptor exploited for transmission and replication *in vivo*. Variants that switch to use CXCR4 and perhaps other co-receptors evolve in some infected individuals and have altered tropism and pathogenic properties. Other cell surface receptors including mannose binding protein on macrophages and DC-SIGN on dendritic cells also interact with gp120 on virus particles but do not actively promote fusion and virus entry. These receptors may tether virus particles to cells enabling interactions with suboptimal concentrations of CD4 and/or co-receptors. Alternatively such receptors may transport cell surface trapped virions into lymph nodes before transmitting them to susceptible cells. Therapeutic strategies that prevent HIV from interacting with receptors are currently being developed. This review describes how the interaction and use of different cellular receptors influences HIV tropism and pathogenesis *in vivo*.

*Correspondence to:
Dr Paul R Clapham,
Center for AIDS Research,
Program in Molecular
Medicine, Department of
Molecular Genetics and
Microbiology, University
of Massachusetts Medical
School, Biotech II,
373 Plantation Street,
Worcester,
MA 01605, USA*

The main cells targeted by HIV *in vivo* are T-cells, macrophages and probably dendritic cells. This narrow tropism is predominantly determined by the cell surface receptors required for HIV to attach to and gain entry into cells. Two different receptors, CD4 and a co-receptor, are usually essential for HIV to infect cells efficiently. The chemokine receptor CCR5 is the co-receptor predominantly used *in vivo*; however, variants that use another co-receptor, CXCR4, evolve during disease in some AIDS patients. *In vitro*, more than a dozen different co-receptors have been identified that support infection of cell lines by different HIV strains. The capacity to exploit alternative co-receptors ought to be advantageous and confer a wider cell tropism; however, current evidence suggests that co-receptors other than CCR5 or CXCR4 have limited use *in vivo*. The factors that preclude the use of a wider range of co-receptors *in vivo* are not known, nor is it clear why such a variable virus as HIV fails to evolve variants capable of exploiting alternative co-receptors and colonizing a broader range of cell types. This article will discuss the cell types infected by HIV and how the use of different receptors influences cell tropism and pathogenesis *in vivo*.

Cell surface receptors for HIV entry into cells

HIV interacts with CD4 and a seven transmembrane (7TM) co-receptor to trigger entry into cells. The envelope glycoprotein spikes on the surface of virus particles comprise an outer surface gp120 (SU) non-covalently linked to a transmembrane gp41 (TM). Each spike on the virus particle comprises a trimer of three gp120 and three gp41 molecules. Binding of CD4 to gp120 triggers a structural change, which exposes a binding site for a co-receptor (Fig. 1). Further structural re-arrangements are initiated when the co-receptor is bound. These changes occur predominantly in gp41 and are thought to be sufficient to trigger fusion of viral and cellular membranes and entry of the virion core into the cell's cytoplasm. In the absence of CD4, infection is

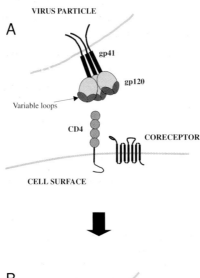

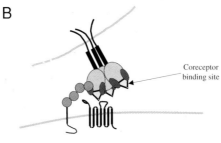

Fig. 1 Receptor interactions involved in HIV entry. (A) HIV virion binds CD4. (B) CD4 binding induces conformation changes in gp120 that result in the movement of the variable loops and exposure of the co-receptor binding site. Flexible regions in CD4 between domains 2 and 3 as well as between domain 4 and the membrane allow orientation of the co-receptor binding site for co-receptor binding.

inefficient and its significance *in vivo*, controversial. Over 14 different 7TM receptors have been identified as potential co-receptors for HIV and SIV by their capacity to support infection of CD4$^+$ cell lines *in vitro* (Table 1). These receptors are members of (or closely related to) the chemokine receptor family. CCR5 and CXCR4 are the major co-receptors and all HIV-1 isolates can use one or both. Several polymorphisms in the CCR5 gene that influence HIV transmission and/or disease progression have highlighted the importance of this co-receptor *in vivo*[1]. The most significant polymorphism is the 32 base pair deletion (Δ32 CCR5) in the coding region that results in a defective CCR5 product that fails to reach the cell surface[2]. Homozygotes are, therefore, effectively CCR5-negative. Their substantial resistance to HIV infection whether the risk to infection is via sex, blood contact[3] or from mother-to-child[4] clearly illustrates a major role for CCR5 during transmission. CCR5, however, is not the only transmission route and a few HIV$^+$ Δ32 CCR5 homozygotes have been identified. These individuals (where tested) appear to carry CXCR4-using viruses[5]. The defective Δ32 CCR5 gene product can still form oligomers with wild-type CCR5 in the endoplasmic reticulum and thus hetero-zygotes are likely to lose more than 50% of cell surface CCR5[2]. HIV$^+$ Δ32 CCR5 heterozygous individuals suffer a significantly slower disease course demonstrating the importance for CCR5 in HIV pathogenesis. No significant CXCR4 polymorphisms have been reported probably because CXCR4 is an essential requirement in development and the 'knockout' phenotype in mice is lethal. The faster disease progression and rapid loss of CD4$^+$ T-cells associated with the emergence of CXCR4-using viruses indicate an important *in vivo* role for CXCR4 in some individuals[6]. The

Table 1 Co-receptors that function for HIV and SIV on CD4$^+$ cell lines. Only CCR5 and CXCR4 have so far been shown to function as co-receptors *in vivo*

Co-receptors	Ligands	Role for viral replication	
		In vitro	*In vivo*
CCR1	MIP-1α, RANTES, MPIF-1, MCP-3	+	
CCR2b	MCP-1, MCP-2, MCP-3	+	
CCR3	Eotaxin, Eotaxin-2, MCP-3, MCP-4, RANTES	++	
CCR5	MIP-1α, MIP-1β, RANTES, MCP-2	++++	++++
CCR8	I-309	+	
CCR9	TECK	+	
CXCR4	SDF-1	+++	++
CX3CR1/V28	Fractalkine	+	
STRL-33/BONZO/CXCR6	CXCL16	+	
GPR1	?	+	
GPR15/BOB	?	+	
APJ	Apelin	+	
ChemR23	?	+	
RDC1	?	+	
Leukotriene B$_4$ receptor	Leukotriene B$_4$	+	

significance of other co-receptors for HIV-1 replication *in vivo* and patho-genesis remains unclear. Recent evidence, however, has demonstrated that STRL-33 (now termed CXCR6) is associated with infection of a subset of primary T-cells *in vitro*[7], while CCR8 supports infection of thymocytes[8]. The capacity of these co-receptors to support infection of such primary cell cultures (rather than indicator cell lines where recombinant CD4 and co-receptors are often expressed at unnaturally high levels) provides stronger support of a possible role *in vivo*.

The interaction between gp120 and co-receptors

The interaction between CD4 and gp120 is conserved among all primate lentiviruses. Some of the amino acids on gp120 that form the CD4 binding site are variable, however, for these residues, the peptide backbone rather than their side chains are involved in contacting CD4[9]. The co-receptor binding site on gp120 is not usually fully exposed until CD4 is bound. The variable V1/V2 loops are probably the main cover for the co-receptor binding site and these loops become repositioned when CD4 is bound[9]. Mutations that expose the co-receptor binding site, therefore, confer a more CD4-independent phenotype[10,11].

The regions of gp120 implicated in the interaction with co-receptors are thought to involve the relatively conserved 'bridging sheet' that lies between the protruding and variable V1/V2 and V3 loops, as well as some amino acids in V3 itself[9]. The V3 loop has long been known to be a major determinant of cell tropism and now co-receptor use. Positively charged amino acids in V3 that confer a syncytium inducing (SI) phenotype correlate with CXCR4 use. The role of the V1/V2 loops in the co-receptor interaction is less clear since an HIV-1 mutant with V1/V2 deleted was infectious[12], while recombinant gp120 similarly deleted for V1 and V2 also bound co-receptors[13]. When present, however, V1 and V2 influence both cell tropism and co-receptors used[14].

Chemokine receptors form rods in the cell membrane with a central pore surrounded by the seven transmembrane regions. Four domains are exposed on the cell surface, the N-terminus, and three extracellular loops (E1, E2 and E3). Co-receptors take up different conformations on cell surfaces and on different cell types[15] that influence their ability to support HIV infection. Such conformations may result from the formation of dimers[16] or association with other cell surface molecules as reported for CCR5 and CD4[17]. Two sites on co-receptors centred around the N-terminus and E2 are involved in HIV entry. Mutagenesis studies showed the N-terminal domain of CCR5 is important for co-receptor activity for CCR5-using (R5) HIV-1s[18]. R5 strains, however, differ considerably in their use of CCR5 as highlighted by a wide variation in their capacity to infect cells expressing different chimeric human/mouse CCR5s[19]. For SIV$_{MAC}$, both macrophage-tropic and T-cell tropic strains use CCR5; however, the former require the N-terminus of CCR5, while E2 is crucial for T-tropic SIVs[20]. It is unclear if there are HIV-1 CCR5-using strains with the properties of T-tropic SIVs.

For CXCR4-using (X4) strains, E2 is critical and deletion of the N-terminus of CXCR4 has little affect on some but not all strains[21,22]. Chimeric co-receptors, therefore, support X4 virus entry as long as E2 of CXCR4 is present; however, Brelot et al[23] showed that X4 strains vary in their use of CXCR4 E2 with different isolates dependent on distinct E2 residues for activity.

Electrostatic charge interactions are also involved and likely to enhance gp120/co-receptor interactions. The N-terminal region of CCR5 (and often other co-receptors) is negatively charged due to 3 acidic amino acids and 4 (potentially) sulphated tyrosine residues which are important for co-receptor function[24]. These negative residues may aid interactions with positive amino acids in and around the bridging sheet on gp120[9]. Moreover, the V3 loops of X4 strains are highly positively charged while E2 of CXCR4 contains five negatively charged amino acids and it is likely that these oppositely charged faces interact. Mutagenesis of all five acidic residues, however, does not completely eliminate HIV infection[25]. Thus, negatively charged residues at the N-terminus of CCR5 and in E2 of CXCR4 may enhance the gp120/coreceptor interaction by electrostatic interactions with R5 and X4 strains respectively, however, they do not determine the specificity of the interaction.

Sites in the V1/V2 loop, the bridging sheet and V3 loop on gp120 may thus contribute to at least two specific interactions with co-receptors centred on the N-terminus and E2. A 'high affinity' interaction at both sites may not be needed to trigger infection, explaining why the specificity of the co-receptor interaction can be predominantly mapped to either the N-terminus or to E2. In summary, diverse virus strains vary considerably in the regions and specific amino acids of co-receptors that they exploit for recognition and triggering fusion. The capacity of HIV to vary the envelope and co-receptor residues involved in their interaction will be a major mechanism of immune evasion.

Cell tropism of HIV in immune and non-immune tissues

In vivo, HIV mainly infects haematapoietic cells that express CD4 and either CCR5 or CXCR4. These include T-helper lymphocytes, macrophages and probably dendritic cells. Many reports describe the infection of CD4-negative non-haematapoietic cell types in vitro.

Generally this type of infection is inefficient and its significance for pathogenesis and viral reservoirs *in vivo* remains controversial. *In vitro*, R5 viruses infect primary cultures of both lymphocytes and macrophages, while X4 isolates also infect T-cell lines. The capacity of X4 strains to infect macrophages is controversial[26]; however, we and others have shown that primary X4 isolates infect at least some populations of macrophages[27]. In the blood of individuals that carry R5 viruses, the CD4+ CD45RO+ memory T-cells carry most of the proviral load, although CD45RA+ naïve cells are also infected. When CXCR4-using strains emerge, their tropism for different T-cell populations is broader. On T-cells, CCR5 expression is mainly restricted to memory cells, while CXCR4 expression is more widespread but predominates on naïve T-cells[28]. Symptomatic, X4-carrying individuals thus have an increased proviral load in naïve T-cells consistent with an expanded T-cell tropism[29]. Early studies suggested that monocytes were infrequently colonized *in vivo*[30]; however, more recent reports indicate that monocytes may harbour replication competent virus in patients treated by HAART[31,32]. Whether dendritic cells are infected has been controversial; however, the current consensus suggests that they are likely to support at least some level of HIV replication *in vivo*, and may play a significant role in transferring newly transmitted virus from mucosa to T-cells in lymph nodes[33]. Suggestions that the capacity to replicate in dendritic cells reflected a mucosal route of transmission and was dependent on HIV-1 subtype[34] have been refuted by others[35]. The extent dendritic cells support full replication may depend on their state of maturation[36]. Immature dendritic cells were reported to selectively support replication by R5 viruses[37], while more mature cells are permissive to R5 and X4 virus entry, but less supportive of post-entry events[37]. Dendritic cells can also trap virus particles by high affinity interactions between sugar groups on gp120 and lectin-like domains on the receptor DC-SIGN[38]. DC-SIGN may, therefore, enable dendritic cells to trap HIV particles and pass them to T-cells while also presenting antigen. *In vitro*, conjugates of T-cells and purified dendritic cells provide a rich environment for intensive replication and production of new viral particles and may also trigger full replication in cells harbouring a restricted infection. Immature dendritic cells, *e.g.* Langerhans' cells at mucosal membranes, are likely to be the first cells encountered by HIV following transmission. These cells may carry HIV either as by DC-SIGN-trapped virus or as an infected cell to lymph nodes where association with T-cells provides a potent medium for rapid amplification of virus.

Chemokines also influence the types of cells that become infected. Saha *et al* showed that several CD4+ CCR5+ T-cell clones derived from non-progressing HIV-1+ individuals and transformed by Herpes Saimiri virus (HSV) were resistant to infection by R5 HIV-1 strains due to the production of endogenous β-chemokines[39]. Saha's study also showed that T-cell clones made from patients who had advanced to AIDS were substantially more sensitive to R5 virus replication consistent with the increasing sensitivity and colonization of CD4$^+$ CCR5$^+$ T-cells as disease progresses. Extensive expression of SDF-1 along mucosal membranes has been detected as well as down-regulation of CXCR4 on T-lymphocytes in the vicinity[40]. These observations suggest a mechanism for the blocked transmission of X4 viruses across mucosal membranes and may explain why dendritic cells *in vitro* and away from the SDF-1 rich environment of mucosa[40] support at least the early entry stages of X4 viruses. Other mechanisms, however, are required to explain the selective transmission of R5 viruses directly into the blood. Thus, soluble factors, *e.g.* chemokines in the tissue milieu or produced endogenously by target cells, can have a major influence on tropism.

In non-immune tissues and organs, the resident specialized macrophage cells carry the viral load. For example, HIV antigens can be detected in the liver macrophages known as Küppfer cells, while alveolar macrophages are infected in the lung. The brain is physically isolated from the blood by the blood–brain barrier, a system of tight gap junctions between endothelial cells in the blood capillaries. The brain is colonized by HIV-1 early in infection and probably seeded by HIV carried in by infected monocytes or macrophages. The main cell types infected in the brain are perivascular macrophages and microglia[41]. Non-haematapoietic astrocytes that do not express CCR5 or CD4 may also become infected, but do not efficiently support production of new virus particles[42]. The extent of astrocyte infection and its significance for brain pathology is controversial. Infection of brain microvascular endothelial cells (BMVECs) is even more contentious but supported in some studies[43], and would represent a simple route of entry into the brain across the blood–brain barrier.

Variation of co-receptor use *in vivo*

The extent HIV-1 adapts to replicate in different cell types or to exploit co-receptors other than CCR5 or CXCR4 *in vivo* is not known. The growing number of different 7TM receptors that support HIV and SIV infection of cell lines *in vitro* does not accurately predict co-receptor usage *in vivo*. High level expression of alternative co-receptors 'out of context' on cell lines seems to deliver them to the cell surface in an active form that can confer virus entry. Additional factors *in vivo* that may prevent many of the same alternative co-receptors from functioning are not known. Nor is it known what factors and/or selective pressures operate *in vivo* that prevent CXCR4-using (SI) strains from emerging until late in disease and often not at all. Both immune (*e.g.* neutralizing antibodies) and non-immune (*e.g.* SDF-1 blockade and/or down-regulation of CXCR4) mechanisms have been suggested to contribute (reviewed by Michael and Moore[44]). The R5 to X4 switch usually occurs via an evolution through an R5X4 stage[6]. The capacity to exploit both CCR5 and CXCR4, however, compromises the interaction with CCR5 and such strains are often ultrasensitive to inhibition by β-chemokines[45]. This reduced CCR5 interaction probably explains why R5X4 viruses cannot follow the CCR5 route for transmission and like SI strains in general are transmitted infrequently.

The evolution of R5 to R5X4 and X4 strains in about 50% of symptomatic individuals, however, illustrates the capacity of HIV-1 to switch co-receptors *in vivo*. Data from SIVs also show the potential of primate lentiviruses to adapt to use alternative co-receptors. For instance, an SIV that predominantly uses CCR2b is present in red capped mangabeys that carry defective CCR5 genes[46]. Alternative unidentified co-receptors are frequently found to support HIV-2 and SIV infection of primary T-cells and macrophages *in vitro*[47] and, as already discussed, evidence is now emerging that implicates CXCR6 (STRL-33/BONZO) for HIV-1 infection of a T-cell subset and CCR8 for thymocytes[7,8].

Co-receptor switching (analogous to an R5 to X4 switch for HIV-1) has not been demonstrated *in vivo* for SIV, although an evolution from macrophage-tropism (M-tropic) to T-cell tropism (T-tropic) has been implicated[48], while neurotropic and neurovirulent SIV$_{MAC}$ strains that rapidly cause brain disease have also been isolated[49]. The switch from M- to T-tropism involves a change in how CCR5 is exploited as a co-receptor rather than the use of an alternative co-receptor. Thus, two potential pathways for envelope evolution exist *in vivo*; one involves a switch to a new co-receptor, while the second involves a change in how a particular co-receptor is exploited to trigger infection.

Are there HIV-1 variants tropic for specialized cells in different tissues?

It is not known if specific variants evolve that have an increased capacity to infect and replicate in the specialized cells of different tissues or if such variants are linked with particular AIDS pathologies, *e.g.* dementia. As already discussed, neurovirulent SIV$_{MAC}$ variants can be isolated and their properties are conferred by determinants that include sequences in the envelope gene[50]. This precedent demonstrates the real possibility that similar neurotropic HIV-1 strains exist that are associated with dementia. Moreover, specific amino acids at particular sites in the V3 loop (or motifs) have also been associated with envelopes in the brain[51,52]. Such motifs are highly controversial, but could be associated with the use of alternative brain encoded co-receptors or adaptation to use CCR5 conformations expressed on brain cells. To date, all brain-derived viruses, support the predominant use of CCR5 in brain tissue[53]. The possibility that viruses in the brain broaden their co-receptor usage from R5 to include an unknown co-receptor expressed on specialized brain cells has not been excluded. Furthermore, most SIV_{MAC} strains use several co-receptors including CCR5, STRL-33, GPR1 and GPR15, thus raising the possibility that one or more are preferentially used to infect specialized cells in different tissues. Further investigation of the tropisms and co-receptors used by envelopes present in the brain and other tissues is clearly needed.

HIV variation in different tissues

Independent HIV variation in different body compartments has been well documented, *e.g.* in the brain[51,54] and in semen[55,56]. This variation is distinct from that seen in blood or lymphatic organs and may represent selection for tissue-adapted variants, or just random but independent evolution. Regardless, variation in the envelope will help the virus to escape from neutralizing antibodies; however, too much divergence is constrained since it will weaken the envelope's interactions with CD4 and co-receptors, reducing the efficiency of infection and probably increasing sensitivity to inhibition by chemokines. Selection pressures in different compartments will vary greatly. For example, the brain is a relatively 'immunoprivileged' environment and viruses replicating there will not be exposed to the same constraints imposed by neutralizing antibodies in lymphoid tissue. Viral strains in the brain may, therefore, adopt a more 'open' envelope conformation that allows enhanced interactions with CD4 and co-receptors, as seems to occur with T-cell line adapted (TCLA) strains that have been cultured *in vitro* in the absence of neutralizing antibodies[57]. Moreover, concentrations of inhibitory chemokines are likely to vary considerably depending on the tissue and levels of cellular activation. CCR5 may also be expressed in distinct tissue or cell type specific conformations that support infection of some R5 variants over others, as we reported for particular R5 viruses that failed to enter primary CCR5+ macrophages[58].

Envelope/co-receptor interactions may also influence early post-entry events[59] in some cell types favouring some strains over others. For instance, the observations that both M-tropic and T-tropic SIV_{MAC} strains enter macrophages[60], while only M-tropic envelopes signal *via* CCR5[61] has raised the possibility that co-receptor signalling events induced by a virus entering at the cell surface may be a requirement for replication in some cell types. Signalling during virus entry, however, is controversial and recent data showing that increased expression of CCR5 on the surface of macrophages fully rescues T-tropic SIV replication probably argue against, in this instance[62].

Thus different cell types in distinct environments will select for or against particular R5 viruses or quasispecies; however, the extent this happens and its impact on pathogenesis is unclear.

The role of other receptors

HIV viral particles interact with a range of other cell surface receptors *via* interactions that involve gp120. These interactions do not actively support HIV entry but aid attachment of HIV virions to cell surfaces that contain suboptimal levels of CD4 or co-receptors, *e.g.* on macrophages and astrocytes. Some of these interactions are mediated by the sugar groups on the envelope glycoprotein associating with other sugars or with receptors that contain lectin-like domains on the cell surface, *e.g.* the mannose specific macrophage endocytosis receptor[63] and DC-SIGN (see above)[38]. HIV envelope gp120 also binds the glycolipid, galactocerebroside (gal-C) and its sulphated derivative, sulphatide[64,65]. These molecules are expressed on neuronal and glial cells in the brain[64], colon epithelial cell lines[65] and importantly also on macrophages[66]. Both DC-SIGN and Gal-C bind gp120 with a high affinity (Kd of 11.6 nM), similar to the binding affinity of monomeric gp120 for CD4 (Kd of 2–5 nM). Gal-C supports suboptimal entry of particular HIV-1 strains without CD4, although infection of the colorectal cell line HT29 requires both gal-C and CXCR4[67]. Mondor *et al*[68] have shown that HIV virions attach to the surface of HeLa/CD4 cells *via* an interaction between gp120 and the glycosaminoglycan moiety (heparan sulphate) on the cell surface. This interaction can be demonstrated for X4 and R5X4 but is less strong for R5 envelopes since it is mediated mainly by positively charged V3 loops interacting with negatively charged sulphate groups on glycosaminoglycans[69]. Although these receptors may aid HIV attachment, fusion will not occur until sufficient CD4 and co-receptor molecules are recruited to trigger formation of a fusion pore. Thus direct and early interactions with CD4 are likely to lead to the most efficient infection process with the fastest kinetics.

Therapies targeted at HIV receptors

Highly active anti-retroviral treatment (HAART) has been very effective in many HIV+ individuals in reducing viral load and often resulting in dramatic recovery from disease. There is still a need to develop new approaches to therapy that will provide alternative drugs when resistant virus variants emerge or particular drugs are not well tolerated. Many novel strategies that interfere with the entry pathway are being developed. Intervention of the interaction between CD4 and the HIV envelope is an attractive therapeutic approach since all HIV and SIV strains can bind CD4, while infection without CD4 is probably insignificant *in vivo*. A soluble form of CD4 containing the four extracellular domains was shown to be an excellent inhibitor of infection by TCLA HIV-1 strains[70]. The sensitivity of TCLA viruses was probably due to the capacity of sCD4 to tear gp120 molecules off the surface off virus particles[71]. Sadly, it turned out that primary isolates of HIV-1 (R5 or X4) were substantially more resistant to sCD4 inhibition[72], because they had a lower affinity for CD4 and gp120 was more stably attached to virions[73]. Clinical trials showed that sCD4 was not toxic and well tolerated, but failed to have a major influence on viral load or the decline in CD4 cell numbers in peripheral blood[74,75] except at very high doses[76]. Chimeric CD4 and immunoglobulin (immunoadhesin) molecules consisting of the N-terminal 2 domains of CD4 joined to the Fc region of an antibody (human IgG$_1$) substantially increased the half life *in vivo* and also conferred antibody functions. CD4-IgG prevented infection of chimpanzees by the prototype TCLA HIV-1 IIIB strain[77]; however, in clinical trials, it had little effect on viral load and declining CD4 cell numbers[78]. Chimeric CD4-*Pseudomonas* exotoxin (CD4-PE40) constructs were also excellent inhibitors *in vitro*, targeting and killing cells infected with patient isolates that resisted sCD4 neutralization[79]. In clinical trials, CD4-PE40 was too toxic to be used at concentrations effective against HIV[80]. Faced with such failure in the clinic, the drive to develop CD4-based therapies has waned. One surviving approach is a version of CD4-IgG, where the Fv portions of both heavy and light chains have been replaced with D1D2 of CD4. This construct, a heterotetramer of CD4 D1D2, is effective against diverse primary HIV-1 strains[81] as well as plasma virus taken straight from patients (*ex vivo*)[82]. Clinical trials with this CD4-IgG have not yet been reported. New strategies will come from the reported crystal structure of gp120/CD4 complexes[9]. For instance, a cavity at the surface of gp120 was revealed that accommodates the phenyl ring of F43 on CD4. Agents designed to block this cavity would be predicted to interfere with the interaction between gp120 and CD4 and so block infection.

The identification of HIV co-receptors has provided an exciting new therapeutic opportunity. Drugs aimed at blocking envelope interactions with both CCR5 and CXCR4 are being developed. CCR5 is an excellent target for therapy since individuals homozygous for the 32 base pair deletion in CCR5 are effectively CCR5-negative but healthy. Agents that specifically block the natural CCR5 receptor activity should, therefore (at least in theory), not be harmful. There has been much debate about whether inhibitors of R5 strains will select for the more pathogenic X4 variants[44], or for variants that exploit alternative co-receptors. Extensive evidence that shows Δ32 CCR5 heterozygotes progress more slowly to AIDS bodes well for CCR5 inhibitors that will also decrease the level of functional CCR5 for HIV infection. One report, however, suggested caution and showed that CXCR4-using viruses may be present more frequently in Δ32 CCR5 heterozygotes[83] Moreover, variation in use of CCR5 by different R5 strains[19] may mean that variant viruses will emerge that escape CCR5 inhibitors but still use CCR5 as a co-receptor. Regardless, co-receptor drugs will be used in combination with agents that target other events in the virus life cycle, *e.g.* RT or protease inhibitors. In these situations, virus replication should be driven down to very low levels minimizing the chances of accruing mutations that confer escape from CCR5 inhibitors.

In the early days after co-receptors were discovered, it was hoped that the chemokines themselves or their antagonist derivatives might be exploited in therapy. We reported that a recombinant form of RANTES modified at the N-terminus (amino-oxy-pentane-RANTES, or AOP-RANTES) potently inhibited infection by R5 strains of HIV[84]. The potency of AOP-RANTES was due to its capacity to induce CCR5 internalization and retention in endosomes, a property that effectively removed CCR5 from the cell surface[85]. Small positively charged peptides have also been reported that interact with CXCR4 and block infection of X4 strains of HIV[86,87]. It is unlikely that such peptides or other protein-based drugs can be widely used for treatment of infected individuals since they are costly to manufacture and are likely to require intravenous administration. One great hope for drug therapies that target co-receptors lies in small organic molecules that are less expensive to synthesize and can be taken orally. The optimism comes from past successes in targeting 7TM, GPCRs, where small organic molecules specific for particular 7TMs have been exploited to treat a range of diseases including schizophrenia and asthma. Many pharmaceutical companies hold large collections or libraries of small organic molecules that are currently being screened for activity to CCR5 or CXCR4. Once molecules that interact with CCR5 or CXCR4 have been identified, then further manipulations of the structure can increase specificity, affinity and other properties. Already an antagonist of CCR5 has been reported (TAK-779) that inhibits R5 strains HIV *in vitro*[88], while AMD3100, a bicyclam derivative, binds CXCR4 and blocks X4 viruses[89]. It is certain that several more are currently the subject of patent applications but will be in clinical trials soon. Whether such molecules will be successful in the treating HIV+ patients will become clear within only a few years.

Acknowledgements

We wish to thank the UK Medical Research Council for supporting our HIV research over many years as well as the NIBSC Centralised Facility for AIDS Reagents for providing many of the reagents we have used. Thanks also to Robin Weiss for continued encouragement. PRC is now an Elizabeth Glaser Pediatric AIDS Foundation Research Scientist. ÁMcK is a Welcome Trust Research Fellow (ref no. 060758).

References

1 Michael NL. Host genetic influences on HIV-1 pathogenesis. *Curr Opin Immunol* 1999; **11**: 466–74

2 Benkirane M, Jin DY, Chun RF, Koup RA, Jeang KT. Mechanism of transdominant inhibition of CCR5-mediated HIV-1 infection by CCR5 delta32. *J Biol Chem* 1997; **272**: 30603–6

3 Wilkinson DA, Operskalski EA, Busch MP, Mosley JW, Koup RA. A 32-bp deletion within the CCR5 locus protects against transmission of parenterally acquired human immunodeficiency virus but does not affect progression to AIDS-defining illness. *J Infect Dis* 1998; **178**: 1163–6

4 Philpott S, Burger H, Charbonneau T *et al*. CCR5 genotype and resistance to vertical transmission of HIV-1. *J Acquir Immune Defic Syndr* 1999; **21**: 189–93

5 Michael NL, Nelson JA, KewalRamani VN *et al*. Exclusive and persistent use of the entry coreceptor CXCR4 by human immunodeficiency virus type 1 from a subject homozygous for CCR5 delta32. *J Virol* 1998; **72**: 6040–7

6 Scarlatti G, Tresoldi E, Bjorndal A *et al*. *In vivo* evolution of HIV-1 co-receptor usage and sensitivity to chemokine-mediated suppression. *Nat Med* 1997; **3**: 1259–65

7 Sharron M, Pohlmann S, Price K *et al*. Expression and coreceptor activity of STRL33/BONZO on primary peripheral blood lymphocytes. *Blood* 2000; **96**: 41–9

8 Lee S, Tiffany HL, King L, Murphy PM, Golding H, Zaitseva MB. CCR8 on human thymocytes functions as a human immunodeficiency virus type 1 coreceptor. *J Virol* 2000; **74**: 6946–52

9 Kwong PD, Wyatt R, Robinson J, Sweet RW, Sodroski J, Hendrickson WA. Structure of an HIV gp120 envelope glycoprotein in complex with the CD4 receptor and a neutralizing human antibody. *Nature* 1998; **393**: 648–59

10 Hoffman TL, LaBranche CC, Zhang W *et al*. Stable exposure of the coreceptor-binding site in a CD4-independent HIV-1 envelope protein. *Proc Natl Acad Sci USA* 1999; **96**: 6359–64

11 Reeves JD, Schulz TF. The CD4 independent tropism of HIV-2 involves several regions of the envelope protein and correlates with a reduced activation threshold for envelope mediated fusion. *J Virol* 1997; **71**: 1453–65

12 Cao J, Sullivan N, Desjardin E *et al*. Replication and neutralization of human immunodeficiency virus type 1 lacking the V1 and V2 variable loops of the gp120 envelope glycoprotein. *J Virol* 1997; **71**: 9808–12

13 Wu L, Gerard NP, Wyatt R *et al*. CD4-induced interaction of primary HIV-1 gp120 glycoproteins with the chemokine receptor CCR-5. *Nature* 1996; **384**: 179–83

14 Cho MW, Lee MK, Carney MC, Berson JF, Doms RW, Martin MA. Identification of determinants on a dual tropic human immunodeficiency virus type 1 envelope glycoprotein that confer usage of CXCR4. *J Virol* 1998; **72**: 2509–15

15 Lee B, Sharron M, Blanpain C *et al*. Epitope mapping of CCR5 reveals multiple conformational states and distinct but overlapping structures involved in chemokine and coreceptor function. *J Biol Chem* 1999; **274**: 9617–26

16 Lapham CK, Zaitseva MB, Lee S, Romanstseva T, Golding H. Fusion of monocytes and macrophages with HIV-1 correlates with biochemical properties of CXCR4 and CCR5. *Nat Med* 1999; **5**: 303–8

17 Xiao X, Wu L, Stantchev TS *et al*. Constitutive cell surface association between CD4 and CCR5. *Proc Natl Acad Sci USA* 1999; **96**: 7496–501

18 Rucker J, Samson M, Doranz BJ *et al*. Regions in beta-chemokine receptors CCR5 and CCR2b that determine HIV-1 cofactor specificity. *Cell* 1996; **87**: 437–46

19 Picard L, Simmons G, Power CA, Meyer A, Weiss RA, Clapham PR. Multiple extracellular domains of CCR-5 contribute to human immunodeficiency virus type 1 entry and fusion. *J Virol* 1997; **71**: 5003–11

20 Edinger AL, Amedee A, Miller K *et al*. Differential utilization of CCR5 by macrophage and T cell tropic simian immunodeficiency virus strains. *Proc Natl Acad Sci USA* 1997; **94**: 4005–10

21 Picard L, Wilkinson DA, McKnight A *et al*. Role of the amino-terminal extracellular domain of CXCR-4 in human immunodeficiency virus type 1 entry. *Virology* 1997; **231**: 105–11

22 Brelot A, Heveker N, Pleskoff O, Sol N, Alizon M. Role of the first and third extracellular domains of CXCR-4 in human immunodeficiency virus coreceptor activity. *J Virol* 1997; **71**: 4744–51

23 Brelot A, Heveker N, Adema K, Hosie MJ, Willett B, Alizon M. Effect of mutations in the second extracellular loop of CXCR4 on its utilization by human and feline immunodeficiency viruses. *J Virol* 1999 **73**: 2576–86

24 Farzan M, Choe H, Vaca L *et al*. A tyrosine-rich region in the N terminus of CCR5 is important for human immunodeficiency virus type 1 entry and mediates an association between gp120 and CCR5. *J Virol* 1998; **72**: 1160–4

25 Wang ZX, Berson JF, Zhang TY *et al*. CXCR4 sequences involved in coreceptor determination of human immunodeficiency virus type-1 tropism. Unmasking of activity with M-tropic Env glycoproteins. *J Biol Chem* 1998; **273**: 15007–15

26 Stent G, Joo GB, Kierulf P, Asjo B. Macrophage tropism: fact or fiction? *J Leukoc Biol* 1997; **62**: 4–11

27 Simmons G, Wilkinson D, Reeves JD *et al*. Primary, syncytium-inducing human immunodeficiency virus type 1 isolates are dual-tropic and most can use either Lestr or CCR5 as coreceptors for virus entry. *J Virol* 1996; **70**: 8355–60

28 Bleul CC, Wu L, Hoxie JA, Springer TA, Mackay CR. The HIV coreceptors CXCR4 and CCR5 are differentially expressed and regulated on human T lymphocytes. *Proc Natl Acad Sci USA* 1997; **94**: 1925–30

29 Ostrowski MA, Chun TW, Justement SJ *et al*. Both memory and CD45RA⁺/CD62L⁺ naive CD4(⁺) T cells are infected in human immunodeficiency virus type 1-infected individuals. *J Virol* 1999; **73**: 6430–5

30 Schnittman SM, Psallidopoulos MC, Lane HC *et al*. The reservoir for HIV-1 in human peripheral blood is a T cell that maintains expression of CD4. *Science* 1989; **245**: 305–8

31 Lambotte O, Taoufik Y, de Goer MG, Wallon C, Goujard C, Delfraissy JF. Detection of infectious HIV in circulating monocytes from patients on prolonged highly active antiretroviral therapy. *J Acquir Immune Defic Syndr* 2000; **23**: 114–9

32 Sonza S, Mutimer HP, Oelrichs R *et al*. Monocytes harbour replication-competent, non-latent HIV-1 in patients on highly active antiretroviral therapy. *AIDS* 2001; **15**: 17–22

33 Rowland-Jones SL. HIV: The deadly passenger in dendritic cells. *Curr Biol* 1999; **9**: R248–50

34 Soto-Ramirez LE, Renjifo B, McLane MF *et al*. HIV-1 Langerhans' cell tropism associated with heterosexual transmission of HIV. *Science* 1996; **271**: 1292–3

35 Pope M, Ho DD, Moore JP, Weber J, Dittmar MT, Weiss RA. Different subtypes of HIV-1 and cutaneous dendritic cells. *Science* 1997; **278**: 786–8

36 Patterson S, Robinson SP, English NR, Knight SC. Subpopulations of peripheral blood dendritic cells show differential susceptibility to infection with a lymphotropic strain of HIV-1. *Immunol Lett* 1999; **66**: 111–6

37 Granelli-Piperno A, Delgado E, Finkel V, Paxton W, Steinman RM. Immature dendritic cells selectively replicate macrophage tropic (M-tropic) human immunodeficiency virus type 1, while mature cells efficiently transmit both M- and T-tropic virus to T cells. *J Virol* 1998; **72**: 2733–7

38 Geijtenbeek TB, Kwon DS, Torensma R *et al*. DC-SIGN, a dendritic cell-specific HIV-1-binding protein that enhances trans-infection of T cells. *Cell* 2000; **100**: 587–97

39 Saha K, Bentsman G, Chess L, Volsky DJ. Endogenous production of beta-chemokines by CD4⁺, but not CD8⁺, T-cell clones correlates with the clinical state of human immunodeficiency virus type 1 (HIV-1)-infected individuals and may be responsible for blocking infection with non-syncytium-inducing HIV-1 *in vitro*. *J Virol* 1998; **72**: 876–81

40 Agace WW, Amara A, Roberts AI *et al*. Constitutive expression of stromal derived factor-1 by mucosal epithelia and its role in HIV transmission and propagation. *Curr Biol* 2000; **10**: 325–8

41 Nottet HS, Gendelman HE. Unraveling the neuroimmune mechanisms for the HIV-1-associated cognitive/motor complex. *Immunol Today* 1995; **16**: 441–8

42 Saito Y, Sharer LR, Epstein LG *et al*. Overexpression of nef as a marker for restricted HIV-1

infection of astrocytes in postmortem pediatric central nervous tissues. *Neurology* 1994; **44**: 474–81

43 Moses AV, Nelson JA. HIV infection of human brain capillary endothelial cells – implications for AIDS dementia. *Adv Neuroimmunol* 1994; **4**: 239–47

44 Michael NL, Moore JP. HIV-1 entry inhibitors: evading the issue. *Nat Med* 1999; **5**: 740–2

45 Kledal TN, Rosenkilde MM, Coulin F *et al.* A broad-spectrum chemokine antagonist encoded by Kaposi's sarcoma-associated herpes virus. *Science* 1997; **277**: 1656–9

46 Chen Z, Kwon D, Jin Z *et al.* Natural infection of a homozygous delta24 CCR5 red-capped mangabey with an R2b-tropic simian immunodeficiency virus. *J Exp Med* 1998; **188**: 2057–65

47 Simmons G, Reeves JD, Hibbitts S *et al.* Co-receptor use by HIV and inhibition of HIV infection by chemokine receptor ligands. *Immunol Rev* 2000; **177**: 112–26

48 Mori K, Ringler DJ, Kodama T, Desrosiers RC. Complex determinants of macrophage tropism in env of simian immunodeficiency virus. *J Virol* 1992; **66**: 2067–75

49 Sharma DP, Zink MC, Anderson M *et al.* Derivation of neurotropic simian immunodeficiency virus from exclusively lymphocytotropic parental virus: pathogenesis of infection in macaques. *J Virol* 1992; **66**: 3550–6

50 Anderson MG, Hauer D, Sharma DP *et al.* Analysis of envelope changes acquired by SIVmac239 during neuroadaption in rhesus macaques. *Virology* 1993; **195**: 616–26

51 Korber BT, Kunstman KJ, Patterson BK *et al.* Genetic differences between blood- and brain-derived viral sequences from human immunodeficiency virus type 1-infected patients: evidence of conserved elements in the V3 region of the envelope protein of brain-derived sequences. *J Virol* 1994; **68**: 7467–81

52 Power C, McArthur JC, Johnson RT *et al.* Demented and non-demented patients with AIDS differ in brain-derived human immunodeficiency virus type 1 envelope sequences. *J Virol* 1994; **68**: 4643–9

53 Gabuzda D, Wang J. Chemokine receptors and mechanisms of cell death in HIV neuropathogenesis. *J Neurovirol* 2000; **6** (**Suppl 1**): S24–32

54 Ball JK, Holmes EC, Whitwell H, Desselberger U. Genomic variation of human immunodeficiency virus type 1 (HIV-1): molecular analyses of HIV-1 in sequential blood samples and various organs obtained at autopsy. *J Gen Virol* 1994; **75**: 67–79

55 Delwart EL, Mullins JI, Gupta P *et al.* Human immunodeficiency virus type 1 populations in blood and semen. *J Virol* 1998; **72**: 617–23

56 Kiessling AA, Fitzgerald LM, Zhang D *et al.* Human immunodeficiency virus in semen arises from a genetically distinct virus reservoir. *AIDS Res Hum Retroviruses* 1998; **14** (**Suppl 1**): S33–41

57 Moore JP, Cao Y, Qing L *et al.* Primary isolates of human immunodeficiency virus type 1 are relatively resistant to neutralization by monoclonal antibodies to gp120, and their neutralization is not predicted by studies with monomeric gp120. *J Virol* 1995; **69**: 101–9

58 Dittmar MT, Simmons G, Donaldson Y *et al.* Biological characterization of human immunodeficiency virus type 1 clones derived from different organs of an AIDS patient by long-range PCR. *J Virol* 1997; **71**: 5140–7

59 Chackerian B, Long EM, Luciw PA, Overbaugh J. Human immunodeficiency virus type 1 coreceptors participate in post entry stages in the virus replication cycle and function in simian immunodeficiency virus infection. *J Virol* 1997; **71**: 3932–9

60 Mori K, Ringler DJ, Desrosiers RC. Restricted replication of simian immunodeficiency virus strain 239 in macrophages is determined by env but is not due to restricted entry. *J Virol* 1993; **67**: 2807–14

61 Weissman D, Rabin RL, Arthos J *et al.* Macrophage-tropic HIV and SIV envelope proteins induce a signal through the CCR5 chemokine receptor. *Nature* 1997; **389**: 981–5

62 Bannert N, Schenten D, Craig S, Sodroski J. The level of CD4 expression limits infection of primary rhesus monkey macrophages by a T-tropic simian immunodeficiency virus and macrophagotropic human immunodeficiency viruses. *J Virol* 2000; **74**: 10984–93

63 Larkin M, Childs RA, Matthews TJ *et al.* Oligosaccharide-mediated interactions of the envelope glycoprotein gp120 of HIV-1 that are independent of CD4 recognition. *AIDS* 1989; **3**: 793–8

64 Harouse JM, Bhat S, Spitalnik SL *et al.* Inhibition of entry of HIV-1 in neural cell lines by antibodies against galactosyl ceramide. *Science* 1991; **253**: 320–3

65 Fantini J, Cook DG, Nathanson N, Spitalnik SL, Gonzalez Scarano F. Infection of colonic epithelial cell lines by type 1 human immunodeficiency virus is associated with cell surface expression of galactosylceramide, a potential alternative gp120 receptor. *Proc Natl Acad Sci USA* 1993; **90**: 2700–4

66 Seddiki N, Ramdani A, Saffar L, Portoukalian J, Gluckman JC, Gattegno L. A monoclonal antibody directed to sulfatide inhibits the binding of human immunodeficiency virus type 1 (HIV-1) envelope glycoprotein to macrophages but not their infection by the virus. *Biochim Biophys Acta* 1994; **1225**: 289–96

67 Delezay O, Koch N, Yahi N *et al*. Co-expression of CXCR4/fusin and galactosylceramide in the human intestinal epithelial cell line HT-29. *AIDS* 1997; **11**: 1311–8

68 Mondor I, Ugolini S, Sattentau QJ. Human immunodeficiency virus type 1 attachment to HeLa CD4 cells is CD4 independent and gp120 dependent and requires cell surface heparans. *J Virol* 1998; **72**: 3623–34

69 Moulard M, Lortat-Jacob H, Mondor I *et al*. Selective interactions of polyanions with basic surfaces on human immunodeficiency virus type 1 gp120. *J Virol* 2000; **74**: 1948–60

70 Clapham PR, Weber JN, Whitby D *et al*. Soluble CD4 blocks the infectivity of diverse strains of HIV and SIV for T cells and monocytes but not for brain and muscle cells. *Nature* 1989; **337**: 368–70

71 Moore JP, McKeating JA, Weiss RA, Sattentau QJ. Dissociation of gp120 from HIV-1 virions induced by soluble CD4. *Science* 1990; **250**: 1139–42

72 Daar ES, Li XL, Moudgil T, Ho DD. High concentrations of recombinant soluble CD4 are required to neutralize primary human immunodeficiency virus type 1 isolates. *Proc Natl Acad Sci USA* 1990; **87**: 6574–8

73 Moore JP, McKeating JA, Huang YX, Ashkenazi A, Ho DD. Virions of primary human immunodeficiency virus type 1 isolates resistant to soluble CD4 (sCD4) neutralization differ in sCD4 binding and glycoprotein gp120 retention from sCD4-sensitive isolates. *J Virol* 1992; **66**: 235–43

74 Husson RN, Chung Y, Mordenti J *et al*. Phase I study of continuous-infusion soluble CD4 as a single agent and in combination with oral dideoxyinosine therapy in children with symptomatic human immunodeficiency virus infection. *J Pediatr* 1992; **121**: 627–33

75 Kahn JO, Allan JD, Hodges TL *et al*. The safety and pharmacokinetics of recombinant soluble CD4 (rCD4) in subjects with the acquired immunodeficiency syndrome (AIDS) and AIDS-related complex. A phase 1 study. *Ann Intern Med* 1990; **112**: 254–61

76 Schooley RT, Merigan TC, Gaut P *et al*. Recombinant soluble CD4 therapy in patients with the acquired immunodeficiency syndrome (AIDS) and AIDS-related complex. A phase I–II escalating dosage trial. *Ann Intern Med* 1990; **112**: 247–53

77 Ward RH, Capon DJ, Jett CM *et al*. Prevention of HIV-1 IIIB infection in chimpanzees by CD4 immunoadhesin. *Nature* 1991; **352**: 434–6

78 Hodges TL, Kahn JO, Kaplan LD *et al*. Phase 1 study of recombinant human CD4-immunoglobulin G therapy of patients with AIDS and AIDS-related complex. *Antimicrob Agents Chemother* 1991; **35**: 2580–6

79 Kennedy PE, Moss B, Berger EA. Primary HIV-1 isolates refractory to neutralization by soluble CD4 are potently inhibited by CD4-*Pseudomonas* exotoxin. *Virology* 1993; **192**: 375–9

80 Ramachandran RV, Katzenstein DA, Wood R, Batts DH, Merigan TC. Failure of short-term CD4-PE40 infusions to reduce virus load in human immunodeficiency virus-infected persons. *J Infect Dis* 1994; **170**: 1009–13

81 Trkola A, Pomales AB, Yuan H *et al*. Cross-clade neutralization of primary isolates of human immunodeficiency virus type 1 by human monoclonal antibodies and tetrameric CD4-IgG. *J Virol* 1995; **69**: 6609–17

82 Gauduin MC, Allaway GP, Maddon PJ, Barbas 3rd CF, Burton DR, Koup RA. Effective *ex vivo* neutralization of human immunodeficiency virus type 1 in plasma by recombinant immunoglobulin molecules. *J Virol* 1996; **70**: 2586–92

83 D'Aquila RT, Sutton L, Savara A, Hughes MD, Johnson VA. CCR5/delta (ccr5) heterozygosity: a selective pressure for the syncytium-inducing human immunodeficiency virus type 1 phenotype. NIAID AIDS Clinical Trials Group Protocol 241 Virology Team. *J Infect Dis* 1998; **177**: 1549–53

84 Simmons G, Clapham PR, Picard L *et al.* Potent inhibition of HIV-1 infectivity in macrophages and lymphocytes by a novel CCR5 antagonist. *Science* 1997; **276**: 276–9

85 Mack M, Luckow B, Nelson PJ *et al.* Aminooxypentane-RANTES induces CCR5 internalization but inhibits recycling: a novel inhibitory mechanism of HIV infectivity. *J Exp Med* 1998; **187**: 1215–24

86 Doranz BJ, Grovit Ferbas K, Sharron MP *et al.* A small-molecule inhibitor directed against the chemokine receptor CXCR4 prevents its use as an HIV-1 coreceptor. *J Exp Med* 1997; **186**: 1395–400

87 Murakami T, Nakajima T, Koyanagi Y *et al.* A small molecule CXCR4 inhibitor that blocks T cell line-tropic HIV-1 infection. *J Exp Med* 1997; **186**: 1389–93

88 Baba M, Nishimura O, Kanzaki N *et al.* A small-molecule, nonpeptide CCR5 antagonist with highly potent and selective anti-HIV-1 activity. *Proc Natl Acad Sci USA* 1999; **96**: 5698–703

89 Donzella GA, Schols D, Lin SW *et al.* AMD3100, a small molecule inhibitor of HIV-1 entry via the CXCR4 co-receptor. *Nat Med* 1998; **4**: 72–7

The pathogenesis of HIV-1 infection

Jonathan Weber

Jefferiss Research Laboratories, Wright-Fleming Institute, Imperial College School of Medicine, London, UK

Epidemiologists have long established beyond all reasonable doubt that infection by the human immunodeficiency virus type 1 (HIV-1) leads to the acquired immune deficiency syndrome (AIDS). Natural history cohorts have demonstrated that the median time from infection to development of AIDS is approximately 12 years, and that this long duration is broadly similar in all populations infected by HIV-1, in all risk groups, in all ethnic groups and in all geographical areas. These epidemiological observations suggest that HIV-1 causes AIDS largely independently of human major histocompatibility complex (MHC) and HIV-1 sequence polymorphisms, as great diversity of both these factors exist world-wide. This is not to say that HLA and HIV diversity do not affect the natural history of HIV disease, but these observations support a common mechanism of HIV-1 pathogenesis which is largely independent of human and viral diversity.

The genome of HIV-1 is small, less than 10 kb, and hundreds of full-length HIV-1 sequences have been studied. All nine HIV-1 genes and their products are characterised, mostly in great detail. The molecular basis of viral entry and tropism is known, and the humoral and cellular immune responses to infection characterised at the level of the individual epitopes. Given that there is greater understanding of the biology of HIV-1 than for any other pathogen, it is frustrating that the pathogenesis of HIV disease is still so difficult to fully define at a molecular level.

The essence of HIV-1 infection is a slow decline in CD4+ T-cells over time, such that once a threshold of approximately 200×10^9 CD4 cells/l is passed, immune deficiency and virally-induced tumours are increasingly liable to occur. It has been known for 17 years that the primary receptor for HIV-1 is the CD4 molecule, expressed on the surface of mature T-helper lymphocytes in peripheral blood and lymph node, and also on macrophages and dendritic cells[1,2]. More recently, the HIV-1 co-receptors have been defined as the 7-transmembrane spanning chemokine receptors, principally CCR5 and CXCR4[3–5]. The distribution of these co-receptors on primary, activated CD4+ T-lymphocytes defines the tropism of HIV *in vitro*, and almost certainly *in vivo*. Only

*Correspondence to:
Prof. Jonathan Weber,
Jefferiss Research
Laboratories, 4th Floor
Wright-Fleming Institute,
Imperial College School
of Medicine, St Mary's
Hospital, Norfolk Place,
London W2 1PG, UK*

CD4+/CCR5+ T-lymphocytes are infectable by primary HIV-1 isolates taken directly from patients.

The central question of HIV-1 pathogenesis is through what mechanism does HIV-1 destroy CD4+ T-cells? Is the virus directly lytic for these cells through infection and viral replication, or is the mechanism indirect? For example, are HIV+/CD4+ T-cells killed through the action of HIV-specific cytotoxic T-lymphocytes (CTLs), or through the action of toxic soluble viral products such as gp120, or even through induction of apoptosis leading to the death of virally infected cells?

The loss of CD4+ cells begins during primary HIV-1 infection, and continues, not necessarily at a constant rate, throughout the course of infection. In late HIV disease, after the decline of CD4+ T-cells to below 200×10^9/l, there is some evidence that CD4+ cells decline more rapidly. In this review, I shall focus in turn firstly on primary HIV-1 infection, secondly the 'chronic' phase of asymptomatic HIV infection and finally on late HIV disease, and review the data on the mechanisms affecting the loss of CD4+ cells at these periods. The natural history of HIV-1 infection is shown diagrammatically in Figure 1.

Primary HIV infection

The early events of HIV infection are likely to be important to the later course of the disease, and are, therefore, the most appropriate starting point to consider pathogenesis. The very earliest events in the entry of HIV-1 *in vivo* are impossible to study in humans. Our knowledge of the mechanism of infection is thus mostly inferred from experimental infections of rhesus macaques with $SIV_{mac}251$. In this model, animals can be sacrificed at intervals after mucosal exposure in order to

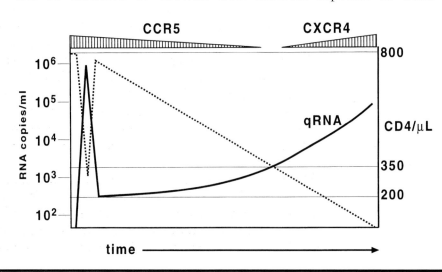

Fig. 1 Diagram of the natural history of HIV-1

determine the localisation of the virus over time. As SIV shares a very similar genetic structure to HIV and also uses CD4 as the primary receptor, it is probably a legitimate model for the study of viral entry *in vivo*. However, there is little evidence that mucosal transmission is the dominant route of transmission for primate lentiviruses in natural infection. As with any animal model, therefore, caveats as to exact applicability to human disease must be borne in mind.

After mucosal exposure to $SIV_{mac}251$, for example across the vagina of the rhesus macaque, HIV-1 appears to first infect mucosal Langerhans' cells (mLc)[6,7]. These cells are migratory within mucosa, and possess long processes which interdigitate among the mucosal epithelial cells, and thus sub-mucosal Lc may be present on the surface of epithelia. Langerhans' cells are a modified macrophage, are fundamental to antigen presentation and attract CD4+ T-cells to their dendritic processes. Mucosal Lc weakly express CD4 and CCR5, and hence are infectable by HIV-1[8]; however, these Langerhans' cells also express a cell surface lectin, DC-SIGN, which is capable of binding the HIV-1 gp120 with a high affinity[9]. The most plausible mechanism for infection across a mucosal surface is that free infectious virions are bound to DC-SIGN on the surface of mLc, which interdigitate and migrate within the vaginal mucosa. Virus bound to mLc is then moved away from the mucosal surface, and is brought in close proximity to CD4+ T-cells. The DC-SIGN bound virus is then able to infect CD4+/CCR5+ T-cells, and these infected T-cells then migrate to their regional lymph nodes (reviewed by Mascola[10]).

The HIV-infected T-cells remain sequestered in regional lymph nodes until a threshold of replication is reached within 2–6 weeks, following which a burst of plasma viraemia occurs. This is termed primary HIV infection (PHI). Following PHI, virus is disseminated within days throughout the body and seeds local, peripheral and distal reservoir sites. PHI is associated with a very high plasma viral burden, and levels of viral RNA detected by quantitative RT-PCR may exceed 5×10^6 copies RNA/ml. PHI may be accompanied by either symptoms of a 'seroconversion illness', comprising rash, painful lymphadenopathy, arthropathy and fever, or more often this period is clinically asymptomatic. The viraemic peak resolves spontaneously after 2–4 weeks, associated with a primary immune response to HIV. Although plasma viraemia is suppressed after seroconversion, HIV-1 is never eliminated and the HIV genome can be found in T-cells in all subjects at all stages of disease, and in varying quantities as virion-associated RNA in the plasma.

The viraemic peak of PHI is invariably associated with a transient reduction in CD4+ T-cells in peripheral blood. This is generally modest and short-lived, but may occasionally lead to a reduction of CD4+ T-cells below 200×10^9/l, which in turn may lead to overt clinical immunosuppression. Indeed, cases of opportunistic infections such as *Pneumocystis carinii* pneumonia and oesophageal candidiasis have been reported from this period of acute, reversible immunosuppression. Once the viraemic peak has been resolved, CD4+ cell levels return towards baseline levels, but remain lower than that seen pre-infection.

This observation of an acute loss of CD4+ T-cells associated temporally with the rapid appearance of plasma viraemia, and the recovery of CD4 count once the plasma viraemia is reduced, would appear to support the capacity of HIV-1 to directly kill CD4+ T-cells through lysis. Certainly, high levels of primary virus replication in activated peripheral blood mononuclear cells (PBMCs) *in vitro* can lead to syncytial formation (multinucleated giant cells) and consequent cell death, and HIV-1 is ultimately lytic in primary cell culture, even if syncytia are not observed. However, viraemic levels are higher in PHI than at any other time in the course of HIV-1 infection, and there is no immune response against the virus at PHI. It is possible, therefore, that the transient reduction in CD4+ T-cells at PHI represents the unopposed effect of high level HIV replication, which is curtailed by the immune response. Thus, the direct viral cause of CD4 T-cell destruction at PHI may not represent a common mechanism throughout the rest of the course of HIV-1 infection, when an immune response is always present.

The initial viraemic peak falls to a set 'steady state' within several weeks or months of infection, the level of which varies considerably between individuals and is predictive of prognosis[11]. Coincidentally with the peak of viraemia there is a vigorous HIV-specific immune response involving cell mediated immunity, CD8+ CTL and CD4+ T-helper HIV-specific responses, in addition to antibody production, all of which are believed to play an important role in controlling the initial plasma viraemia. The study of neutralising antibodies to the autologous primary isolates at PHI suggest that these are relatively slow to develop, and are rarely detectable until 6 months after infection[12]. By contrast, HIV-specific, CD8+, HLA-restricted CTLs do appear to be related temporally to the reduction in viraemia[13]. Furthermore, a number of groups have documented the emergence of escape mutations within CTL epitopes following the immune response in PHI[14,15]. These observations have been taken as evidence that CTLs are the major effector of the immune containment of HIV-1 following PHI. Certainly, it would be attractive to consider that the slow progression of HIV-1 disease is related to the balance between viral replication and the cellular immune response mediated through CD8+ CTL. However, other hypotheses exist for the control of viraemia at PHI. Following the appearance of the plasma viraemia, non-neutralising antibodies appear at the same time as CTL, principally to the core (p24), matrix (p17) and envelop (gp120) proteins[16]. These non-neutralising antibodies may bind to virions to generate circulating immune complexes, which are subsequently cleared through Fc-receptor binding in the spleen, a mechanism of viral clearance thought to be relevant to enterovirus viraemia. Furthermore, availability of activated CD4+ T-cells may become limiting during the viraemia of PHI; exhaustion of the CD4+ substrate for HIV replication may lead to reduction of viraemia without an immune mechanism being involved[17]. This hypothesis has some experimental support from the observation that treatment with low dose cyclosporin-A at PHI reduces T-cell activation and leads to reduction in viraemia and preservation of CD4 cells[18].

When the immune system first responds to HIV-1, the outcome is thought to determine much of the subsequent natural history of the disease. The titre of the antibody response to p24 at seroconversion is associated with disease outcome[16]. Acute primary infection activates the HIV-1 specific CD4+ T-helper response. However, this HIV-specific CD4+ T-helper response is generally lost during the course of untreated HIV-1 infection. In untreated patients with high levels of plasma viraemia after PHI, the HIV-specific T-helper response is undetectable within the first year of infection. When anti-retroviral drugs are given 6 months or later after seroconversion, HIV-specific T-helper responses do not return if already lost, and cytotoxic T-lymphocytes directed against HIV continue to decline. However, early anti-retroviral therapy, during PHI, is associated with preservation of both CD8+ CTL and CD4+ T-helper lymphocyte responses to HIV[19]. Most studies have failed to detect HIV specific CD4+ T-helper responses in untreated patients except for those with very slow progression and low viral loads[20].

Summary

Primary HIV-1 infection is manifest by a viraemic peak associated with a temporally related decline in CD4+ T-cells; the viraemia is probably curtailed by an HIV-specific CD8+ CTL response. There is some evidence that the reduction in CD4+ T-cells in PHI may be a direct and unopposed effect of HIV-1 replication which is curtailed and then controlled by cellular immunity.

Chronic asymptomatic HIV-1 infection

As shown diagrammatically in Figure 2, following PHI the CD4 count returns towards baseline but does not regain pre-infection levels. CD4 counts decline slowly, and in a linear manner, during the chronic asymptomatic stage of HIV-1 infection. During this period, HIV-1 RNA levels as determined by RT-PCR are highly variable between individuals, and may

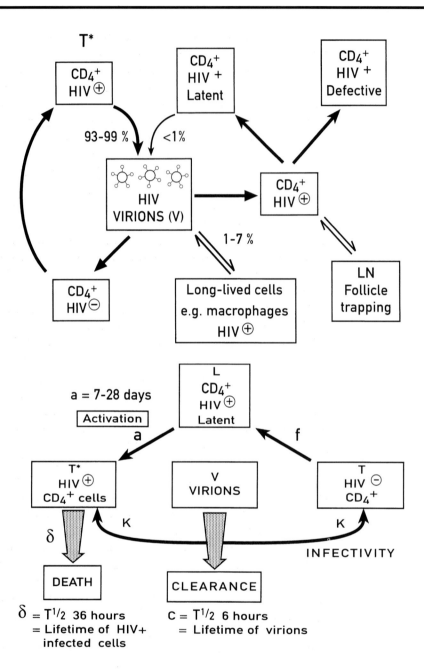

Fig. 2 Diagram of the dynamics of HIV-1 replication *in vivo*.

range from <50 copies RNA/ml, to >1,000,000 copies RNA/ml[11]. However, HIV-1 proviral DNA is always detectable in PBMCs, even if plasma viraemia is undetectable. The small number of infected cells in peripheral blood, generally 1:50,000 PBMCs, has suggested that direct viral lysis is an unlikely mechanism for the decline of CD4 cells in this period of infection.

The breakthrough in the investigation of the pathogenesis of CD4⁺ T-cell loss in this period of HIV infection came from careful multi-disciplinary observations of the effect of potent, combination anti-retroviral chemotherapy. Use of anti-retroviral drugs leads to suppression of viral replication, a reduction of plasma viraemia and an increase in CD4 count. Two landmark papers from Ho and Shaw revealed that starting anti-retroviral therapy altered the steady state of HIV-1 replication, where viral replication and clearance were in balance[21,22]. The drug therapy strongly suppressed viral replication and lead to an exponential decline in plasma viraemia over 1–2 weeks, followed by a slower second phase decline after 2–4 weeks. Mathematical modelling of the plasma viraemia decay slope enabled the production rate of HIV-1 virions to be determined, as 10^7–10^8 virions/day. The rapid replication of virions is from within the peripheral CD4⁺ T-cell compartment, and leads to a greatly reduced T-cell life expectancy of approximately 24–36 h, against an expected life-time in the absence of HIV infection of 100 days. The slower second phase decline represents HIV-1 replication in long-lived cells such as macrophages and dendritic cells. The model also accounted for the loss of CD4⁺ T-cells by assessing the rate of CD4 turnover as 70-fold over baseline, caused by the viral replication within this compartment leading to premature cell death.

These models of HIV dynamics and pathogenesis have been termed the 'bath-tub' analogy. The loss of CD4⁺ T-cells is the result of greatly increased turnover through HIV-1 driven CD4 death; new CD4⁺ T-cell production fails to match the increased CD4 cell loss, and hence a slow, continuous reduction in CD4 cells is seen. As with a bath-tub, the level of water can be maintained if the taps are on full, even if the plug is out. However, over time the taps will fail to keep up with the rate of water going down the plug, and a gradual loss of water level will be observed, until the bath is nearly empty.

There have been a number of objections to this simple model of HIV pathogenesis. Firstly, Miedema's group studied the telomere length in CD4 and CD8 lymphocytes from HIV-infected subjects[23]. Telomeres are repetitive DNA sequences at the end of all chromosomes which are cut by about 50 bp with each cell division. Although there is an enzyme which can re-extend telomeres (telomerase), the enzyme is only expressed in germ cells and tumours. Hence, telomere length should be an estimate of the number of times a cell has divided. Miedema showed that there was telomere shortening in HIV infection, but that it occurred in CD8⁺ cells, and not in CD4⁺ cells. He concluded that there was evidence for increased CD8⁺ cell turnover in HIV infection, but no evidence for increased CD4⁺ turnover.

Subsequently, a number of techniques to label lymphocytes *in vivo* have been developed, using bromodeoxyuridine (BrdU), [6-²H]-glucose or [¹³C]-

glucose. A summary of all these studies supports increased turnover (2–6-fold) of both CD4[+] and CD8[+] T-cells in HIV infection, with a reduction in half-life of about 60% compared to HIV-negative subjects (reviewed by Johnson[24]). The mechanism for the effect of anti-retroviral therapy on raising CD4[+] lymphocyte counts could, therefore, be either through reducing the rate of cell death (as in the bath-tub model), or through increasing CD4[+] cell production. Unfortunately, there are conflicting data supporting both these hypotheses. Interestingly, studies from sooty mangabeys, an old-world monkey species naturally infected with SIVsm, a virus which is non-pathogenic in this host, show that T-cell turnover is normal in this model despite high levels of plasma viraemia[25]. This observation, if reproduced, would suggest that indirect mechanisms for T-cell loss are more likely to account for the observations in HIV-infected subjects.

The unexpected, but reproducible, observations that CD8[+] lymphocytes have a higher turnover and shorter half-life in HIV-infected subjects re-focuses attention on the role of CTL in HIV infection. Potent drug treatment in chronic asymptomatic infection produces impressive restoration of immunity as judged by rise in CD4 count and loss of disease progression. However, distortions in the CD4[+] repertoire are not corrected and the HIV-specific CD8[+] CTL populations decline. Although this decline has been attributed to a loss of antigenic drive, because potent therapy is so effective at suppressing viral replication, very early use of anti-retroviral drugs preserves CD8 populations at a low but easily detectable level (reviewed by Siliciano[26]). Since it is becoming clearer that there is on-going viral turnover even in patients on continuous efficient treatment, the decline in CD8[+] numbers may be attributable, at least in part, to loss of HIV-1 specific T helper function[19]. There is good evidence that the preservation of CD8[+] CTL function and numbers in animal models is intimately dependent on T helper function.

A synthesis of these data supports HIV replication leading to loss of CD4[+] T-lymphocytes both by direct (or indirect) cell killing, and through the action of HIV-specific CTL killing of CD4[+]/HIV[+] T-cells. This would also account for the observed increase in CD8[+] T-cell turnover in HIV infection, as the action of CTL killing also increases the killing of the effector cells. The relative roles of alterations in T-cell production induced by HIV-infection and anti-retroviral therapy require further experimental study.

Summary

Chronic asymptomatic HIV infection is associated with highly dynamic, persistent viral replication, with the production of approximately 10^8

virions/day. Viral replication leads to loss of CD4⁺ T-cells, which could be due either to increased cell death, or to reduced production, or both. The increased turnover of both CD4⁺ and CD8⁺ T-cells in HIV-1 infected subjects compared to controls supports the killing of virally infected cells by HIV-specific CTL as a leading hypothesis for CD4⁺ T-cell decline in HIV infection. However, the direct relationship between plasma viral load and rate of CD4 decline suggests that viral replication also contributes, directly or indirectly, to CD4 loss.

Late stage HIV-1 infection

The decline in CD4 count during the course of HIV-1 infection is not constant over time. There is a very rapid, transient decline in CD4⁺ T-cells at primary HIV infection, as noted above. The decline in CD4 count in the chronic asymptomatic phase of HIV-1 infection is variable, and related principally to the 'steady state' level of plasma viraemia. However, the decline in this phase appears to be approximately linear, and hence constant over time. However, in late stage HIV disease, when the CD4 count is $< 200 \times 10^9/l$, there is evidence of an increase in the rate of CD4 decline.

It was observed early in the HIV epidemic that the phenotype of HIV-1 isolates grown from patients at different stages of HIV infection were different. Asjo and Levy showed independently that viral isolates taken early in the course of infection were slow growing, producing low titres of reverse transcriptase in culture (slow, low). These isolates could grow in fresh primary peripheral blood mononuclear cells (PBMCs), but were not able to infect transformed, immortalised T-cell lines such as H9, CEM or MT2[27,28]. By contrast, isolates made from patients with advanced HIV disease were able to grow rapidly to high titre in PBMCs and a wide range of T-cell lines (fast, high). Subsequently, Tersmette showed that the viral phenotype could be defined by the ability to produce syncytia (multinucleated giant cells) in the MT-2 cell line; this allowed viral isolates to be characterised as non-syncytial (NSI slow/low) or syncytial (SI fast/high)[29]. Fouchier then showed that the viral phenotype NSI/SI could be defined genetically through the charge of the V3 loop in the gp120 envelop[30]. Since the discovery of the chemokine receptors as HIV co-receptors, it has been possible to understand these phenomena at a molecular level.

NSI viruses are associated with primary HIV infection and early chronic disease. These viruses use CCR5 as their co-receptor. In late disease, viral isolates use CXCR4 as their co-receptor, or have dual tropism for both CCR5 and CXCR4[31,32]. CCR5 is expressed principally on activated T-lymphocytes and macrophages, and is not highly expressed on resting T-cells. This is part explains the association between T-cell activation and susceptibility to HIV-1 infection *in vitro*. By contrast, CXCR4 is more widely expressed on resting and activated immune cells. With the switch in viral phenotype from NSI to SI, and from CCR5 to CXCR4 usage, the capacity exists for HIV-1 infection of a broader range of target cells. Furthermore, SI/CXCR4 viruses are more cytopathic *in vitro*, and replicate to higher levels than NSI/CCR5 viruses, which may lead in turn to more efficient T-cell killing.

The difference between NSI/CCR5 usage and SI/CXCR4 usage can be shown to reside in 2 amino acid substitutions in the V3 loop of gp120. The mutation rate of HIV-1 is high, at 1:10,000 bases substituted per replication, and as the HIV genome is approximately 10,000 bases, and 10^8 virions are produced/day, the capacity to generate the two SI/CXCR4 mutations in V3 must occur on a daily basis. Yet, throughout the course of early and chronic HIV infection, it is only possible to isolate NSI viruses. Genetic studies of HIV+ subjects who have died from unrelated causes during this period show no evidence of SI/CXCR4 mutations. If these SI/CXCR4 mutations are being generated, then they are strongly selected against in favour of NSI/CCR5 using envelopes[32].

One hypothesis for the continued selection of NSI/CCR5 viruses is that the SI/CXCR4 mutations are under strong cellular immune control. Thus, whenever these mutations appear, the dominant immune response against the mutant form leads to maintenance of the NSI/CCR5 form. In late HIV disease, the loss of cellular immune regulation which leads to AIDS also suppresses the regulation of the SI/CXCR4 variants. Thus, late stage HIV-1 infection may see an increased rate of CD4 loss through broadening of the viral tropism, mediated by a switch in co-receptor usage from CCR5 to CXCR4. Presumably, CD4+ T-cell loss is this period of infection is entirely mediated through the direct (or indirect) effects of viral replication, as there is no remaining cellular immune response.

The critical role of the CCR5 co-receptor in defining the entry of HIV-1 into activated T-cells can be demonstrated through the impact of CCR5 polymorphisms. A deletion mutation of 32 base pairs of CCR5 has been described, Δ-32, where the co-receptor is synthesised but is unable to be expressed on the cell surface[33]. Subjects who are homozygous for the Δ-32 mutation appear to be immunologically normal, yet are resistant to HIV-1 infection, at least by NSI/CCR5 using primary isolates. Approximately 1% of Caucasian populations are homozygous for this mutation, and 17% heterozygous. Heterozygosity for Δ-32 does not prevent HIV-1 infection, but is associated with a slower rate of CD4 decline, and hence a better prognosis in HIV-1 infection[34]. Other polymorphisms, such as in the SDF-1 promotor region, also impact on the rate of CD4 decline. Presumably, these polymorphisms affect the relative infectability of activated CD4+ T-cells, and further support the central role of viral replication in the destruction of CD4⁺ lymphocytes.

Summary

The natural history of HIV-1 infection is marked by a prolonged asymptomatic period with a continuous slow decline in CD4⁺ T-lymphocytes. While this period is clinically quiet, the virus is highly dynamic, with large numbers of virions produced every day. The rate of CD4 decline is directly related to the quantity of virus detected in plasma, suggesting a direct relationship between viral replication and CD4⁺ T-cell destruction. A direct viral T-cell killing mechanism may indeed be dominant in the absence of an effective cellular immune response to HIV-1, as seen prior to seroconversion (primary HIV infection) and at late stage disease when HIV-specific cellular immunity is exhausted. However, during the chronic asymptomatic phase of HIV-1 infection, which is characterised by an active HIV-specific humoral and cellular immune response, turnover of both CD4⁺ and CD8⁺ T-lymphocytes is elevated. The most plausible explanation for this is that HIV-specific CD8⁺ CTL are the main effectors of HIV⁺/CD4⁺ T-cell destruction.

References

1   Dalgleish A, Beverley P, Clapham P et al. The CD4 (T4) antigen is an essential component of the receptor for the AIDS retrovirus. Nature 1984; 312: 20–4
2   Klatzmann D, Champagne E, Chamaret S et al. T-lymphocyte T4 molecule behaves as the receptor for human retrovirus LAV. Nature 1984; 312: 24–7
3   Alkhatib G, Combadiere C, Broder C et al. CC CKR5: A RANTES, MIP-1α, MIP-1β receptor as a fusion cofactor for macrophage-tropic HIV-1. Science 1996; 272: 1955–8
4   Dragic T, Litwin V, Allaway G et al. HIV-1 entry into CD4⁺ cells is mediated by the chemokine receptor CC-CKR-5. Nature 1996; 381: 667–73
5   Deng H, Liu R, Ellmeier W et al. Identification of a major co-receptor for primary isolates of HIV-1. Nature 1996; 381: 661–6
6   Spira A, Marx P, Patterson B et al. Cellular targets of infection and route of viral dissemination after an intravaginal inoculation of simian immunodeficiency virus into rhesus macaques. J Exp Med 1996; 183: 215–25
7   Zaitseva M, Blauvelt A, Lee S et al. Expression and function of CCR5 and CXCR4 on human Langerhans cells and macrophages: Implications for HIV primary infection. Nat Med 1997; 3: 1369–75
8   Dittmar M, Clapham P, Weber J et al. Langerhans cell tropism of human immunodeficiency virus type 1 subtype A through F isolates derived from different transmission groups. J Virol 1997; 71: 8008–13
9   Geijtenbeek T, Kwon D, Torensma R et al. DC-SIGN, a dendritic cell-specific HIV-1-binding protein that enhances trans-infection of T cells. Cell 2000; 100: 587–97
10 Mascola J, Schlesinger Frankel S, Broliden K. HIV-1 entry at the mucosal surface: role of antibodies in protection. AIDS 2000; 14 (Suppl 3): S167–75

11   Mellors J, Rinaldo C, Gupta P *et al*. Prognosis in HIV-1 infection predicted by the quantity of virus in plasma. *Science* 1996; **272**:1167–70

12   Ariyoshi K, Harwood E, Chiengsong-Popov R, Weber J. Is clearance of HIV-1 viraemia at seroconversion mediated by neutralising antibodies? *Lancet* 1992ii; **340**: 1257–8

13   Koup R, Safrit J, Cao Y *et al*. Temporal association of cellular immune responses with the initial control of viraemia in primary human immunodeficiency virus type 1 syndrome. *J Virol* 1994; **68**: 4650–5

14.   Borrow P, Lewicki H, Hahn B *et al* Virus-specific CD8⁺ cytotoxic T-lymphocyte activity associated with control of viraemia in primary human immunodeficiency virus type 1 infection. *J Virol* 1994; **68**: 6103–10

15   Phillips R, Rowland-Jones S, Nixon D *et al*. Human immunodeficiency virus genetic variation that can escape cytotoxic T cell recognition. *Nature* 1991; **354**: 453–9

16   Cheingsong-Popov R, Pangliotidi , Weber J *et al*. Humoral immune response to HIV antigens at seroconversion define outcome of HIV infection. *BMJ* 1991; **302**: 23-26

17   Phillips A. Reduction of HIV concentration during acute infection: independence from a specific immune response. *Science* 1996; **271**: 497–9

18   Pantaleo G. Immune-based therapy and therapeutic vaccines. *5th International Conference on Antiretroviral Therapy*, Glasgow, November 2000

19   Rosenberg E, Billingsley J, Caliendo A *et al*. Vigorous HIV-1-specific CD4⁺ T cell responses associated with control of viraemia. *Science* 1997; **278**: 1447–50

20.   Oxenius A, Price D, Easterbrook P *et al*. Early highly active antiretroviral therapy for acute HIV-1 infection preserves immune function of CD8⁺ and CD4⁺ T lymphocytes. *Proc Natl Acad Sci USA* 2000; **97**: 3382–7

21   Ho D, Neumann A, Perelson A *et al*. Rapid turnover of plasma virions and CD4 lymphocytes in HIV-1 infection. *Nature* 1995; **373**: 123–6

22   Wei X, Ghosh S, Taylor M *et al*. Viral dynamics in human immunodeficiency virus type 1 infection. *Nature* 1995; **373**: 117–22

23   Wolthers K, Wisman G, Otto S *et al*. T cell telomere length in HIV-1 infection: No evidence for increased CD4+ T cell turnover. *Science* 1996; **274**: 1543–7

24   Johnson RP. The dynamics of T-lymphocyte turnover in AIDS. *AIDS* 2000; **14 (Suppl 3)**: S3–9

25   Chakrabarti L, Lewin S, Zhang L *et al*. Normal T-cell turnover in Sooty Mangabeys harbouring active simian immunodeficiency virus infection. *J Virol* 2000; **74**: 1209–23

26   Siliciano RF. Latency and reservoirs for HIV-1. *AIDS* 1999; **13 (Suppl A)**: S49–58

27   Asjo B, Albert J, Karlsson A *et al*. Replicative capacity of human immunodeficiency virus from patients with varying severity of HIV infection. *Lancet* 1986; **ii**: 660–2

28   Cheng-Mayer C, Seto D, Levy J. Biologic features of HIV-1 that correlate with virulence in the host. *Science* 1988; **240**: 80–2

29   Tersmette M, de Goede M, Al B *et al*. Differential syncytium-inducing capacity of human immunodeficiency virus isolates: Frequent detection of syncytium-inducing isolates in patients with acquired immunodeficiency syndrome (AIDS) and AIDS-related complex. *J Virol* 1988; **62**: 2026–32

30   Fouchier R, Groenink M, Koostra N *et al*. Phenotype-associated sequence variation in the third variable domain of the human immunodeficiency virus type 1 gp20 molecule. *J Virol* 1992; **66**: 3183–7

31   Schuitemaker H, Koostra N, Koot M *et al*. Monocytotropic human immunodeficiency virus type 1 (HIV-1) variants detectable in all stages of HIV-1 infection lack T-cell line tropism and syncytium-inducing ability in primary T-cell culture. *J Virol* 1991; **65**: 356–63

32   Schuitmaker H. Biological properties of HIV-1 and their relevance for AIDS pathogenesis. (Chapter 3) In: Dalgleish A, Weiss R. (eds) *HIV and the New Viruses*, 2nd edn. London: Academic Press, 1999; 43–58

33   Liu R, Paxton W, Choe S *et al*.Homozygous defect in HIV-1 coreceptor accounts for resistance some multiply-exposed individuals to HIV-1 infection. *Cell* 1996; **86**: 367–77

34   Huang Y, Paxton W, Wolinsky S *et al*. The role of a mutant CCR5 allele in HIV-1 transmission and disease progression. *Nat Med* 1996; **2**: 1240–3

Demography and economics of HIV/AIDS

Alan Whiteside

Health Economics and HIV/AIDS Research Division, University of Natal, Durban, South Africa

The rapid spread of HIV in the 1980s and 1990s in the non-industrialised world is now leading to an AIDS epidemic. This in turn is having a demographic and economic impact on these societies. This article assesses the most recent evidence for these impacts. It concludes that, while there is already a real and measurable impact, there is far worse to come. The demographic consequences will be particularly serious. Economic impact is rather more uncertain, and the article looks at the macro-economic impact as well as that on firms. In addition, it is postulated that economics may not be the most appropriate discipline to assess the true effects of the disease.

In late 2000, as it rained on England's Yorkshire moors, the inhabitants on the banks of the Rivers Nidd and Ouse braced themselves for the flood that they knew would follow. So it is with HIV and AIDS. However, unlike those unfortunate Yorkshire folk, the deluge the non-industrialised world faces will follow in years rather than days and its impact will be carried through generations. Furthermore, the signals of impending catastrophe are not clear for many.

Since the 1970s and 1980s, HIV has been spreading in much of the non-industrialised world. Worst affected is sub-Saharan Africa. UNAIDS estimates that 24.5 million of the 34.3 million global infections are here. An estimated 8.57% of adults (defined as those aged 15–49 years) are infected in the region. In numbers, the next highest total is that of South and South East Asia, with 5.6 million infected people. There are smaller but worrying epidemics in a number of Latin American countries; adult HIV prevalence is 5.17% in Haiti, 4.13% in the Bahamas and 3.01% in Guyana[1]. In addition, there is concern that HIV may spread beyond the drug-using populations in Eastern Europe, creating a generalised epidemic[2]; already Ukraine is estimated to have 240,000 infections and the Russian Federation 130,000.

The epidemic in Africa, and particularly Southern and Eastern Africa, is the most advanced and serious. In Botswana, it is estimated that 35.8% of adults are HIV positive. Swaziland and Zimbabwe are both thought to have more than a quarter of adults infected. In this region only Tanzania and Uganda have an adult prevalence rates of less than 10%. In Tanzania it is 8.09%, while Uganda provides the sole example on the African continent of an epidemic where prevalence has actually fallen – here it is estimated to be 8.3%.

Correspondence to:
Prof. Alan Whiteside,
Health Economics and
HIV/AIDS Research
Division, University of
Natal, Durban 4041,
South Africa

As the epidemic is further advanced in Africa, it is here we must look in order to assess the actual and potential impact of AIDS. There are, however, problems in doing this.

Firstly, HIV/AIDS is a new epidemic. Nowhere, apart from in Uganda, has the HIV epidemic run its course through a population, peaked and begun to decline. Even in Uganda, the data are confined to a limited number of sites which exclude the war-torn North. The significance of this, given the period between HIV infection and AIDS, is that the AIDS epidemic – the illnesses and deaths that result from HIV infection – is still to appear. AIDS is a long wave disaster[3]; it takes time for the impact to develop and be felt, and even longer for it to work its way through society.

Secondly, how do we measure the impact? Demographers rely on censuses and surveys. Censuses are held only every 10 years and frequently it takes 3 or more years for the results to be analysed and released. Increasing numbers of countries are carrying out demographic and health surveys; these provide some additional data, but they are limited in coverage and frequency. The reality is that most statements about the demographic impacts of HIV/AIDS are based on modelled, rather than observed, data.

Economists collect data on economic output and income and expenditure patterns at various levels, from the household to the national economy (although the data in this paper presented will be for the national economy and firms). The data are usually reasonably robust, but have limitations – they measure what happens in the formal economy not the informal. Furthermore, economists have great difficulty in disentangling causality. For example, they are hard put to explain why Uganda, the country affected both first and most severely by HIV/AIDS, should have recorded an annual average economic growth rate of 7.2% between 1990 and 1999, while Botswana's growth was 4.2% (the world average was 2.5% and that of Africa 2.4%)[4]. Economics is perhaps not the right lens through which to examine the situation.

Demographic impact

What demographic events get measured and reported? Most countries conduct censuses to measure key demographic indicators such as the number of people by age and gender. These and occasional household censuses are used to calculate other indicators such as total fertility rates, growth, age structure, dependency ratios, life expectancy and infant, child and maternal mortality rates.

The major demographic processes, mortality and fertility, are affected by AIDS. Direct effects on mortality occur because AIDS causes the deaths of adults and children. The effects on fertility are indirect and less well understood. The accumulation of these direct and indirect effects causes changes in other demographic indicators.

Mortality

The most direct demographic consequence is an increase in mortality. Without effective treatment of HIV infection, people will die of AIDS. The period from infection to illness, in the absence of effective treatment, is estimated to be 7.5–10 years[5]. In the medium term, therapy is unlikely to make a difference to life expectancy in the non-industrialised world. It is too expensive, requires a fairly sophisticated delivery system, and people need to know they are infected in order to access it. None of these conditions apply in the non-industrialised world.

Since AIDS is primarily spread through sexual transmission, the peak ages of HIV infection are 20–40 years, and the peak ages of AIDS death are 5–10 years later. Thus, AIDS increases mortality in adult age groups that typically have the lowest mortality rates. Mother-to-child transmission, which is estimated to occur, in the absence of interventions, in about 30% of births to infected mothers, accounts for increased infant and child mortality.

A review of data on the impact of AIDS on mortality, using data from national household surveys and censuses, was carried out by Timæus in 1998[6]. He notes that measuring the impact of HIV on mortality is fundamental for developing programmes to mitigate the impact of the disease. However, 'no mainland country in sub-Saharan Africa has an adequate vital registration system. South Africa is the only country that registers sufficient deaths to attempt to produce national estimates of mortality from this source. Even in this country coverage is far from complete. Thus apart from research studies of localised populations the main sources on mortality in Africa are national censuses and household surveys[6].' The conclusion he draws from the limited data is that mortality of adults and children has risen, but he also notes that this mortality reflects the state of the HIV epidemic a decade ago.

Data are available for some specific sites and are modelled at the national level. Recent information on excess mortality for subnational locations comes from Uganda. In Rakai, Uganda, a cohort of 19,983 adults aged 15–59 years was followed for four surveys at 10 monthly intervals. HIV prevalence in this cohort was 16.1%. Mortality in HIV positive people was 132.6 per 1000 person years, while in HIV negative people it was only 6.7[7].

The most comprehensive data are those from South Africa's vital registration. Readers will be aware that South Africa has gone through a divisive and unnecessary period of questioning accepted wisdom around HIV/AIDS. As a result, a Presidential AIDS Advisory Panel was established.

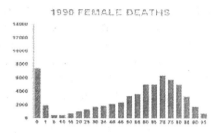

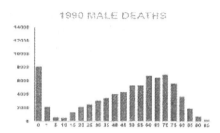

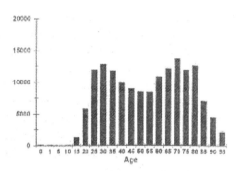

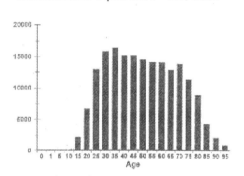

Fig. 1 Female and male deaths, South Africa, 1990 and 1999/2000.

Among the 'dissident' members there were those who questioned the existence of HIV, those who said HIV did not cause AIDS, and others who argued that while AIDS existed, the illness and deaths arose from the drugs. One of the major contentions was that there was no evidence of increased mortality in South Africa. In order to address this, the Medical Research Council and the Actuarial Society of South Africa collected and analysed mortality data from the Department of Home Affairs Population register (the author was a member of the Presidential AIDS Advisory Panel). The data for male and female deaths in 1990 and 1999/2000 in South Africa are shown in Figure 1 [These data were published in the South African edition on *The Sunday Times* just before the AIDS Conference in July 2000. They are being reworked by the South African Medical Research Council, but at the time of writing this report had been blocked.].

It will not come as a surprise to learn that the response of the dissidents, when these data were presented, was to say that they were not comparable, as in 1990 the homelands were not counted while in 2000 they were! While being true, the expected effect would be to show higher young adult mortality in South Africa excluding homelands due to the migration patterns created by apartheid. Thus, if anything, the data provided an even stronger case for increased mortality as the result of a new infectious disease.

Given the problems with official data, one of the questions we recently tried to answer is whether there are alternative data sources[8]. Swaziland's first survey of ante-natal clinic attenders was in 1992 when 4.3% of women attending the clinics were infected. By 1998, the prevalence had risen to over 30%[1]. We would expect mortality to have begun increasing from about 1997. As in Swaziland there is no vital registration, and stigma and prejudice are particularly marked, we set out to look at the one possible source of data. A feature of the society is that many people place bereavement notices in the local press. Increasingly, these notices will include a photograph and some biographical detail of the deceased. The study reviewed death notices in the *Swazi Times* for every Thursday, Friday and Saturday, the days most death notices appear, from 1 July 1994 to 30 June 1999.

The total number of deaths reported rose substantially during the observed period. Furthermore, the reported deaths track the deaths projected by The Futures Group (data provided by John Stover of The Futures Group International). This is shown in Figure 2.

When the deaths are assessed by age it is apparent that the majority of those dying are aged 26–40 years, and that the numbers have risen rapidly. This pattern of mortality is common to all the data on AIDS deaths, but is generally not available at a national level. Since AIDS deaths are concentrated in this age group, there are important consequences for the number of AIDS orphans, and for economic growth.

Infant and child mortality
Transmission of infection from mother to child will increase infant and child mortality. In the Rakai cohort study, it was found that the infant

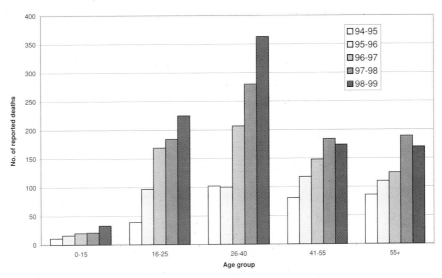

Fig. 2 Reported deaths by age, Swaziland.

mortality rate was 225 per 1000 for children born to HIV positive mothers, and 97.7 for children born to HIV negative mothers[7]. The impact on the under five mortality rate will be more severe, as many infected infants will live beyond their first birthdays but few will survive beyond their fifth. The actual effects could be larger if children who are orphaned when their mothers die receive worse care than other children.

The international agencies have been projecting child mortality, and show a worsening picture in a number of countries with high HIV prevalence. When the latest projections from the US Bureau of the Census are examined, it is evident that the situation will deteriorate further. We should remind ourselves that these are all modelled rather than observed data. In addition this reflects the estimated actual mortality. When mortality in the absence of AIDS is projected this shows how wide the gap has become and how serious the impact of the disease is – for Botswana in 2000, child mortality would have been only 38.9 per thousand in the absence of AIDS instead of the 136 modelled; in Kenya 70.1 per thousand instead of the 110 predicted.

Child mortality data from the UNDP and US Bureau are shown in Table 1. This table also shows that the UNDP is not considering AIDS consistently, for there is no deterioration shown for Botswana in their figures!

The reduction of infant and child mortality by two-thirds by 2015 is, of course, one of the international development goals (these goals were set by the Development Assistance Committee of the OECD[9]). In order to achieve this goal for infant mortality, sub-Saharan Africa needs to move from the 1990 rate of 101 per thousand to 33 in 2015. In 1998 the rate was 92 and set to rise[9].

Life expectancy

Life expectancy at birth is particularly sensitive to AIDS, as deaths occurring to young adults and young children result in a large number

Table 1 Child mortality for selected African countries

	1996 HDR data for 1994	1998 HDR data for 1996	2000 HDR data for 1998	2000 US Bureau of the Census	2010 US Bureau of the Census
Botswana	54	50	48	136	169.5
Kenya	90	90	117	110.1	107.4
South Africa	68	66	83	119.6	146.6
Zambia	203	202	202	168.8	145.7
Uganda	185	141	134	163	129.7

Source: United Nations Development Programme, Human Development Reports 1996, 1998 and 2000, and US Bureau of the Census

Table 2 Life expectancy for selected countries

	1996 HDR data for 1993	1998 HDR data for 1995	2000 HDR data for 1998	2000 US Bureau of the Census	2010 US Bureau of the Census
Botswana	65	51.7	46.2	39.3	29
Haiti	58.6	54.6	54	49.2	51.5
Kenya	55.5	53.8	51.3	48	44.3
South Africa	63.2	64.1	53.2	51.1	35.5
Zambia	48.6	42.7	40.5	37.2	38.9
Uganda	44.7	40.5	40.7	42.9	46.6

Source: United Nations Development Programme, Human Development Reports 1996, 1998 and 2000, and US Bureau of the Census.

of years of life lost. Again, data are available from both the UNDP and the US Bureau of the Census. This is shown in Table 2. Effectively, some of these life expectancies have not been seen since the Stone Age. How individuals and societies will react to this remains to be seen.

Fertility

It is clear that the number of births may be affected if many women die before reaching the end of their child-bearing years. Most births, however, occur to women at young ages. The average age at the time of death from AIDS is usually around 30 years or higher for women. In Africa, only about one-third of life-time births occur to women over the age of 30 years. Recent data, however, suggest that HIV infection may substantially reduce fertility. In Uganda, it was found that HIV infected women had lower fertility rates than HIV negative women. One study in rural Rakai district found that age-specific fertility rates for HIV-infected women were 50% less than those for women who were not infected[10]. Another study among a rural population in Masaka[11] found that fertility rates were 20–30% less among HIV-infected women. Since most women did not know their sero-status, the reduced fertility rates are due to biological rather than behavioural factors.

Population size and growth

There has been much speculation about the effect AIDS will have on population size and growth rates. Work done early in the epidemic, particularly by Anderson, warned it was likely that populations would be relatively smaller than they would have been in the absence of AIDS, and it was possible there might even be declines in absolute numbers[12–14]. This view has not been held by the UN agencies but increasingly modelling, done for non-industrialised country governments and by the US Bureau of the Census, suggests that population growth might well turn negative in some countries. By the year 2003, Botswana, South Africa and Zimbabwe will be experiencing negative population growth – down to –0.1 to –0.3 from +1.1 to +2.3 in the absence of AIDS[15].

Dependency ratio and orphaning

The dependency ratio is the number of dependants, usually children under the age of 15 years and adults over the age of 64 years, per 100 adults 15–64 years of productive age. It might seem that the dependency ratio should become worse due to AIDS because of the increased number of deaths to young adults. AIDS, however, also leads to an increase in the number of child deaths. These two factors tend roughly to balance each other, with the result that the dependency ratio does not change dramatically in the presence of an AIDS epidemic[16]. The dependency situation is adversely affected in other ways. AIDS increases the number of widows and widowers[17]. When parents die, children are often left in the care of grandparents and/or other members of the extended family or community. AIDS will produce population structures never seen before, as is shown in Figure 3[18].

One of the worst consequences of the AIDS epidemic is the fact that it creates a number of AIDS orphans. UNAIDS estimates that about 2% of all children in non-industrialised countries were orphans before AIDS. By 1997 the proportion with one or both parents dead had risen to 7% in many African countries, and rose to 11% in some[1].

The economic impact of AIDS

As has already been alluded to, measuring the economic impact of AIDS is even more difficult than measuring the demographic effects. One of the key questions is at what level do we wish to measure these economic impacts? The national economy; households; firms; sectors; somewhere in between; or at all levels? Perhaps the best way to begin is to ask how AIDS will affect economies, and then assess what impacts can be seen.

At the simplest level AIDS reduces income and increases expenditure. It also requires choices to be made as to what money is spent on. This is as true at the national level as it is for the household.

When people fall ill they are no longer able to be productive, and, obviously, when they die their production is lost. Illness, however, will have consequences beyond the individual. Other family members may have to make hard choices between tending the fields or looking after

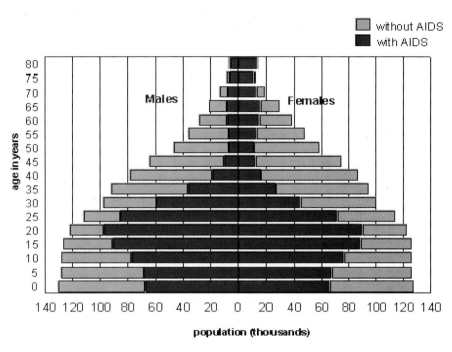

Fig. 3 Projected population structure with and without the AIDS epidemic, Botswana, 2020.

the sick family member. Funerals take time and resources. Thus, an increase in illness has a detrimental effect on any household. In the recent work on poverty, the World Bank[19] found 'the most important trigger for downward mobility was illness and injury – everywhere, illness was dreaded'.

Does this matter to the national economy or even the private sector? The answer is – it depends! It depends on how many people are ill and who they are, in the sense of what they contribute to the measured national economy and what claims they can make on government services. If the majority of people who fall ill with AIDS are poor rural farmers who market few of their crops and buy little from the formal economy, then their deaths will, in economic terms, count for little. On the other hand, if the deaths from AIDS are among skilled urban workers, who are hard to replace, then the impact on measures such as gross domestic product and the output of firms could be significant.

Increases in expenditure are important because money used in the care of AIDS patients or on funerals is not available for other uses, some of which might be more productive. For example, purchase of health care may mean education is neglected. Households may sell assets in order to cope with the shock of the illness and death of an adult. Firms may see profits decrease as productivity falls and the cost of employee benefits rises.

Recent work is beginning to give a picture of some of the economic impacts of the epidemic. We will examine this for macro-economies and the private sector.

Macro-economic impacts

Early studies suggested that national economic growth would slow as a result of the epidemic. It was estimated that over a 25 year period economies could be up to 25% smaller than they would have been in the absence of AIDS. The impact on *per capita* incomes was projected to be somewhat smaller, as the population growth rates would also slow. Recent work has also looked at the broader impact of ill health. It is estimated that low life expectancy – a proxy for health-related problems – reduces growth by 1.3%[19].

A number of studies into the impact of AIDS on the South African economy were completed in 2000. These use different methodologies and assumptions but agree on the outcomes. The South African economy will grow more slowly because of AIDS[20,21]. Across the border in Botswana, it is estimated that the rate of GDP growth will fall from a projected 3.9% a year without AIDS to 2.0–3.1% a year with AIDS, and after 25 years the economy will be 24–38% smaller with AIDS than it would have been without AIDS[22]. The only non-African recent study (from the Caribbean) suggests that by 2005 the GDP in Trinidad and Tobago would be 4.2% lower than it would have been in the absence of AIDS. In Jamaica the figure is 6.4%. In addition savings, investment, labour supply and employment in all sectors is predicted to decrease[23].

Unbelievably, virtually no work appears to have been done on the impact of AIDS on the government budget. In Botswana, as part of the macro-economic modelling, estimates were made of the effects of AIDS on government revenue and expenditure. By 2010, the government is projected to need to increase spending by 7–18% with the bulk of the expenditure being on health, poverty alleviation and employment. The health spending does not allow for any form of anti-retroviral therapy; provision of double therapy at current prices to all those infected would cost P3.9 billion per annum, which is 17% of the total GDP in Botswana and 56% of the recurrent budget. Government revenue is expected to fall by about 9.6%.

The macro-economic models do not take into account the full complexity of the impact of the disease. For example, how do we measure the effects on government efficiency, which is expected to decrease as civil servants take increasing amounts of time off and their posts are not filled? What is the effect on investment flows, and do international fund managers factor HIV/AIDS into their decision making processes? In addition, it is worth stressing that the macro-economic models do not take into consideration the suffering caused by HIV/AIDS. Even in the scenario where *per capita* incomes are said to rise as a result of the epidemic, they rise only for the survivors.

AIDS and the private sector

The business sector is increasingly aware of the threat posed by HIV/AIDS. The major concerns for businesses are reduced productivity and increased costs. Productivity will fall and costs rise because of:

1   Increased absenteeism not only be because of the ill health experienced by the employees, but also because staff, particularly women, take time off to care for sick members of their families. Attendance at funerals is potentially a major source of lost time, especially in cultures where colleagues are expected to attend the funeral of the deceased co-worker.

2   Workers who are beginning to experience failing health will be less productive at work and unable to carry out more demanding physical jobs.

3   Employees who die or retire on medical grounds have to be replaced and their replacements may be less skilled and experienced, and require training.

4   Employers may increase the size of the workforce, and hence payroll costs, to provide for absenteeism.

5   As skilled workers become scarcer, wages may increase. Preliminary estimates from Southern African indicate that these skilled wages may rise. (By as much as 17% in Botswana and up to 45% by 2010 in South Africa, the two countries where these estimates have been made.)

What do we actually know? Despite the problems with data there does seem to be a consistency in impacts in companies (across Southern Africa at least). As Table 3 shows, the death rates attributable to HIV/AIDS in Swaziland, Zimbabwe and Zambia are all similar[24]. (The slightly lower rates in Zambia and Zimbabwe may be due to the fact that this was 7 years earlier in the epidemic.)

The question asked by the managing directors and financial directors is: 'what is the effect of this disease on the bottom line?' Again there

Table 3 Comparison of AIDS attributable death rates

Industry	Year	HIV/AIDS attributable death rate
Fridgemaster (manufacturing), Swaziland	1999	7.5/1000
Hippo Valley (sugar), Zimbabwe	1997	5.0/1000
Nakambala Sugar Estate, Zambia	1992	6.75/1000
RSSC (sugar), Swaziland	1999	9.41/1000

Table 4 The impact of AIDS on the 'bottom line' in the private sector

Date	Country	Company	Impact
1994	Cote d'Ivoire	3 manufacturing companies	0.8–3.2% of the wage bill (Aventin & Huard 1997[28])
1996	Malawi	Makandi Tea Estate	6% of operating profit (Jones 1996[29])
1999	South Africa	Company A	7.2% of salaries (Thea *et al* 2000[30])
1999	Swaziland	Royal Swaziland Sugar Corporation	1.1% of operating profits, 3.4% of pre-tax profits and 4.6% of after tax profits (Coutinho 2000[31])
1999	Botswana	Hypothetical company	25–250% of company's current salary roll

were, in the early stages of the epidemic, a number of attempts to estimate and project impact, and these suggested that the cost could be 5–20% of profits. Other work, however, has suggested that the costs are small and manageable. The World Bank study of 992 firms in the manufacturing sector of Zambia, Zimbabwe, Kenya, Tanzania and Ghana in 1994 found[25]:

1 The average attrition rates from all causes were 8–30 times larger than those due to (any) sickness or death.

2 The replacement time for deceased workers ranged between 2 weeks for unskilled to 24 weeks for skilled – but noted that even the latter did not seem long to search for a skilled professional.

3 The departure of a worker is estimated to reduce the value-added per worker by a statistically significant but small amount.

A summary of recent findings is shown in Table 4.

Collecting information on costs does not go far enough. In particular, it ignores the question as to whether there are key posts or functions in an organisation that are critical. A methodology for this is the institutional audit which attempts to judge whether an organisation is vulnerable to the impact of HIV and AIDS[26]. Critical functions are those that must be filled for a company to be able to operate.

Estimates of the impact of HIV/AIDS on markets is under-researched. AIDS could reduce the absolute number of potential customers, making markets that are relatively saturated and which depend critically on population size the most vulnerable. This impact is evident from the first part of the article. The effect of the epidemic on specific markets will depend on the demographic profile (age, sex, geographic location) of consumers. Because of the demographics of HIV/AIDS, consumers in the 25–49 year age group are likely to be most affected. In countries where demand for goods is far from saturated, many of the consumers who die or have their disposable income reduced by HIV/AIDS will be replaced by new earners and consumers, but only if overall GDP and consumption expenditure remain unaffected by the pandemic.

South African furniture and household appliance retailer the JD Group (JDG) actually commissioned a study looking at the potential impact of AIDS on their consumers and operations. This suggested that the overall HIV (1998) prevalence rate among JDG's customers was 15%, and that this would rise to 27% by 2015. The report concluded that the South African customer base would grow slowly until 2010. Thereafter, the demographic impact of AIDS would kick in, resulting in an 18% decline in customers by 2015 in all provinces bar the Western Cape. Other countries such as Swaziland, Lesotho and Botswana would experience a reduction in market size by 2010 of about 14%. The increase in illness and death meant that consumption patterns would change as disposable income is re-allocated. JDG concluded that:

1 AIDS would influence consumption patterns as households divert expenditure to AIDS care.

2 The previous relationships between GDP, personal consumption expenditure and durable consumption expenditure would change.

3 Considerable social impact is expected.

4 The impacts by age group and market region are anticipated to differ substantially.

5 A strategic repositioning of JD Group would be required before 2005.

As a result of the study, the group introduced personal services as part of the product range it offers, and has expanded into Eastern Europe, opening stores in Poland and the Czech Republic[27].

Private companies do not operate in isolation of what is happening in the societies around them. The macro-economic trends will affect them, as will the investment climate and the relative efficiency (or inefficiency) of government. Some companies have been looking at the impact AIDS will have on their markets, but there is no recorded evidence of them assessing the effect on wage rates, government efficiency, capital flows or other factors. Perhaps it would not be possible for an individual company to address these complex issues but certainly they need to be considered. The way these issues are being considered is as part of the overall business environment, and they are more implicit than explicit.

Other impacts

Space does not allow a discussion of other economic impacts. Of particular concern would be the effects of the disease on the households, and specific sectors such as health and education. However, as shown above, if there is limited information on the macro and private sector impacts, there is even less for these areas. Nonetheless, we should re-iterate that economic impact is only part of the story. Increased morbidity and mortality will affect all aspects of society in many complex ways. Indeed, it is possible that the sum of the parts may even be greater than the whole.

Conclusions

AIDS is a crisis for much of the non-industrialised world. In this article we have examined the demographic trends that are developing and will continue. We have looked at the economic impact in terms of the national economies and the private sector. We have to conclude that the disease will have long-term adverse effects and that these are neither understood nor appreciated. Furthermore, we are only at the beginning of the impact.

Unfortunately, in many non-industrialised countries demographers do not consider AIDS and its current or potential impacts. The reasons are not clear – but we speculate that they do not understand the likely effect, are in denial about it, or do not have the conceptual framework or tools to take it into account. However, even in the few countries where serious demographers are considering AIDS, other sectors have been slow to incorporate these figures into their planning.

Economics shows an impact, but we suggest that this reflects only part of the picture. It cannot measure the true misery that this disease is causing, and will cause. Finally, while prevention remains the target, the reality is that impact is not properly measured and no serious attempts are being made to respond to impact on a national basis.

Acknowledgements

Comments on an earlier draft were made by John Stover of The Futures Group International. Jaine Roberts of HEARD assisted in the preparation of the manuscript for publication. The manuscript was prepared while the author was being funded by the Association François – Xavier Bagnoud, writing with Prof. Tony Barnett. The opportunity this gave to think, read and write is gratefully acknowledged.

References

1   UNAIDS. Report on the Global HIV/AIDS Epidemic. Geneva: UNAIDS, 2000
2   Barnett T, Whiteside A, Khodakevich L, Kruglov Y, Steshenko V. The HIV/AIDS epidemic in Ukraine: its potential social and economic impact. *Soc Sci Med* 2000; **51**: 1387–403
3   Barnett T, Blaikie P. *AIDS in Africa: Its Present and Future Impact*. New York: Guildford, 1992
4   The World Bank. *World Development Report 2000/2001 Attacking Poverty*. New York:

Oxford University Press, 2000

5   Stover J, Way P. Projecting the impact of AIDS on mortality. *AIDS* 1998; **12 (Suppl 1)**: S29–39

6   Timæus IM. Impact of the HIV epidemic on mortality in sub-Saharan Africa: evidence from national surveys and censuses. *AIDS* 1998; **12 (Suppl 1)**: S15–27

7   Sewankambo NK, Gray RH, Ahmad S *et al*. Mortality associated with HIV infection in rural Rakai district, Uganda. *AIDS* 2000; **14**: 2391–400

8   Whiteside A, Desmond C, King J, Tomlinson J. Evidence of AIDS mortality from an alternative source. Swaziland case study. 2001; Submitted

9   The World Bank. *World Development Indicators*. Washington DC: World Bank, 2000

10 Gray RH, Serwadda D, Wawer MJ *et al*. Reduced fertility in women with HIV infection: a population-based study in Uganda. *The Socio-Demographic Impact of AIDS in Africa Conference*. Durban: International Union for the Scientific Study of Population and University of Natal, Durban, February 1997

11 Carpenter LM, Nakiyingi JS, Ruberantwari A *et al*. Estimates of the impact of HIV-1 infection on fertility in a rural Ugandan cohort. *The Socio-Demographic Impact of AIDS in Africa Conference*. Durban: International Union for the Scientific Study of Population and University of Natal, Durban, February 1997

12 Garnett GP, Anderson RM. No reason for complacency about the potential demographic impact of AIDS in Africa. *Trans R Soc Trop Med Hyg* 1993; **87**(Suppl 1): 19–22

13 Anderson RM, May RM, Boily MC, Garnett GP, Rowley JT. The spread of HIV-1 in Africa: sexual contact patterns and the predicted demographic impact of AIDS. *Nature* 1991; **352**: 581–9

14 Rowley JT, Anderson RM, Ng TW. Reducing the spread of HIV infection in sub-Saharan Africa: some demographic and economic consequences. *AIDS* 1990; **4**: 47–56

15 Anon. *Monitoring the AIDS Pandemic: Status and Trends of the HIV/AIDS Epidemics in the World, Provisional Report*. Durban, South Africa, 5–7 July 2000, Published by Monitoring the AIDS Pandemic

16 Stover J, Way PO. Impact of interventions on reducing the spread of HIV in Africa: computer simulation applications. *Afr J Med Pract* 1995; **2**: 110–20

17 Ntozi JPM. Widowhood, remarriage and migration during the HIV/AIDS epidemic in Uganda. *The Socio-Demographic Impact of AIDS in Africa Conference*. Durban: International Union for the Scientific Study of Population and University of Natal, Durban, February 1997

18 US Bureau of the Census. *World Population Profile 2000*. Washington DC, US Bureau of the Census, 2000

19 The World Bank. *Can Africa claim the 21st century?* Washington DC: World Bank, 2000: 85

20 Arndt C, Lewis J. The macro implications of HIV/AIDS in South Africa: a preliminary assessment. *S Afr J Econ* 2000; **68**(1): 856–87

21 Quattek K. The economic impact of AIDS in South Africa: a dark cloud on the horizon. In: Konrad-Adenauer Stiftung. *HIV/AIDS: A Threat to the African Renaissance*. Occasional Papers. Johannesburg: Konrad-Adenauer Stiftung 2000

22 Botswana Institute for Development Policy Analysis. *Macroeconomic Impacts of the HIV/AIDS Epidemic in Botswana Final Report*. Gaborone: Botswana Institute for Development Policy Analysis, 2000

23 Nicholls S, McLean R, Theodore K, Henry R, Camara B and team. *Modelling the Macroeconomic Impact of HIV/AIDS on the English Speaking Caribbean: The Case of Trinidad and Tobago and Jamaica*. Paper presented at the IAEN, Durban 2000

24 Coutinho AG. *An Assessment of the Economic Impact of HIV/AIDS on the Royal Swaziland Sugar Corporation*. A research report submitted in partial fulfilment of the award of Masters Degree in Public Health, Department of Community Health, University of Witwatersrand, Johannesburg, August 2000

25 World Bank. *Confronting AIDS Public Priorities in a Global Epidemic*. New York: Oxford University Press, 1997

26 Barnett T, Whiteside A. *Guidelines for Studies of the Social and Economic Impact of HIV/AIDS*. UNAIDS Best Practice Collection. Geneva: UNAIDS, 2000

27 Whiteside A, Sunter C. *AIDS The Challenge for South Africa*. Cape Town: Human and Rosseau, 2000

28   Aventin L, Huard P. HIV/AIDS and manufacturing in Abidjan. *AIDS Analysis Africa* 1997; **7**(3)

29   Jones C. *The Microeconomic Implications of HIV/AIDS*. Masters dissertation submitted to the School of Development Studies, University of East Anglia, September 1996

30   Thea D, Rosen S, Vincent JR, Singh G, Simon J. *Economic Impact of HIV/AIDS in Company A's Workforce*. Session D14, XIII International Conference of AIDS, Durban, South Africa, 11 July 2000

31   Coutinho AG. An Assessment of the Economic Impact of HIV/AIDS on the Royal Swaziland Sugar Corporation. A research report submitted in partial fulfilment of the Award of a Masters Degree in Public Health, Department of Community Health, University od Witwatersrand, Johannesburg, August 2000

Paediatric HIV infection: correlates of protective immunity and global perspectives in prevention and management

Philip JR Goulder*,†, Prakash Jeena‡, Gareth Tudor-Williams§
and **Sandra Burchett****

*Partners AIDS Research Center, Massachusetts General Hospital, Harvard Medical School, Charlestown, Massachusetts, USA
†Department of Paediatrics, Nuffield Department of Medicine, John Radcliffe Hospital, University of Oxford, Oxford, UK
‡Department of Paediatrics, King Edward VIII Hospital, University of Natal, South Africa
§Department of Paediatrics, St Mary's Hospital, Imperial College of Science Technology and Medicine, London, UK
**Division of Infectious Diseases, The Children's Hospital, Boston, Massachusetts, USA

Correspondence to:
Dr Philip JR Goulder,
Partners AIDS Research
Center, Massachusetts
General Hospital, Harvard
Medical School, 13th St,
Bldg 149, Rm 5219,
Charlestown,
MA 02129, USA

The impact of the HIV epidemic on child health globally is beginning to be appreciated. With the burden of new infections falling on young women, there is a skyrocketing number of AIDS orphans, and a rapidly increasing number of children infected *via* mother-to-child-transmission (MTCT). An estimated 600,000 new paediatric infections occur each year, of which some 1500/day (> 90%) occur in sub-Saharan Africa. But whereas children account for only 4% of those currently living with HIV infection, 20% of AIDS deaths have been in children. This reflects the rapid progression to disease in paediatric HIV infection. Whereas a dramatic reduction in viraemia follows acute adult infection, corresponding to the appearance of a vigorous anti-HIV cytotoxic T lymphocyte response, virtually no impact of the immune response is observed in acute paediatric infection following MTCT. Two specific challenges for the paediatric immune response are: (i) infection occurs before the immune system itself is fully developed; and (ii) the viruses transmitted by MTCT have already evaded an immune system sharing close genetic relatedness to that of the child. Accumulating evidence indicates that the immune system is potentially capable of effective control of HIV infection, and that events occurring in acute infection critically determine the ultimate outcome. Technological advances that have transformed the study of T-cell immunity now enable the developing immune system in childhood to be better understood. *Via* novel immunotherapeutic approaches described, it may be possible to modulate the infant's immune response to reach effective and durable suppression of HIV, as can be achieved by the rare long-term non-progressors of HIV infection. The feasibility of adopting these approaches globally are as yet untested. Finally, the striking disparity between the burden of paediatric HIV infection and access to the necessary infrastructure and therapeutic options required for its optimal management is addressed in a comparison between three sites of paediatric HIV care: Durban, South Africa; London, UK; and Boston, USA.

In 1998, an estimated 5.8 million new HIV infections occurred world-wide, of which 10% were in perinatally infected children[1]. The figures are similar for the years 1999 and 2000. This translates into more than 1600 infants newly infected each day. But only 4% of the world's population who are currently infected with HIV are children, whereas 20% of the AIDS deaths have been in children. This reflects the rapid progression to disease that is a hallmark of paediatric HIV infection, especially in the non-industrialised world where access to antiretroviral therapy is limited at best. Approximately 90% of the 3 million live children infected are in sub-Saharan Africa, where the HIV prevalence in antenatal clinics was typically between 15–30% in the mid-1990s[2] and today approaches 50% in the worst-hit regions[3–5]. Even taking into account the potential impact of prophylactic antiretroviral therapy instituted peripartum[6], and other approaches – notably influencing infant breast-feeding patterns[7] – to reduce mother-to-child-transmission (MTCT), it is likely that 10–15% of children born to infected mothers will be infected. In the children who are not perinatally infected with HIV, the incidence of new infection when they reach teenage begins to rise rapidly, up to levels of 20% per year for women aged 20–24 years[8]. Avoiding exposure to HIV infection in some regions of the world is extremely difficult. The clear and logical conclusion is that an HIV vaccine that is effective in early childhood is most vitally needed.

The first part of this review will focus on the extent of our under-standing to date of what constitutes protective immunity against HIV in paediatric infection and how these research studies might translate into effective new immunomodulatory approaches or vaccine design in the future. The second part of the review describes the practicalities of preventing paediatric infection and of managing children infected with HIV. The approaches available in the non-industrialised world are contrasted with those in countries such as the US and the UK, where there is accessibility to highly active antiretroviral therapy (HAART) in paediatric infection.

Natural history of paediatric HIV infection

Perinatally infected children generally progress to disease more rapidly than infected adults[9–12]. Early studies of perinatally infected children, before the era of HAART, from the European Collaborative and US groups indicated that a subset of approximately 25% of perinatally infected children progress very rapidly to AIDS within 1 year. The median time to AIDS for the remaining 75% was approximately 7 years. Recent data from a cohort in Malawi appear to indicate an even more dismal prognosis for perinatally infected children in parts of sub-Saharan Africa, with 89% mortality by 3 years of age[13]. Since the median age at enrolment was 8 months, by which time a proportion of infants would have already died (the recorded infant mortality being only 7%), it is possible that this figure of 89% may even underestimate the impact of HIV on childhood mortality in the first 3 years of life. Some of the more dramatic and intriguing data from this study are that the majority of the infected children died in the short period between 2.0 and 2.7 years of age. Whether HIV infected children progress more rapidly to disease and death as a result of HIV *per se* in non-industrialised countries than they would do in industrialised countries in the absence of antiretroviral therapy it is only possible to speculate. A recent review argued that adult HIV-1 infection progresses to disease no more rapidly in Africans than in industrialised nations[14]. However, the observation that infants are more vulnerable than adults to HIV disease is beyond dispute. Importantly, the reasons for this are not yet established.

Successful control of HIV in adult infection

The immune system is capable of effective control of chronic virus infections such as herpes virus infections and HIV. Whereas successful containment of chronic herpes virus infections is the rule, control of HIV is exceptional. However, a very small subset of HIV-infected persons have now been infected for over 20 years with successful suppression of virus. Early studies revealed that cytotoxic T lymphocytes (CTL) play a central role in reducing HIV replication, both by killing virus-infected cells and by the production of antiviral factors[15-17]. A critical difference between the immune response towards HIV in 'long-term non-progressors (LTNP)' and the 'progressors' is that anti-HIV T helper activity is required to enable CTL to maintain suppression of virus long-term[18].

Investigators in Boston recently set out to determine why the majority of HIV-infected adults fail to control virus long-term[19]. It was reasoned that, during acute infection, T helper cells are specifically targeted by the virus and thus in most cases rapidly become eliminated; and that early institution of highly active antiretroviral therapy (HAART) would protect against this loss of T helper cells. Acutely infected adults were, therefore, recruited and treated immediately with HAART. The T helper responses in these early-treated subjects reached very high levels, similar to those in LTNP subjects. However, since HAART had so quickly switched off virus replication, the CTL responses in this group were relatively low. After stopping HAART for short periods, the CTL responses increased substantially, and the T helper responses were augmented even further. At this stage, it was possible for these subjects to discontinue HAART altogether and yet maintain control of HIV to low levels for more than a year.

The value of these studies in terms of the global epidemic are 3-fold. First, the view that HIV infection inevitably leads to AIDS and death is discredited, since, with the appropriate immune responses intact, control of the virus by the immune system is clearly possible. Second, the specific immune responses that are associated with effective containment of HIV are identifiable more clearly as the CTL and T helper responses. Third, the acute immune response as key[20–29] is underlined. Similar interventions in chronically infected adults have not had measurable impact[30]. The next step is to expand on these studies of B clade HIV infection in the US and apply the work to C clade infection dominating the sub-Saharan African and the growing Asian epidemics[31,32].

Mechanisms of progression to disease at different rates

The causes of HIV pathogenesis in adult as well as paediatric infection are not well understood. In adult infection, as described above, Gag-specific T helper activity and CTL activity[33] have been associated with successful control of viraemia. But what determines whether some individuals maintain the critical helper responses whilst the majority lose them in acute infection? Factors unconnected with the immune response such as chance, the amount of virus transmitted, the fitness of the transmitted virus, and host genetic factors affecting viral entry all may play a role[34,35]. However, a strong clue that specific components of the immune response play an important part in determining HIV outcome derives first from the finding that HLA class I homozygositiy is strongly associated with more rapid progression to disease[36]; and, second, from the associations of particular class I molecules with slow or rapid progression[35].

The class I molecule that stands out as being associated with rapid progression is HLA-B35[36,37]]. Detailed analysis of this effect revealed that the commonest subtype, B*3501, is not in fact associated with rapid progression, and the association with rapid progression comes from the strong effect of the less common subtypes[37]. Structurally, the difference between these subtypes lies in the size of the residue that can be accommodated in the F pocket of the peptide-binding groove, into which binds the C-terminal anchor residue of the B35-binding peptide.

HLA-B*3501 has a more capacious F pocket and preferentially binds large residues such as Tyr in this C terminal anchor position of the peptide. The less common subtypes of B35, such as B*3502 and B*3503, carry smaller F pockets only capable of binding smaller residues. One can hypothesise that there is less choice in the peptides that can bind to B*3502 and B*3503, since small residues can be accommodated within a large pocket in the peptide-binding groove, with water molecules adequately filling the remaining space available[38].

The class I molecule most strongly associated with slow progression in HIV infection is HLA-B57[39–41]. In this case, again, the F pocket admits a large residue, preferentially Trp[42]. Notably, HLA-B57 is able to bind peptides of quite variable lengths, from 8-mers to 11-mers[43], whereas the class I alleles associated with rapid progression such as B35 or B8 tend to bind shorter peptides of 8 or 9 amino acids in length only[44]. Closely related to B57 is HLA-B*5802, a subtype that would be expected to have difficulty accommodating Trp in C-terminal position of the peptide[32]. HLA-B58 is, interestingly, not associated with slow progression from preliminary studies[45]. HLA B57 and B58 are important in sub-Saharan Africa since, in HIV-affected populations such as Zulu, South Africa, 35–40% of persons express one or other of these class I molecules[46,47]. Further studies are needed to test this hypothesis, that a large choice in peptide is important in mounting an effective response to a virus such as HIV.

An alternative hypothesis to explain the association of particular class I molecules with slow progression is that, by chance, the immunodominant epitopes that are targeted happen to be situated in regions of fundamental importance to viral fitness. One good example of this is the HLA-B27-restricted epitope in p24 Gag, KRWIILGLNK (KK10). With very few exceptions, all B27-expressing adults so far studied generate a strong response to this epitope KK10[48]. This is sometimes the only detectable HIV-specific response[49]. HLA-B27 is associated with slow progression in adult infection[39,50]. Thus the mechanism of this association of slow progression is may be through this KK10-specific response. Loss of recognition of the KK10 epitope arises through mutation in the anchor position 2 in the B27-binding peptide: this position has to be occupied by Arg for adequate binding to B27[51–53]. The mutations arising in this normally highly conserved epitope are largely restricted to persons with B27 and arises late in the infection[52].

This epitope lies in the centre of the helix-7 that forms the interface between one p24 molecule and its partner in the formation of the homodimeric p24 Gag structure[54,55]. Loss of this homodimeric structure leads to failure of new virion formation[56]. It happens that a mutation in the second position of the KK10 epitope involves a residue that is critically participating in the homodimer binding. In fact this mutation does not appear to be accommodated within this helix-7 in the absence of other compensatory mutations developing previously[57]. In some instances, these compensatory mutations arise elsewhere within the KK10 epitope, in others they occur far outside the epitope in the linear sequence but very close within the p24 structure[58]. Thus the association of B27 with slow progression may derive from the chance happening of the dominant epitope being situation in a region of critical importance to viral replicative fitness.

Studies to characterise further the role of CTL escape in HIV pathogenesis need to be undertaken in persons expressing alleles such as B8 and B35 that are associated with rapid progression and comparative evaluations made of CTL escape in persons expressing alleles such as B27 and B57 that are associated with slow progression. The most illuminating data will come from investigations of acute infection where, as described above, the immune events to a great extent set the ultimate course for the infection as a whole. However, identification of acute HIV infection in adults is problematic unless there are symptoms, and emerging evidence is that adults with acute infection who express HLA-B27 or HLA–B57 are less likely to present with acute HIV syndrome[59]. One may hypothesise that effective B27- and B57-restricted CTL responses are generated early in acute infection, bringing about more rapid control of viraemia and reducing symptomatic acute infection. In contrast, B8- and B35-restricted responses may arise later or may be easily evaded by immune escape, in either case failing to bring about effective early control of virus replication (Fig. 1). The limited data available support this hypothesis[24,60]. What is beyond dispute is that quite distinct CTL specificities may operate in acute

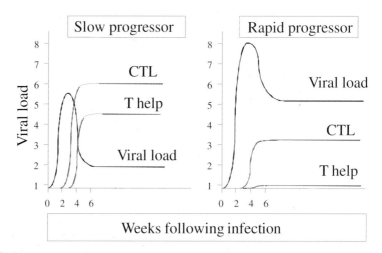

Fig. 1 Schematic view of hypothesised changes in viral load, HIV-specific CTL and T helper cell responses during the course of HIV infection in slow and rapid progression. Viral load shown in $\log_{10}$ RNA copies/ml plasma.

and chronic HIV infection[60]. Further evaluation of early immune events will be invaluable.

Specific problems in control of paediatric HIV infection

There are two particular problems for children infected with HIV. The first is the timing of infection, in that in the great majority of cases transmission occurs perinatally and, therefore, at a time when the immune system is not fully developed. If, as indicated above, T cell immunity plays the central part in successful containment of HIV, and the critical time for an effective immune response to kick in is in acute infection, then the infected infant is very vulnerable to HIV infection around the time of birth. An immature immune response would certainly fail to contain the virus, and would also expose the thymus to HIV-mediated destruction, as has clearly been observed[61]. Studies of the effectiveness of the neonatal immune response in humans to perinatal virus infection have not been made, however, largely because of the unavailability of assay systems sensitive enough to obtain useful information from small amounts of blood. The advent of Elispot and flow cytometry-based assays (reviewed by Goulder[32]) has transformed what is now possible in studies of childhood T cell immunology[62].

The second particular problem for children infected with HIV is that the virus is transmitted from their mother. The degree of HLA class I

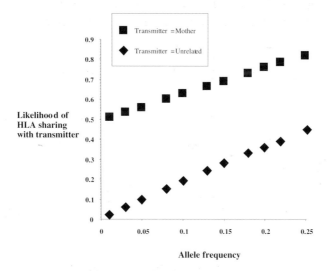

Fig. 2 Likelihood of sharing a particular HLA class I allele expressed in the transmitter of HIV, if the transmitter is the mother of the infected subject (squares) or unrelated to the infected subject (diamonds). These calculations assume random mating irrespective of HLA allele expression and Hardy-Weinberg distribution in the population of heterozygotes and homozygotes.

sharing between mother and child is higher than might initially be appreciated since, for a given allele expressed in the mother, the chances are only as low as 50% if the prevalence of that allele in the population is < 0.5% (Fig. 2). For alleles that have a frequency of as high as 25%, such as A*0201 in many Caucasoid populations[63], the chances of a mother with that allele sharing it with her child is > 80%. This is because there is a substantial chance of the mother being homozygous for that highly frequent allele, and also because the child also has a high chance of inheriting that same allele from the father. Furthermore, it is certain that the child will share at least 3 of the 6 HLA-A, HLA-B and HLA-C class I molecules expressed by the mother, whereas the chances that any individual shares more than one allele with an unrelated person is low – the precise likelihood depending on the particular alleles expressed by the mother. The potential significance of this HLA class I sharing between mother and child is that virus that has evaded the maternal HLA class I restricted CTL response will already be equipped to evade the child's CTL response, since the identical epitopes would be targeted by the child's immune response.

In order to determine whether this HLA sharing is actually significant in limiting the CTL activity against HIV available to children infected by MTCT, we investigated further[48] the HLA-B27-KK10 response described above which has been associated with protection against progression to disease in adult infection[39,49,50]. Comparison of the frequency with which HIV-infected children and infected adults with B27 target this KK10 epitope showed a significant difference, with > 85% of adults (19/22 studied) targeting this epitope and only 33% (2/6) children with B27 showing responses to this epitope ($P = 0.02$, Fisher's exact test). When the virus in the non-responding children was compared with the virus present in the mothers, in each of the 3 cases where the mother and the child shared B27, the same KK10-escape sequence (Arg to Thr in each instance) was also common to the mother and child. In the single case where transmission to a child with B27 occurred from a mother who was B27-negative, there was no mutated KK10 epitope transmitted. That child in fact resembles an adult with HLA-B27, since at 7.8 years of age he is a long-term non-progressor, with a CD4 count of > 800 cells/mm^3, strong p24 Gag-specific T helper activity[18] (data not shown) and an undetectable viral load since first measured at 4 years of age (< 400 or < 50 RNA copies/ml plasma) on ddI/AZT therapy. This is exceptional by paediatric standards[9,64,65], with levels this low seen in only 5/130 infected children being treated at The Children's Hospital, Boston out-patient clinics (Burchett S and McIntosh K, personal communication).

Thus, there are additional challenges to the immune system in perinatal HIV infection to those that are posed by HIV in adult infection. As described above, the early immune events are critical to the outcome from HIV infection. An effective and multifaceted early CTL response is likely to be the key to limiting the damage that occurs to the immune system in acute infection. Evasion of this early CTL response by epitope mutation is one of the principal methods by which the virus can maintain a foothold and inflict this irreparable damage. Work to compare the timing and role of escape in the adult and infant is underway, but from the preliminary data that are available, one may hypothesise that CTL escape plays a far more extensive part in preventing the paediatric immune response from containing early viraemia (Fig. 3). Two principal reasons for this, as described above, may be the immaturity of the paediatric immune response at the time of infection and the transmission of preformed CTL escape viruses from the HLA class I sharing mother. Determining the relative importance of these two factors in the more rapid progression to disease that is observed in paediatric infection is vitally important, as the approaches to achieving successful containment of HIV in paediatric infection depend on first understanding the cause of failure to control viraemia.

Augmenting HIV-specific immunity in paediatric infection

The ultimate goal for the prevention of paediatric HIV infection is an effective vaccine that can be administered at birth. Even then, it may be

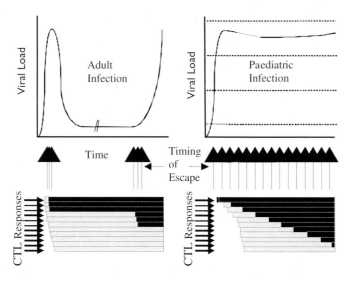

Fig. 3 Hypothesised model of CTL escape in paediatric versus adult HIV infection. The majority of escape in adult infection occurs in acute infection and then late in chronic infection prior to progression to AIDS. In paediatric infection CTL escape occurs prior to transmission, and then post-transmission occurs continuously during the course of infection without effective control being attained.

envisioned that this vaccine would be needed to be given in conjunction with a period of HAART in infected neonates in order to prevent the immune destruction that follows persistently high levels of viral replication. In the absence of a vaccine, similar approaches to the one that has been utilised so effectively in acute adult infection in the US[19] may be adopted. In the case of paediatric as opposed to adult acute infection, there is the great advantage that it is possible to anticipate early infection in infants by antenatal testing of mothers. Having determined whether MTCT has occurred by determining plasma viral RNA levels in the first 1–2 months of life, HAART may be instituted with the goal of limiting to a minimum any HIV-mediated damage to the developing immune system. This can be achieved in the setting of the US healthcare system, as demonstrated by Luzuriaga and colleagues[66]. As the understanding of which particular antiretroviral drugs are suitable for use in infants, and as formulations of the drugs are developed to facilitate adherence, it may be possible to construct effective regimens of HAART that can be adopted also in non-industrialised countries for infected infants. This will buy a period of time during which the developing immune system is protected from HIV-mediated damage, and during which the immune system itself can mature to generate a more effective suppression of viraemia. At this point, HAART may then be discontinued for short periods of supervised treatment interruption (STI) to enable the infant's immune response against the virus to be boosted, but with HAART restarted before viraemia can reach the levels at which damage can be done, in particular to the developing virus-specific T helper responses. The long-term aim of this approach would be to augment the virus-specific immunity sufficiently via these STIs to enable HAART ultimately to be discontinued altogether. One particular advantage of STI as a form of autovaccination is that the immune system is being boosted with the autologous virus sequence. The theoretical disadvantage is that, having cleared viral reservoirs of virus via long-term HAART, that these will be filled rapidly by STI. However, against this there is now strong evidence that viral reservoirs are never completely eradicated by HAART, either in adult or paediatric infection[67–69].

An alternative method of inducing HIV-specific immunity in infected children whose virus is suppressed by HAART is to use HIV vaccines. A variety of candidate HIV vaccine approaches are presently being developed (reviewed by Letvin *et al*[70]). Other forms of immunotherapy currently being developed include the infusions of peptide-pulsed dendritic cells to induce primary CTL responses[71,72], and approaches using inactivated whole virus vaccines specifically designed to induce HIV-specific T helper activity[73]. However, the distinction should be emphasised again between interventions that are made in children or adults whose immune systems have been protected by HAART instituted in acute infection, as opposed to HAART instituted in chronic infection, after the damage of acute infection has been done. Also, it is expected that attempts to boost T helper activity in chronic infection will be fruitless in the absence of effective HAART cover[73].

In summary, the options available to augmenting anti-HIV immunity in paediatric infection are growing, although their accessibility in countries worst afflicted by the epidemic at present are limited and even in industrialised countries progress is at an early stage. However, the transformation of what is possible in studies of T cell immunity has been so startling over the past 2–3 years that dramatic advances in our understanding of neonatal and older paediatric T cell immunity are likely rapidly to follow. These will inevitably bring new approaches to supplement those promising immunotherapeutic avenues already being developed.

Prevention of paediatric HIV infection

Prevention of paediatric HIV infection has centred until very recently on the belief that HAART is unaffordable for people infected with HIV in non-industrialised countries. Prophylactic drugs used in pregnancy or simply in labour[6] are effective in reducing MTCT. The use of a single drug, nevirapine, that is given once to the mother and once to the new-born child, in reducing MTCT by close to 50% is difficult to argue against at $4 a treatment. However, high prevalence of HIV infection in children depends particularly on two factors – high prevalence of HIV in antenatal mothers, and high viral loads in the antenatal mothers. The peripartum administration of nevirapine reduces the viral load to which the new-born is exposed by ensuring therapeutic drug levels in the baby during the first few days of life. However, these therapeutic drug levels are only maintained for a few days, and this intervention neither protects fully against peripartum MTCT, nor at all against post-partum (breast-milk) transmission. The MTCT rate remains in the region of 10–15% in spite of prophylactic nevirapine. Clearly more needs to be achieved.

One intriguing approach being developed in Durban, South Africa by Coutsoudis and colleagues[74] is the idea that exclusive breast-feeding might reduce MTCT. Most studies (for example see Dunn et al[75]) previously described the risk of breast milk transmission without reference to the feeding pattern of the infant, in particular whether breast-feeding was exclusive or mixed with formula or other forms of nutrition. The initial observations in Durban[7] were that the rate of MTCT was 18.8% in children whose mothers did not breast feed, was 24.1% in children whose mothers mixed breast- and other feeding, and was only 14.6% in the children whose mothers exclusively breast-fed for > 3 months. The mothers in these different groups did not differ in their viral loads or CD4 counts[74]. These data appeared to be inconsistent with a concurrent study by Miotti *et al* in Malawi[76], but this latter study did not distinguish between exclusive and mixed breast-feeding. Further studies with longer follow-up are underway. However, a distinctly sobering caveat to any recommendation that HIV-infected mothers should exclusively breast-feed has emerged from work in Kenya, where a greatly increased mortality was observed in mothers who breast-fed[77]. As many as 69% of the deaths observed in HIV-infected mothers could be attributable to breast-feeding alone. This cost to HIV-infected mothers who are evidently at the limit of their metabolic reserves is an additional factor that clearly needs to be fully taken into account before the optimal infant feeding patterns can be determined.

Equally controversial is the issue of availability of HAART for all adults and children[78,79] infected with HIV. Clearly, HAART accessibility would have a huge impact on preventing paediatric infection for at least two reasons. Transmission between adults as well as from mother-to-child is more likely in the setting of a high viral load in the donor[80–82], and thus reducing viral load via HAART would be likely not only to reduce the prevalence of HIV in antenatal mothers but also to reduce the viral load in those infected mothers throughout pregnancy. This might be expected to reduce MTCT by closer to 67%[78] than the 47%[6] reported for nevirapine alone.

Is making HAART available for all infected persons world-wide a realistic prospect? Certainly Attavan and Sachs have served to highlight how little assistance is being given towards dealing with the problem of the global HIV epidemic, and how static this level of support has remained (approximately $200 million per year in total development assistance from 1994–1998, latest figures available) in the face of the rapidly expanding numbers of HIV infection[79]. These authors estimate that to treat 10 million infected persons with HAART would cost $5 billion a year, provided drugs can be obtained at ~5% of the usual costs of $10,000 per person per year. Whether this can be achieved remains to be seen. Suffice it to say that this appears to be a new option that has hitherto been overlooked, and one that would have a real chance of making a significant impact on the global epidemic, while work to develop vaccines and other immunomodulatory approaches can continue apace.

Management of paediatric HIV infection

The contrast between management of paediatric infection in resource-rich countries and resource-poor countries could not be more stark.

Table 1 Numbers of HIV infected children at the 3 study sites and infrastructure available to provide necessary care

	King Edward VIII Hospital, Durban, South Africa	St Mary's Hospital, London, UK	The Children's Hospital, Boston, USA
Total country population	40 million	59 million	285 million
Number of deliveries to HIV infected women per year	300,000/year (SA-wide)	350/year (UK-wide)	5,000/year (US-wide)
Number of infected infants per year	40–75,000/year (SA-wide)	~50/year (UK-wide)	200–500/year (US-wide)
Antenatal HIV testing	Not routine: voluntary testing at 2 sites in KwaZuluNatal	Strongly recommended (UK-wide): low uptake	Strongly recommended (US-wide): high uptake
Antenatal management of infected mother	Mothers given nevirapine to take with onset of labour	Aim for maternal VL < 50 if needing HAART on basis of VL/CD4*. Otherwise, AZT monoRx from 28–30/40 and elective C/S at 38/40	Aim for maternal VL < 50. Infant Rx AZT x 6 weeks. Maternal VL > 1,000: add NVP or d4T
Follow-up of children born to infected mothers	Clinic visits 3 monthly; serology at 18 months	Seen at dl, 2–4 weeks, 3 months and 18 months – PCR at dl, 2–4 weeks and 3 months; serology at 18 months	Minimum 5 clinic visits in first 6 months
Total number of infected children regularly attending the clinic	240	118	130
Age of infected children	Range 0–12 years	Range 0–17 years	Range 0–24 years
Family clinics	Towards integration (adults seen in same hospital)	Completely integrated (adults seen in paediatric clinic)	Adult hospitals adjacent to TCH
Who looks after the children at home?	40% with biological parents, 50% with extended family, 5% adopted, 5% in foster care	90% with biological parents, 7% with extended family, 2% adopted, 1% in foster care	53% with biological parents, 33% with extended family, 9% adopted, 6% in foster care
Non-healthcare support for HIV-infected families	Voluntary support only (minimal)	Statutory and voluntary sector support	Daycare, after school programme, respite care
Healthcare support system	ID attending, registrar, nurse practitioner	Multidisciplinary team: ID attending, ID fellow, SHV, CNS, psych, dietician, physio, OT	HIV ID attending + ID fellow, nurse practitioner, social worker
Nurse practitioners or equivalent (e.g. clinical nurse specialist) per clinic	0/240 patients	0/118 patients	5 (1/26 patients)
Social workers per clinic	0/240 patients	1/118 patients	2 (1/65 patients)
Nurse home visits	Nil	Telephone contacts; home visits not routine	Daily x 2 weeks for new therapy; then weekly

*Criteria for starting therapy in UK.

While this relates in part to access to HAART, it reflects also the disparity in the infrastructure and supportive networks that underpin paediatric HIV management in countries such as the US, where there are perhaps 200 new cases of perinatally acquired HIV infection each year,

Table 2 Clinical presentation of paediatric HIV infection at each study site

Age of child	King Edward VIII Hospital, Durban, South Africa	St Mary's Hospital, London, UK	The Children's Hospital, Boston, USA
< 1 year	< 2 months: congenital TB, CMV, syphilis 2–6 months: PCP, HSM, chronic gastroenteritis, candidiasis 6–12 months: FTT, recurrent LRTIs, thrush, chronic diarrhoea, neurodevelopment delay	PCP, FTT, neurodevelopment regression, CMV retinitis, refractory candidiasis	PCP, FTT, neurodevelopment regression
Toddler age group	Lymphoid interstitial pneumonitis (LIP), TB, chronic gastroenteritis, recurrent bacterial sepsis (skin/ears/chest), zoster, malignancies	Persistent adenopathy ± HSM, LIP, bilateral parotid enlargement, Extensive molluscum contagiosum	Persistent adenopathy
Older children	recurrent LRTI, LIP, bronchiectasis, chronic lung disease, TB, otitis media, impetigo, CNS infection – toxoplasmosis, cryptococcal meningitis	Asymptomatic (family member diagnosed), recurrent LRTI, LIP, bacteraemia, zoster, candidiasis, (MAI/PCP end-stage)	PCP, oral candidiasis, MAI, zoster, recurrent severe HSV

CMV, cytomegalovirus; PCP, *Pneumocystis carinii* pneumonia; HSM, hepatosplenomegaly; FTT, failure-to-thrive; LRTIs, lower respiratory tract infections; LIP, lymphoid interstitial pneumonitis; MAI, *Mycobacterium avium* intracellulare; HSV, herpes simplex virus.

and in countries such as South Africa, where the figure would be currently approximately 75,000 per year[3–6]. The differences in infrastructure and management are summarised in Tables 1–3.

The most striking differences in the management of HIV infected children relate to the disparity between burden of infection and infrastructural support (Table 1). It should be noted that King Edward VIII Hospital (KEH) in Durban is distinctly one of the better equipped hospitals in sub-Saharan Africa, and that even more striking disparities would have been evident had a rural hospital in sub-Saharan Africa been included in the comparisons. Although at KEH prophylaxis against MTCT is available in the form of nevirapine in labour and to the child in the first 3 days of life, this is only available currently at a handful of localities in South Africa – hence the wide range in estimated newly infected children in South Africa of between 40,000 and 75,000 each year, depending upon accessibility of nevirapine. Less apparent than might be expected in the KEH is the real impact of HIV in the adult community on AIDS orphans in Africa, with as many of 40% of children attending the clinic being looked after at home by biological parents. However, this may be due to selection bias, with children having living parents more liable to be brought to the KEH clinic.

The clinical presentation of paediatric HIV infection at the three sites is summarised in Table 2, and perhaps the major differences being the broader spectrum of clinical presentation patterns in Durban. This may be reflective of the larger numbers of infected children seen in Durban, and also of the higher background morbidity in the Durban population, with

Table 3 Clinical management of paediatric HIV infection at each study site

	King Edward VIII Hospital, Durban, South Africa	St Mary's Hospital, London, UK	The Children's Hospital, Boston, USA
Stable patients doing well **Frequency of follow-up**	1–2 monthly	3 monthly	2 monthly
Routine investigations	FBC/Diff/LFT	• CD4/VL/FBC/Diff/LFT/ U&E/amylase/lipids/glucose • 4 monthly: also TG/cholesterol (if on PI)	• CD4/VL/FBC/Diff/LFT/ U&E/amylase/lipids/glucose • 4 monthly: also TG/cholesterol (if on PI)
Patients starting therapy or changing therapy **Frequency of follow-up**	Monthly	2, 4 and 8 weeks after start; (also 6 weeks if NVP) then 2–3 monthly	2, 4 and 8 weeks after start; monthly until VL < 50; then 2 monthly
Prophylaxis	• PCP: all children of HIV +ve mothers until 1 year; continue if clinicallyindicated • Anti-TB prophylaxis if TB contact; INH + rifampicin for 3 months after excluding TB • Ketoconzaole (for recurrent candidiasis)	• PCP: all children of HIV +ve mothers until third PCR –ve (at 4 months); prophylaxis until CD4 > 15% • MAI/HSV/VZV/fungal: rarely used only if CD4 < 5% and unresponsive to new HAART • Most common prophylaxis: valaciclovir for recurrent shingles	• PCP: CD4 < 200 or CDC cat 3 or 12 months of age • MAI: CD4 < 75 or CDC cat 3 • Fungal: fluconazole for CDC category 3 symptoms
Treatment **What drugs are used?**	AZT/3TC or ddI/d4T	• Initial: 2 NRTIs + 1 NNRTI (NVP or EFV) • High VL: 3 NRTIs (AZT/3TC/ABC) + NNRTI (NFV or EFV) • Change: 2 new NRTIs + PI (Kaletra) • Salvage change: res testing + e.g. new PI + NNRTI	• Initial: 2 NRTIs + PI/NNRTI (PI usually NFV; NNRTI either NVP or EFV) • High VL: 2 NRTIs + PI + NNRTI • Change: res testing + 2 new NRTIs/2 PIs or 2 new NRTIs/NNRTI/PI(s) • Salvage change: res testing + new PI + NRTIs, NNRTI if susc, 2 new PIs (res testing) • PI preferences: NFV > IDV + RTV, SQV/RTV, APV, LPV, APV/LPV
Treatment **Who is treated?**	If drugs can be afforded by parents of children symptomatic of HIV infection	All new diagnoses, if parents willing Symptomatic older children or CD4 < 25% or falling CD4%	All new infant diagnoses Aim for: normal immune system + VL control
% patients not on ART	> 95% (> 228/240 not on HAART)	> 29% (> 34/118 not on HAART)	> 0% (> 5/130 on only NRTIs)
Monthly IVIG	0%	0%	5%
Gastrostomy tubes	0%	3%	5% (for medication)

Antiretroviral drugs: NRTIs, nucleoside analogue reverse transcriptase inhibitors; AZT, zidovudine; 3TC, lamivudine; ABC, abacavir; NNRTIs, non-nucleoside analogue reverse transcriptase inhibitors; NVP, nevirapine; EFV, efavirenz; PIs, protease inhibitors, Kaletra; NFV, nelfinavir; IDV, indinivir; RTV, ritonavir; SQV, saquinavir; APV, amprenavir.

Investigations: FBC, full blood count; Diff, differential; U&E, urea and electrolytes; LFT, liver function tests; VL, viral load; CD4, T-cell subsets.

factors including overcrowding, limited access to fresh water supplies, and malnutrition contributing to the higher frequency of TB, CMV, gastroenteritis and other infectious disease seen in this population.

Clinical management of infected children at the three sites are summarised in Table 3. As expected, although clinical follow-up is very frequent in Durban and long-term follow-up of children attending the clinic at KEH is exceptionally complete, more investigations are undertaken in the management of children cared for in the UK and in the US, where many more treatment options are available, in particular of course antiretroviral therapy.

Conclusions

The impact of HIV on childhood health world-wide is becoming increasingly apparent. Children infected with HIV progress rapidly to disease for reasons that are not fully established. The immune response mediated through CTL and T helper cell activity plays a central role in control of HIV in adult infection. Technical obstacles to investigating the immune response in infants have been to a large extent overcome by access to Elispot and flow cytometry-based assays, and these on-going studies should bring significant advances to our understanding of the specific problems encountered by the immune system of the neonate and infant confronted by MTCT of HIV infection. Preliminary data would indicate that there is a particularly strong rationale to adopting one or more of a variety of novel immunotherapeutic approaches to augment these HIV-specific T-cell responses in paediatric infection. Considerable challenges would lie in the way of the delivery of any new approach, including antiretroviral therapy itself, to dealing with HIV infection at the site of the epidemic. However, since the critical events determining the course of infection may be concentrated at the very early stages of infection, effective interventions or treatments of short duration can be envisaged that could have a major positive impact on the global paediatric epidemic.

Acknowledgements

This work was supported by grants to PJRG from the Elizabeth Glaser Pediatric AIDS Foundation, the UK Medical Research Foundation (grant G108/274) and the National Institutes of Health (AI46995); PJRG is an Elizabeth Glaser Scientist of the Elizabeth Glaser Pediatric AIDS Foundation.

References

1   UNAIDS/WHO. *AIDS Epidemic Update*. Geneva: WHO, 1988.
     www.unaids.org/wac/2000/wad00/files/WAD_epidemic_report.htm

2   Luo C. Achievable standard of care in low-resource settings. *Ann NY Acad Sci* 2000; **918**:
     179–87

3   UNAIDS web-site: http://www.unaids.org/epidemic_update/report/Epi_report.htm

4   Anonymous. *Department of Health 1998: Ninth Annual National HIV Sero-Prevalence Survey
     of Women attending antenatal clinics in South Africa*. South Africa: Health Systems Research
     and Epidemiology, Department of Health, 1999

5   Wilkinson D, Connolly C, Rotchford K. Continued explosive rise in HIV prevalence among
     pregnant women in rural South Africa. *AIDS* 1999; **13**: 740

6   Guay LA, Musoke P, Fleming T *et al*. Intrapartum and neonatal single-dose nevirapine
     compared with zidovudine for prevention of mother-to-child transmission of HIV-1 in
     Kampala, Uganda: HIVNET 012 randomised trial. *Lancet* 1999; **354**: 795–802

7   Coutsoudis A, Pillay K, Spooner E, Kuhn L, Coovadia HM. Influence of infant-feeding patterns
     on early mother-to-child transmission of HIV-1 in Durban, South Africa: a prospective cohort
     study. South African Vitamin A Study Group. *Lancet* 1999; **354**: 471–6

8   Wilkinson D, Abdool Karim SS, Williams B, Gouws E. High HIV incidence and prevalence
     among young women in rural South Africa: developing a cohort for intervention trials. *J Acquir
     Immune Defic Syndr* 2000; **23**: 405–9

9   Barnhart HX, Caldwell MP, Thomas P. Natural history of HIV disease in perinatally infected
     children: an analysis from the pediatric spectrum of disease project. *Pediatrics* 1996; **97**:
     710–16

10   European Collaborative Study. Natural history of vertically acquired HIV-1 infection.
     Pediatrics 1994; **94**: 815–9

11   Collaborative Group on AIDS Incubation and HIV Survival including the CASCADE EU
     Concerted Action. Time from HIV-1 seroconversion to AIDS and death before widespread use
     of highly antiretroviral therapy: a collaborative re-analysis. *Lancet* 2000; **355**: 1131–7

12   Koblin BA, van Benthem BH, Buchbinder SP *et al*. Long-term survival after infection with HIV-
     1 among homosexual men in hepatitis B vaccine trial cohorts in Amsterdam, New York City
     and San Francisco. *Am J Epidemiol* 1999; **150**: 1026–30

13   Taha TE, Graham SM, Kumwenda NI *et al*. Morbidity among human immunodeficiency virus-
     1 infected and uninfected African children. *Pediatrics* 2000; **106**: 1–8

14   Morgan D, Whitworth JAG. The natural history of HIV-1 infection in Africa. *Nat Med* 2001;
     7: 143–5

15   Walker BD, Chakrabati S, Moss B *et al*. HIV-specific T lymphocytes in seropositive individuals.
     Nature 1987; **328**: 345–8

16   Yang OO, Kalams SA, Rosenzweig M *et al*. Efficient lysis of human immunodeficiency virus
     type 1-infected cells by cytotoxic T lymphocytes. *J Virol* 1996; **70**: 5799–806

17   Goulder PJR, Rowland-Jones S, McMichael AJ, Walker BD. Anti-human immunodeficiency
     virus cellular immunity: progress towards vaccine design. *AIDS* 1999; **13 (Suppl A)**: S121–36

18   Rosenberg ES, Billingsley JM, Caliendo A *et al*. Vigorous HIV-1-specific CD4$^+$ T-cell responses
     associated with control of viraemia. *Science* 1997; **278**: 1447–50

19   Rosenberg ES, Altfeld M, Poon SP *et al*. Immune control of HIV-1 after early treatment of acute
     infection. *Nature* 2000; **407**: 523–6

20   Koup RA, Safrit JT, Cao Y *et al*. Temporal association of cellular immune responses with the
     initial control of viremia in primary HIV infection. *J Virol* 1994; **68**: 4650–5

21   Borrow P, Lewicki H, Hahn BH, Shaw GM, Oldstone MBA. Virus-specific CD8$^+$ CTL activity
     associated with control of viremia in primary HIV infection. *J Virol* 1994; **68**: 6103–10

22   Mellors JW, Rinaldo CR, Gupta P, White RM, Todd JA, Kingsley LA. Prognosis in HIV-1
     infection predicted by the quantity of virus in plasma. *Science* 1996; **272**: 1167–70

23   Borrow P, Lewicki H, Wei X *et al*. Antiviral pressure exerted by HIV-1-specific cytotoxic T
     lymphocytes (CTLs) during primary infection demonstrated by rapid selection of CTL escape
     virus. *Nat Med* 1997; **3**: 205–11

24 Price DA, Goulder PJR, Klenerman P *et al*. Positive selection of HIV-1 cytotoxic T lymphocyte escape variants during primary infection. *Proc Natl Acad Sci USA* 1997; **94**: 1890–5

25. Pantaleo G, Demarest JF, Schacker T *et al*. The qualitative nature of the primary immune response to HIV infection is a prognosticator of disease progression independent of the initial level of plasma viremia. *Proc Natl Acad Sci USA* 1997; **94**: 254–8

26 Schmitz JE, Kuroda M, Santra S *et al*. Control of viremia in simian immunodeficiency virus infection by CD8⁺ lymphocytes. *Science* 1999; **283**: 857–60

27 Jin X, Bauer DE, Tuttleton SE *et al*. Dramatic rise in plasma viremia after CD8⁺ T cell depletion in SIV-infected macaques. *J Exp Med* 1999; **189**: 991–8

28 Allen T, O'Connor D, Jing P *et al*. Tat-specific cytotoxic T lymphocytes select for SIV escape variants during resolution of primary viraemia. *Nature* 2000; **407**: 386–90

29 Goulder PJR, Walker BD. The great escape: AIDS viruses and immune control. *Nat Med* 1999; **5**: 1233–5

30 Oxenius A, Price DA, Phillips RE. Unpublished data

31 Goulder PJR, Brander C, Annamalai K *et al*. Differential narrow focusing of immunodominant HIV Gag-specific CTL responses in infected African and Caucasoid adults and children. *J Virol* 2000; **74**: 5679–90

32 Goulder PJR. Rapid characterization of HIV clade C-specific cytotoxic T lymphocyte responses in infected African children and adults. *Ann NY Acad Sci* 2000; **918**: 330–45

33 Ogg GS, Jin X, Bonhoeffer S *et al*. Quantitation of HIV-1-specific cytotoxic T lymphocytes and plasma load of viral RNA. *Science* 1998; **279**: 2103–6

34 Deacon NJ, Tsykin A, Solomon A *et al*. Genomic structure of an attenuated quasi species of HIV-1 from a blood transfusion donor and recipients. *Science* 1995; **270**: 988–91

35 Hill AV. Genetics and genomics of infectious disease susceptibility. *Br Med Bull* 1999; **55**: 401–13

36 Carrington M, Nelson GW, Martin MP *et al*. HLA and HIV-1: heterozygote advantage and B*35-Cw*04 disadvantage. *Science* 1999; **283**: 1748–52

37 Gao X, Nelson GW, Karacki P *et al*. Effect of a single amino acid change in MHC class I molecules on the rate of progression to AIDS. *N Engl J Med* 2001; **344**: 1668–75

38 Freemont DH, Stura EA, Matsumura M, Peterson PA, Wilson IA. Crystal structure of an H-2Kᵇ-ovalbumin peptide complex reveals the interplay of primary and secondary anchor positions in the major histocompatibility complex binding groove. *Proc Natl Acad Sci USA* 1995; **92**: 2479–83

39 Kaslow RA, Carrington M, Apple R *et al*. Influence of human MHC genes on the course of HIV infection. *Nat Med* 1996; **2**: 405–11

40 Migueles SA, Sabbaghian MS, Shupert WL *et al*. HLA-B*5701 is highly associated with restriction of virus replication in a subgroup of HIV-infected long-term non-progressors. *Proc Natl Acad Sci USA* 2000; **97**: 2709–14

41 Goulder PJR, Crowley S, Krausa P *et al*. Novel, cross-restricted, conserved and immunodominant CTL epitopes in long-term slow progressors in HIV-1 infection. *AIDS Res Hum Retroviruses* 1996; **12**: 1691–8

42 Barber LD, Percival L, Arnett KL, Gumperz JE, Chen L, Parham P. Polymorphism in the α1 helix of the HLA-B heavy chain can have an overriding influence on peptide-binding specificity. *J Immunol* 1997; **158**: 1660–9

43 Goulder PJR, Tang Y, Pelton SI, Walker BD. HLA-B57-restricted CTL activity in a single infected subject towards two optimal HIV epitopes, one of which is entirely contained within the other. *J Virol* 2000; **74**: 5291–9

44 Brander C, Goulder PJR. The evolving field of HIV CTL epitope mapping: new approaches for the identification of novel epitopes. In: Korber BTM, Brander C, Walker BD *et al*. (eds) *HIV Molecular Database*. Los Alamos, NM: Los Alamos National Laboratory, 2000

45 Keet IP, Tang J, Klein MR *et al*. Consistent associations of HLA class I and II and transporter gene products with progression of human immunodeficiency virus type 1 infection in homosexual men. *J Infect Dis* 1999; **180**: 299–309

46 Hammond MG, du Toit ED, Sanchez-Mazas A *et al*. HLA in sub-Saharan Africa: 12th International Histocompatibility Workshop SSAF report. In: Charron D. (ed) *Proceedings of*

the Twelfth International Histocompatibility Workshop and Conference. Paris: EDK, 1997; 345–53

47 Goulder PJR, Brander C, Tang Y et al. Stable evolution and transmission of CTL escape mutants in HIV infection. Nature 2001; **412**: 334–8

48 Goulder PJR, Tang Y, Tremblay C et al. Stable evolution and transmission of CTL escape mutants in HIV infection. Nature 2001; In press

49 Goulder PJR, Phillips RE, Colbert R et al. Late escape from an immunodominant cytotoxic T lymphocyte response associated with progression to AIDS. Nat Med 1997; **3**: 212–7

50 McNeil AJ, Yap PL, Gore SM. Association of HLA types A1-B8-DR3 and B27 with rapid and slow progression of HIV disease. Q J Med 1996; **89**: 177–85

51 Jardetzky TS, Lane WS, Robinson RA, Madden DR, Wiley DC. Identification of self-peptides bound to purified HLA-B27. Nature 1991; **353**: 326–9

52 Guo H-C, Madden DR, Silver ML et al. Comparison of the P2 specificity pocket in three human histocompatibility antigens, HLA-A*6801, HLA-A*0201, and HLA-B*2705. Proc Natl Acad Sci USA 1993; **90**: 8053–7

53 Mear JP, Schreiber KL, Munz C et al. Misfolding of HLA-B27 as a result of its B pocket suggests a novel mechanism for its role in susceptibility to spondyloarthropathies. J Immunol 1999; **163**: 6665–70

54 Momany C, Kovari LC, Prongay AJ et al. Crystal structure of dimeric HIV-1 capsid protein. Nat Struct Biol 1996; **3**: 763–70

55 Gamble TR, Vajdos FF, Yoo S et al. Crystal structure of human cyclophilin A bound to the amino-terminal domain of HIV-1 capsid. Cell 1996; **87**: 1285–94

56 Berthet-Colominas C, Monaco S, Novelli A, Sibai G, Mallet F, Cusack S. Head-to-tail dimers and interdomain flexibility revealed by the crystal structure of HIV-1 capsid protein (p24) complexed with a monoclonal antibody Fab. EMBO J 1999; **18**: 1124–36

57 Kelleher AD, Long C, Holmes EC et al. 1: Clustered mutations in HIV-1 gag are consistently required for escape from HLA-B27-restricted cytotoxic T lypmphocyte responses. J Exp Med 2001; **193**: 375–86

58 Kelleher AD, Goulder PJR, McMichael AJ, Phillips RE, Brander C. 2001; Manuscript in preparation

59 Altfeld M. Unpublished data

60 Goulder PJR, Altfeld M, Rosenberg ES et al. Substantial differences in specificity of HIV-specific cytotoxic T lymphocytes in acute and chronic HIV infection. J Exp Med 2001; **193**: 181–93

61 Kourtis AP, Ibegbu C, Nahmias AJ et al. Early progression of disease in HIV infected infants with thymic dysfunction. N Engl J Med 1996; **335**: 1431–6

62 Vekemans J, Amedei A, Ota MO et al. Neonatal bacillus Calmette-Guerin vaccination induces adult-like IFN-gamma production by CD4+ T lymphocytes. Eur J Immunol 2001; **31**: 1531–5

63 Clayton J, Lonjou C, Whittle D. Allele and haplotype frequencies for HLA loci in various ethnic groups. In: Charron D. (ed) Proceedings of the Twelfth International Histocompatibility Workshop and Conference. Paris: EDK, 1997; 665–820

64 Mofenson LM, Korelitz J, Meyer 3rd WA et al. The relationship between serum human immunodeficiency virus type 1 (HIV-1) RNA level, CD4 lymphocyte percent, and long-term mortality risk in HIV-1-infected children. National Institute of Child Health and Human Development Intravenous Immunoglobulin Clinical Trial Study Group. J Infect Dis 1997; **175**: 1029–38

65 Shearer WT, Quinn TC, LaRussa P et al. Viral load and disease progression in infants infected with human immunodeficiency virus type 1. Women and Infants Transmission Study Group. N Engl J Med 1997; **336**: 1337–42

66 Luzuriaga K, McManus M, Catalina M et al. Early therapy of vertical human immunodeficiency virus type 1 (HIV-1) infection: control of viral replication and absence of persistent HIV-1-specific immune responses. J Virol 2000; **74**: 6984–91

67 Siliciano JD, Siliciano RF. Latency and viral persistence in HIV-1 infection. J Clin Invest 2000; **106**: 823–5

68 Persaud D, Pierson T, Ruff C et al. A stable latent reservoir for HIV-1 in resting CD4(+) T lymphocytes in infected children. J Clin Invest 2000; **105**: 995–1003

69 Finzi D, Blankson J, Siliciano JD *et al.* Latent infection of CD4+ T cells provides a mechanism for lifelong persistence of HIV-1, even in patients on effective combination therapy. *Nat Med* 1999; **5**: 512–7

70 Letvin NL, Bloom BR, Hoffman SL. Prospects for vaccines to protect against AIDS, tuberculosis, and malaria. *JAMA* 2001; **285**: 606–11

71 Dhodapkar MV, Steinman RM, Sapp M *et al.* Rapid generation of broad T-cell immunity in humans after a single injection of mature dendritic cells. *J Clin Invest* 1999; **104**: 173–80

72 Dhodapkar MV, Krasovsky J, Steinman RM, Bhardwaj N. Mature dendritic cells boost functionally superior CD8(+) T-cell in humans without foreign helper epitopes. *J Clin Invest* 2000; **105**: R9–14

73 Kahn JO, Cherng DW, Mayer K, Murray H, Lagakos S. Evaluation of HIV-1 immunogen, an immunologic modifier, administered to patients infected with HIV having 300 to 549 x 10(6)/L CD4 cell counts: a randomized controlled trial. *JAMA* 2000; **284**: 2193–202

74 Coutsoudis A. Influence of infant feeding patterns on early mother-to-child transmission of HIV-1 in Durban. *Ann NY Acad Sci* 2000; **918**: 136–44

75 Dunn DT, Newell ML, Ades AE, Peckham CS. Risk of HIV-1 transmission through breastfeeding. *Lancet* 1992; **340**: 585–8

76 Miotti PG, Taha TE, Kumwenda NI *et al.* HIV transmission through breastfeeding – a study in Malawi. *JAMA* 1999; **282**: 744–9

77 Nduati R, Richardson BA, John G *et al.* Effect of breastfeeding on mortality among HIV-1 infected women: a randomised trial. *Lancet* 2001; **357**: 1651–5

78 Editorial. Grants, not loans, for the developing world? *Lancet* 2001; **357**: 1

79 Attaran A, Sachs J. Defining and refining international donor support for combating the AIDS pandemic. *Lancet* 2001; **357**: 57–61

80 Connor EM, Sperling RS, Gelber R *et al.* Reduction of maternal-infant transmission of human immunodeficiency virus type 1 with zidovudine treatment. Pediatric AIDS Clinical Trials Group Protocol 076 Study Group. *N Engl J Med* 1994; **331**: 1173–80

81 Quinn TC, Wawer MJ, Sewankambo N *et al.* Viral load and heterosexual transmission of human immunodeficiency virus type 1. Rakai Project Study Group. *N Engl J Med* 2000; **342**: 921–9

82 Hisada M, O'Brien TR, Rosenberg P S, Goedert JJ. Virus load and risk of heterosexual transmission of human immunodeficiency virus and hepatitis C virus by men with hemophilia. The Multicenter Hemophilia Cohort Study. *J Infect Dis* 2000; **181**: 1475–8

HIV-1 transmission and acute HIV-1 infection

Pokrath Hansasuta and **Sarah L Rowland-Jones**

Human Immunology Unit, Institute of Molecular Medicine, John Radcliffe Hospital, Oxford, UK

An understanding of the central events in the transmission of HIV-1 infection is critical to the development of effective strategies to prevent infection. Although the main routes of transmission have been known for some time, surprisingly little is known about the factors that influence the likelihood of transmitting or acquiring HIV-1 infection. Once infection has taken place, the series of virological and immunopathological events that constitute primary HIV-1 infection are thought to be closely linked with the subsequent clinical course of the infected person. Recent studies have provided some support for the notion that intervention with aggressive anti-retroviral drug therapy at this stage has the potential to prevent some of the damage to the immune system that will otherwise develop in the vast majority of infected people.

HIV-1 transmission

Routes of HIV-1 transmission

The main routes of HIV-1 transmission are well-known, and are listed in Table 1. On a world-wide scale, the vast majority of new infections are acquired through heterosexual contact. The likelihood of transmission from male to female has been estimated to be as high as 8-fold more likely that from female to male[1], although the biological basis for this is not fully understood. Transmission of HIV-1 through oro-genital contact, although rare, is an increasingly recognised route of infection (reviewed by Caceres and van Griensven[2]).

In non-industrialised countries, as many as 42% of the children born to infected mothers will become infected[3], either at birth or in the postnatal period through exposure to infected breast-milk (reviewed by Nduati[4]). In contrast, vertical transmission of HIV-1 infection is now becoming a rare event in industrialised countries, through a combination of anti-retroviral therapy, obstetric management and the use of alternative infant feeding methods. The high rates of breast-milk transmission to infants of infected mothers emphasise the potential for HIV-1 to establish infection through the oral route. This is further demonstrated by the relative ease in which infant macaques can become infected with SIV through the atraumatic application of virus to the

Correspondence to:
Prof. Sarah Rowland-Jones, Human Immunology Unit, Institute of Molecular Medicine, John Radcliffe Hospital, Oxford OX3 9DS, UK

Table 1 Routes and likelihood of HIV-1 transmission

Study population	Transmission route	Transmission probability	Ref.
Heterosexual			
	US (male to female)	0.0008–0.001	12–14
	US (from male to female, and from female to male)	0.001	15
	Europe (from male to female, and from female to male)	0.0005–0.001	16
	Thailand (from male to female)	0.002	17
	Thailand (from female sex workers to men)	0.03–0.06	18,19
	Kenya 0.1	20	
Homosexual	US (receptive anal sex with ejaculation)	0.005–0.03	21
Perinatal transmission	Thailand		22
	Without AZT	18.9%	
	With AZT	9.4%	
	Cote d'Ivoire		23
	Without AZT	24.9%	
	With AZT	15.7%	
	USA		
	With Caesarean section and anti-retrovirals:		
	All three periods	2%	
	One or two periods	8.2%	
	Zero period	10.4%	
	Without Caesarean section:		
	All three periods	7.3%	
	One or two periods	16.4%	
	Zero period	19.0%	
Newborn	Breastfeeding:		
	6 weeks	3.9%	25
	14 weeks	10.2%	
	6 months	11.3%	
	12 months	14.1%	
	24 months	16.2%	
Healthcare workers	Percutaneous (Thailand)	< 0.5%	26,27
	Percutaneous (Holland)	0.3%	
	Percutaneous (Tanzania)		
	Healthcare workers	0.27%	28
	Surgeons	0.7%	
Blood recipients	Blood transfusion – screened blood	0.003–0.0007%	
	Developed countries		29,30
	Developing countries	5-10%	31
Intravenous drug users	Blood contamination	No reports	
Artificial insemination with contaminated sperm		Case report	32

back of the tongue[5]. Pathological studies in macaques infected by this route show that the infection begins locally in the tonsils, from where it spreads rapidly to other lymphoid tissue[6].

There is little evidence for HIV-1 being transmitted between household contacts in the absence of a recognised route of transmission (reviewed by Gershon et al[7]), although occasional cases have been reported[8,9].

Most countries have implemented screening procedures for donated blood that substantially reduce the risk of blood-borne infection[10]. Where the screening is limited to antibody testing, there is a small risk of using blood from a donor in the 'window' period of acute HIV infection, before antibodies have developed.

The chances of HIV-1 infection in healthcare workers after accidental exposure to contaminated blood is generally very low[11], and no cases have so far been reported in subjects given combination anti-retroviral therapy post-exposure prophylaxis.

What influences the 'infectivity' of the infected person?

The key factor influencing a person's likelihood of transmitting HIV-1 infection appears to be their viral burden – this can be predicted by measuring plasma viral load. A recent study in Rakai, Uganda[33] showed that transmission was rare from people with viral loads of less than 1500 RNA copies/ml. It is likely that genital viral secretion (which is harder to measure) is more relevant to infectivity than plasma viraemia[34]: genital shedding of virus is not always predicted by plasma viral load, and is increased during genital infection and in people with severe vitamin A deficiency[35]. It is becoming clear that HIV can be transmitted by people with apparently good viral suppression on anti-retroviral therapy: for example, when virus persists in relevant body compartments such as semen[36].

Host genetic factors can influence the infectiousness of the contact: it has recently been shown in a cohort of Kenyan HIV-infected women that those with one copy of a mutant allele of the gene encoding the chemokine SDF-1α (which binds to the co-receptor, CXCR4, often used by HIV in late infection) were more likely to transmit the infection to their infants[37]. It is feasible that certain HIV-1 strains are more infectious than others, but this has not been unequivocally demonstrated in vivo (reviewed by Vernazza et al[38]). The E clade strain of HIV, which rapidly outstripped B clade HIV-1 as the major strain in the Thai epidemic, was initially thought to infect Langerhans' cells more readily[39], but this finding could not be reproduced by others[40]. However, it is well-documented that HIV-2 is much less efficiently transmitted by the sexual route than HIV-1 and is hardly ever transmitted from mother to child (reviewed by Whittle et al[41]).

Factors influencing susceptibility and resistance to HIV-1 infection

Mucosal integrity

The likelihood of acquiring HIV infection following sexual contact is most clearly affected by physical factors, such as the presence of genital ulcerating infections[20,42], which have been proposed to be one of the main reasons for the rapid spread of HIV-1 in sub-Saharan Africa[43]. Male circumcision is associated with protection from HIV infection 20 (reviewed by Halperin and Bailey[44]), but this can be difficult to disentangle from cultural and religious factors that determine circumcision practice. One potential explanation for a protective role for circumcision is the high frequency of dendritic cells in the mucosa of the foreskin that could provide an accessible pool of HIV-susceptible target cells[45].

Hormonal factors can also influence mucosal integrity. Macaques treated with depot preparations of progesterone were more susceptible to SIV infection through vaginal exposure[46], whereas oestrogen had a protective effect[47]. Hormonal influences on infection risk have not been well-studied in humans, but the use of depot progesterone contraception is thought to increase the likelihood of infection[48].

Genetic factors

Genetic factors also play a role in susceptibility and resistance to HIV infection. The most important of these is a deletion (CCR5Δ32) in the major co-receptor for entry of primary HIV strains into CD4+ T-cells, a chemokine receptor called CCR5[49,50]. Homozygotes for the deletion (~1% of Caucasians) do not express the receptor at the cell-surface, and, therefore, can only become infected with strains of HIV that are able to use other co-receptors, such as CXCR4. Thus, although CCR5Δ32 homozygotes show a significant degree of resistance to HIV infection, a number of cases of infection with CXCR4-using HIV strains have been reported[51-53]. The CCR5Δ32 mutation is not found in all races, being largely confined to Caucasians, particularly those of Northern European descent[54]. If the relative levels of CCR5 expression are an important determinant of HIV susceptibility, then it might be expected that CCR5Δ32 heterozygotes (who express lower levels of the receptor than most other people[55]) would show a degree of resistance to infection, but this has not been observed in any study. However, cells from highly exposed persistently seronegative (HEPS) donors are often less easy to infect with primary HIV strains, even in the absence of any known CCR5 mutations, and this phenotype is associated with higher production than average of the HIV-suppressing chemokines, MIP-1α, MIP-1β and RANTES 56, which bind to the CCR5 receptor[57].

Two other polymorphisms in the CCR5 gene have been shown to have an effect on HIV susceptibility. One is a rare point mutation in the coding sequence of CCR5, which in combination with the CCR5Δ32 deletion is associated with HIV resistance[58]. The other is a polymorphism in the promoter region (at position 59356), largely confined to people of African descent, which increases the likelihood of infants acquiring HIV infection from their mothers[59]. Although the mechanism is not yet entirely clear, polymorphisms in the promoter region of the gene encoding the HIV-suppressing chemokine RANTES have been recently reported to show an association with HIV susceptibility[60]. Curiously, the same haplotype is linked with prolonged survival in people who do become infected. It has been suggested that this haplotype leads to increased RANTES production which may increase the likelihood of mucosal inflammation and reduced integrity: however, if infection takes place, then higher RANTES levels would suppress HIV replication[60].

A handful of other genetic polymorphisms have been shown to affect HIV susceptibility. HLA class I and II types have been associated with both resistance and susceptibility to HIV infection. In a cohort of highly-exposed Kenyan sex-workers, HIV resistance is associated with HLA-A2, A*6802, B18 and DR1, whilst HLA-A23 is associated with increased HIV infection[61]. A reduced risk of vertical HIV transmission was seen in infants with particular class II alleles (DRB1*1501 and DR13)[62]. A number of other genetic associations with HIV resistance have emerged in relatively small studies, including alleles of the TAP (transporters associated with antigen-processing) genes, namely TAP1.4 and TAP2.3[63] in the MACS cohort and the non-secretor genotype (which is associated with homozygosity for a stop mutation in the enzyme α-(1, 2)-fucosyltransferase, FUT2) in a cohort of Senegalese sex workers (OR 0.18, 95% CI 0.04–0.9)[64]: susceptibility has been associated with variant alleles of the mannose-binding lectin (MBL)[65], although it was not possible to distinguish between a direct effect on HIV susceptibility and an increased risk of other genital infections known to be affected by MBL genotype.

Immunological mechanisms of HIV resistance

The associations between HLA type and HIV resistance imply that immune responses may be playing a part in resistance to HIV infection, for example if the T-cells using these HLA molecules are particularly efficient at controlling HIV replication. In recent years, a great deal of interest has focused on potential immune mechanisms that may be linked with protection from HIV-1 infection in individuals with documented HIV-1 exposure who remain HIV-1 seronegative, often referred to as highly exposed persistently seronegatives (HEPS). If lymphocytes from HEPS donors are used to reconstitute the immune system of mice with severe combined immunodeficiency (the SCID-Hu mouse model), these animals show resistance to HIV infection, but this is not the case when control donors are used: this protection appears to reside in the CD8+ T-cell compartment[66]. A number of studies have shown that a significant proportion of HEPS donors have HIV-specific T-cells in their blood and genital mucosa (reviewed by Kaul and Rowland-Jones[67]). These include CD4+ T-cells which show both proliferation[68] and IL-2 secretion in response to HIV antigens[69–72]. HIV-specific CD4+ T-cells from HEPS individuals may also secrete HIV-suppressing chemokines[73,74]. Many HEPS donors have HLA class I-restricted HIV-specific cytotoxic T lymphocytes (CTL) in both blood (reviewed by Kaul and Rowland-Jones[67]) and genital mucosa[75]. The earliest descriptions of HIV-specific CTL in exposed uninfected individuals came from studies in babies born to infected mothers[76–79], who were likely to have been exposed to HIV for only a brief period around birth. Similar findings came from studies in healthcare workers exposed to HIV-contaminated blood through needlestick injuries[80,81]. Similar immune responses have also been described in people with repeated exposure who appeared to be genuinely resistant to infection, such as couples discordant for HIV infection who continue to have unprotected intercourse[68,82–85], and sex-workers in parts of the world with high HIV seroprevalence and low condom usage[86,87]. These observations suggest that HIV-specific cellular immune responses may be genuinely linked with protection from subsequent infection and has led to efforts to develop HIV-1 vaccines that might induce similar immune responses[88].

Early events in primary HIV-1 infection

A better understanding of the early events of HIV-1 infection would seem to be crucial for designing better strategies to prevent or interrupt HIV-1 transmission, yet there is relatively little data about what happens immediately following acute HIV-1 infection in people (Fig.1). One way of addressing these issues is to study events in macaques experimentally infected with the monkey equivalent of HIV, simian immunodeficiency virus (SIV), although these results cannot necessarily always be extrapolated to the human situation. In one such study, only a small number of infected cells were detected in the first 3 days after endo-cervical infection, close to the site of inoculation. At this stage, the

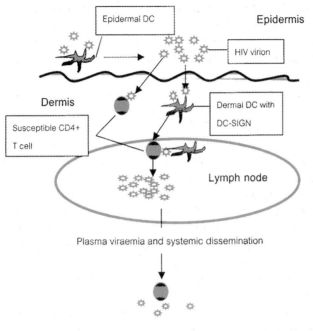

Plasma viraemia and systemic dissemination

Low but persistent replication of HIV in immune priviledged

sites during clinically asymptomatic period

T cell activation

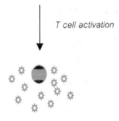

Fig. 1 Diagram to show the likely route of HIV entry and dissemination following primary HIV-1 infection.

Active replication of HIV, burst of viraemia and

consequent immune suppression lead to progression of

HIV disease and AIDS

predominant cell population to be infected were T-cells in the lamina propria. Over the next few days, the infection spread to other cell-types, including macrophages and dendritic cells (DCs), but the majority (> 90%) of the infected cells were CD4+ T-cells, many of which appeared to be resting T-cells[89]. By day 12, the virus could be found disseminated throughout the lymphatic system and bone marrow.

The role of DCs in early HIV-1 infection is controversial. Some investigators have suggested that DCs are the first cells to become infected in SIV infection[90], although this has not been confirmed in other studies. DCs provide a highly specialised mechanism whereby an antigen encountered in peripheral tissues, notably skin and mucosal membranes, can be brought into contact with the T-cells in the lymph node that will generate the immune response against it. The principal form of DC in the tissues, exemplified by Langerhans' cells in epithelial and mucosal surfaces, are immature DCs specialised for antigen capture by phagocytosis or pinocytosis. HIV can enter into immature DCs but undergoes only limited replication until the DCs come into contact with T-cells in lymphoid tissue[91]. However, there is an additional mechanism which HIV-1 may be able to exploit in the form of a unique lectin called DC-SIGN, which binds to the envelope of HIV-1 with high affinity[92]. When bound to DC-SIGN, the virus can remain viable outside the cell for several days. In this way, the virus could be safely transported to the T-cell rich areas of the lymph nodes, where DC-SIGN is thought to play an important role in activating the responding T-cell population. Since HIV-1 replicates preferentially in activated T-cells, this would provide the virus with a pool of highly susceptible target cells and allow the infection to become established in lymphoid tissue. Although it is very plausible that HIV-1 could subvert the DC system in this way, it is not known how important a mechanism this constitutes *in vivo*.

Early reports describing the characteristics of virus isolated very early in primary HIV infection showed a remarkable degree of conservation in the envelope gene prior to seroconversion[93] suggesting that some degree of selection for HIV envelopes with characteristics particularly suited to transmission was taking place. The viral phenotype early in infection was described as uniformly macrophage-tropic and non-syncitium-inducing[94], which we now understand to be characteristics of CCR5-using isolates. The reasons why CCR5 usage is required for virus strains to establish primary infection are not entirely understood, but are thought to be related to co-receptor expression on the primary cellular targets of HIV infection, such as CD4+ T-cells, DCs and macrophages. It has been generally thought that infection takes place with just a single (often minor) variant from the infected contact[94], but this derives predominantly from studies in infected men. When similar studies were carried out in Kenyan women, it became clear that the picture was very different. Shortly after infection, these women were shown to be infected by several distinct strains, the first striking demonstration of a gender-based difference in the biology of HIV infection[95].

Clinical presentation of primary HIV-1 infection

The clinical syndrome of acute HIV-1 infection was first described 16 years ago as an illness resembling infectious mononucleosis[96]. However, not all patients with primary HIV-1 infection present with this typical clinical picture. One cohort study of the clinical features of acute HIV-1 disease demonstrated that only a minority of patients presented with 'typical' mononucleosis-like symptoms[97]. It is estimated that up to 87% of people undergoing acute HIV infection experience recognisable symptoms[98], but this could be an overestimate given that this study was carried out in a clinic in which subjects at risk of contracting HIV infection were followed prospectively. Indeed, only 25% of persons in the same cohort received diagnosis of primary HIV infection at their first clinic visit.

Clinical symptoms usually present within days or weeks after primary HIV infection[99], and may last from a few days up to 10 weeks, although in general the duration is less than 14 days. The most common symptom is fever[98,100,101], which is reported by nearly three-quarters of seroconverting subjects[100,101]. Other non-specific symptoms commonly reported include fatigue, headache, myalgia, lymphadenopathy and cutaneous rash[100]. The last symptom may be particularly suggestive of primary HIV infection: a maculo-papular skin rash, usually involving the trunk, is found in 40–80% of persons with symptomatic HIV-1 infection. Symptoms may differ in different clinical settings. Although there is a high degree of consistency in Western clinics[102], a carefully-conducted study looking prospectively at signs and symptoms during HIV-1 seroconversion in Kenyan female commercial sex workers reported a quite distinct range of clinical signs and symptoms from those reported in Caucasians (see Table 2)[101]. Another study in India showed that 81% of patients attending an STD clinic with primary HIV infection had at least one of these eight symptoms: fever, adenopathy, joint pain, thrush, pharyngitis, rash, diarrhoea, and paraesthesia[103].

There is some debate about the prognostic significance of severe clinical manifestations of primary HIV-1 infection. A number of studies have

Table 2 Comparison of clinical presentations from two large seroconverter cohorts

Signs and symptoms	Frequencies (% patients) Lavreys et al[101] (Kenya)	Frequencies (% patients) Vanhems et al[100] (USA, Switzerland, Australia)
Fever	53.4*	77.1
Headache	43.7*	50.9
Fatigue	26.2	65.6
Arthralgia	24.3	30.7
Myalgia	18.4*	54.6
Vomiting	18.4*	12.4
Diarrhoea	16.5*	22.9
Cutaneous rash	8.7	56.4
Inguinal lymphadenopathy	2.9*	20.2
Oral thrush/candidiasis	0	17

*$P < 0.001$.

suggested that a more severe illness, particularly with a mononucleosis-like syndrome, may predict more rapid disease progression subsequently[104,105].

The non-specific symptoms of acute HIV infection make it difficult to determine the true frequency of symptomatic illness. This presents a major challenge to healthcare providers, and underscores the need to obtain an accurate history of exposure. Some investigators have proposed criteria to assist in the clinical diagnosis of primary HIV-1 infection by developing a scoring system[101]. Algorithms to aid clinical diagnosis in this way should help in the selection of patients who warrant further laboratory investigations to confirm or exclude HIV infection, especially in developing countries where sophisticated diagnostic tests are not readily affordable.

In industrialised countries, laboratory tests help to confirm the diagnosis of acute HIV infection. Conventional serological testing is often negative for a window period of approximately 22–27 days after the initial infection[106]. Detection of either plasma or serum p24 antigen is normally recommended for diagnosis for acute HIV infection and for screening of blood donors who may unintentionally donate contaminated blood if tested by serology during the window period. Rarely, the p24 antigen assays may give false-negative results[107]. In this prospective cohort study, the sensitivity and specificity of p24 antigen detection assays were estimated to be 88.7% and 100%, respectively. Interestingly, the false-negative results from these patients were not because the HIV RNA viral load was low: the mean level of HIV RNA in 5 patients who had primary HIV infection but undetectable p24 antigen was 251,189 copies/ml (range 100,000–630,957 copies/ml). On the other hand, the detection of HIV RNA by viral load assays, which gives a sensitivity of 100% and specificity of 97.4%, may be a more prudent screening method to detect primary HIV infection. This method has also proved to be cost-effective in screening pooled serum or plasma from blood donors[108]. Suspected cases should then be confirmed by p24 antigen detection, which is more specific. However, HIV RNA assays are relatively time-consuming, expensive and need sophisticated technology, which pose significant problems for non-industrialised countries.

Immunopathological events in primary HIV-1 infection

Once infection with HIV-1 has become established in the lymphoid tissues, there is extensive virus replication, which is soon reflected in very high levels of plasma viraemia[109]. The peak viraemia occurs an average of 6–15 days after the onset of symptoms[110], with viral load levels of 1–10 million/copies/ml[111], at which time the donor is probably highly infectious[33]. During this period, extensive viral seeding takes place, so that the virus disseminates widely through lymphoid and other tissues[112]. In lymphoid tissue, the virus particles can become trapped in the follicular dendritic cell (FDC) network[113], so that during the asymptomatic period, the viral burden is much higher in the lymph nodes than in the blood. The very high levels of plasma viraemia are generally short-lived[109,110], suggesting that the host is able to generate an immune response which controls viral replication. Over the next few weeks, the plasma virus load falls by several orders of magnitude, although antibodies with the capacity to neutralise the virus are rarely detected at this stage[114,115]. It is thought that the cellular immune response is largely responsible for the early control of HIV replication[116]. There is a profound CD8+ T-cell lymphocytosis, with massive oligoclonal expansions (representing up to 40% of all T cells), which express activation markers like CD38, CD27 and HLA-DR but are CD28 negative[117]. In culture these CD8+ CD28- cells are primed for apoptosis[118], and are thought to represent terminally differentiated effector cytotoxic T lymphocytes (CTL)[119]. Virus-specific CTL have been described as early as 2 days after clinical presentation, and can generally be detected within weeks of the onset of symptoms[115,120,121]. Using soluble class I HLA-B27 molecules assembled with HIV peptides as 'tetramers', it could be shown that as many as 5% of circulating CD8+ T-cells were specific for a single HIV gag epitope[122]: using other tetramers we have seen responses as high as 10% of CD8+ T-cells in patients undergoing primary HIV-1 infection (unpublished observations). Studies of the T-cell receptor (TCR) repertoire in primary HIV infection have shown that the CD8+ response is represented by large but transient oligoclonal expansions in many patients[119].

In some studies, a few donors failed to make a detectable CTL response, and these patients exhibited a rapidly progressive course of HIV infection without control of virus levels[115,120], suggesting that the early generation of a vigorous HIV-specific CTL response may not only be responsible for the initial control of viraemia but also influence the subsequent disease course. In one study, a high frequency of envelope-specific CTL during acute HIV infection was associated with a significantly lower HIV-1 viral load subsequently[123]. A particularly narrow repertoire of CD8+ expansions is also associated with a poor prognosis[124]: this implies that a relatively limited CD8+ response could facilitate viral escape from the immune system or lead to more rapid immune exhaustion[119,125]. The selection of virus variants that have acquired changes in the epitopes recognised by the dominant acute CTL response, sufficient to abrogate CTL recognition, is now well-described in both acutely infected people[126,127] and monkeys infected with cloned SIV[128]: this may contribute to the ultimate failure of the immune response to contain viral replication in HIV-1 infection.

During primary infection, the CD4 count falls, and occasionally it may be sufficiently depressed to allow the development of opportunistic infections[129,130]. The initial loss of CD4+ T-cells is mainly concentrated in the CCR5 negative subset[131]. CD4+ T cell function is also markedly abnormal[132]. Even though the CD4+ count may rebound with the resolution of primary infection, it rarely returns to baseline. It is then relatively stable during the asymptomatic period, but in untreated HIV infection shows an abrupt decline late in disease, shortly before the onset of symptoms. CD4+ T-cell function remains abnormal throughout the course of HIV infection[133–135]. Qualitative loss of CD4+ T-cell help, first to HIV antigens and then to other recall antigens, is perhaps the most characteristic abnormality detected throughout HIV infection[69,135,136]. The deletion of HIV-specific helper responses seems most likely to occur early in primary HIV infection, when presumably CD4+ T-cells responding to HIV antigens are not only highly activated but also localised to sites of HIV replication, making them prime targets for HIV infection. Following the initial reduction of viraemia, a viral 'set-point' is established at around 12–18 months after infection, the level of which is closely related to the ultimate clinical outcome in HIV disease[137].

Treatment of primary HIV-1 infection

With increasing early diagnosis of primary HIV-1 infection, it has become possible recently to investigate the effect of prompt institution of anti-retroviral therapy. The early reports have been encouraging, with data to show that patients treated very early in infection can recover or retain HIV-specific CD4+ T-cell responses whilst maintaining an effective CD8+ T-cell response[136,138]. Other investigators have raised concerns that if therapy is initiated too early then the immune system does not generate a full response to HIV antigens[139,140]. One promising strategy to counteract these concerns is to allow carefully controlled viral replication using supervised treatment interruptions following initial aggressive therapy: early reports suggest that patients treated in this way develop a broader HIV-specific CTL response and may be able to control viral load without therapy[141].

Key points for clinical practice

- The likelihood of HIV-1 transmission is generally predicted by plasma viral load, but can still occur from people with good viral suppression on therapy.
- Genital ulcer disease is a potent co-factor for HIV-1 transmission
- Antibody tests may be negative for several weeks after primary infection: the best method of diagnosis of acute HIV infection is plasma RNA combined with a p24 antigen test

- Early treatment of primary HIV-1 infection with anti-retroviral therapy appears to provide the best hope of preserving immune function in infected people

Acknowledgements

The authors acknowledge the support of the Medical Research Council and the Elizabeth Glaser Paediatric AIDS Foundation. SR-J is an Elizabeth Glaser Scientist of the Paediatric AIDS Foundation.

References

1 Padian NS, Shiboski SC, Glass SO, Vittinghoff E. Heterosexual transmission of human immunodeficiency virus (HIV) in northern California: results from a ten-year study. *Am J Epidemiol* 1997; **146**: 350–7
2 Caceres CF, van Griensven GJ. Male homosexual transmission of HIV-1. *AIDS* 1994; **8**: 1051–61
3 Datta P, Embree JE, Kreiss J *et al*. Mother-to-child transmission of HIV-1 : report from the Nairobi study. *J Infect Dis* 1994; **170**: 1134–40
4 Nduati R. Breastfeeding and HIV-1 infection. A review of current literature. *Adv Exp Med Biol* 2000; **478**: 201–10
5 Baba TW, Jeong YS, Pennick D, Bronson R, Greene MF, Ruprecht RM. Pathogenicity of live, attenuated SIV after mucosal infection of neonatal macaques. *Science* 1995; **267**: 1820–5
6 Stahl-Hennig C, Steinman RM, Tenner-Racz K *et al*. Rapid infection of oral mucosal-associated lymphoid tissue with simian immunodeficiency virus. *Science* 1999; **285**: 1261–5
7 Gershon RR, Vlahov D, Nelson KE. The risk of transmission of HIV-1 through non-percutaneous, non-sexual modes – a review. *AIDS* 1990; **4**: 645–50
8 Fitzgibbon JE, Gaur S, Frenkel LD, Laraque F, Edlin BR, Dubin DT. Transmission from one child to another of human immunodeficiency virus type 1 with a zidovudine-resistance mutation. *N Engl J Med* 1993; **329**: 1835–41
9 Belec L, Si Mohamed A, Muller-Trutwin MC *et al*. Genetically related human immunodeficiency virus type 1 in three adults of a family with no identified risk factor for intrafamilial transmission. *J Virol* 1998; **72**: 5831–9
10 Schreiber GB, Busch MP, Kleinman SH, Korelitz JJ. The risk of transfusion-transmitted viral infections. The Retrovirus Epidemiology Donor Study. *N Engl J Med* 1996; **334**: 1685–90
11 Cardo DM, Culver DH, Ciesielski CA *et al*. A case-control study of HIV seroconversion in health care workers after percutaneous exposure. Centers for Disease Control and Prevention Needlestick Surveillance Group. *N Engl J Med* 1997; **337**: 1485–90
12 Peterman TA, Stoneburner RL, Allen JR, Jaffe HW, Curran JW. Risk of human immunodeficiency virus transmission from heterosexual adults with transfusion-associated infections. *JAMA* 1988; **259**: 55–8
13 Wiley JA, Herschkorn SJ, Padian NS. Heterogeneity in the probability of HIV transmission per sexual contact: the case of male-to-female transmission in penile-vaginal intercourse. *Stat Med* 1989; **8**: 93–102
14 Padian N, Marquis L, Francis DP *et al*. Male-to-female transmission of human immunodeficiency virus. *JAMA* 1987; **258**: 788–90
15 Fischl MA, Dickinson GM, Scott GB, Klimas N, Fletcher MA, Parks W. Evaluation of heterosexual partners, children, and household contacts of adults with AIDS. *JAMA* 1987; **257**: 640–4
16 Downs AM, De Vincenzi I. Probability of heterosexual transmission of HIV: relationship to the number of unprotected sexual contacts. European Study Group in Heterosexual Transmission of HIV. *J Acquir Immune Defic Syndr Hum Retrovirol* 1996; **11**: 388–95

17 Duerr A, Nagachinta T, Tovanabutra S, Tansuhaj AKN. Probability of male-to-female HIV transmission among married couples in Chiang Mai, Thailand. *Tenth International Conference on AIDS*, Yokohama, Japan 1994; Abstract 105C

18 Mastro TD, Satten GA, Nopkesorn T, Sangkharomya S, Longini IM. Probability of female-to-male transmission of HIV-1 in Thailand. *Lancet* 1994; **343**: 204–7

19 Satten GA, Mastro TD, Longini IM. Modelling the female-to-male per-act HIV transmission probability in an emerging epidemic in Asia. *Stat Med* 1994; **13**: 2097–106

20 Cameron DW, Simonsen JN, D'Costa LJ *et al*. Female to male transmission of human immunodeficiency virus type 1: risk factors for seroconversion in men. *Lancet* 1989; **ii**: 403–7

21 DeGruttola V, Seage 3rd GR, Mayer KH, Horsburgh Jr CR. Infectiousness of HIV between male homosexual partners. *J Clin Epidemiol* 1989; **42**: 849–56

22 Shaffer N, Chuachoowong R, Mock PA *et al*. Short-course zidovudine for perinatal HIV-1 transmission in Bangkok, Thailand: a randomised controlled trial. Bangkok Collaborative Perinatal HIV Transmission Study Group. *Lancet* 1999; **353**: 773–80

23 Wiktor SZ, Ekpini E, Karon JM *et al*. Short-course oral zidovudine for prevention of mother-to-child transmission of HIV-1 in Abidjan, Cote d'Ivoire: a randomised trial. *Lancet* 1999; **353**: 781–5

24 The International Perinatal HIV Group. The mode of delivery and the risk of vertical transmission of human immunodeficiency virus type 1 – a meta-analysis of 15 prospective cohort studies. *N Engl J Med* 1999; **340**: 977–87

25 Nduati R, John G, Mbori-Ngacha D *et al*. Effect of breastfeeding and formula feeding on transmission of HIV-1: a randomized clinical trial. *JAMA* 2000; **283**: 1167–74

26 Pungpapong S, Phanuphak P, Pungpapong K, Ruxrungtham K. The risk of occupational HIV exposure among Thai healthcare workers. *Southeast Asian J Trop Med Public Health* 1999; **30**: 496–503

27 de Graaf R, Houweling H, van Zessen G. Occupational risk of HIV infection among western health care professionals posted in AIDS endemic areas. *AIDS Care* 1998; **10**: 441–52

28 Gumodoka B, Favot I, Berege ZA, Dolmans WM. Occupational exposure to the risk of HIV infection among health care workers in Mwanza Region, United Republic of Tanzania. *Bull World Health Organ* 1997; **75**: 133–40

29 Cohen ND, Munoz A, Reitz BA *et al*. Transmission of retroviruses by transfusion of screened blood in patients undergoing cardiac surgery. *N Engl J Med* 1989; **320**: 1172–6

30 Gerst PH, Fildes JJ, Rosario PG, Schorr JB. Risks of human immunodeficiency virus infection to patients and healthcare personnel. *Crit Care Med* 1990; **18**: 1440–8

31 Lackritz EM. Prevention of HIV transmission by blood transfusion in the developing world: achievements and continuing challenges. *AIDS* 1998; **12**: S81–6

32 Matz B, Kupfer B, Ko Y *et al*. HIV-1 infection by artificial insemination. *Lancet* 1998; **351**: 728

33 Quinn TC, Wawer MJ, Sewankambo N *et al*. Viral load and heterosexual transmission of human immunodeficiency virus type 1. Rakai Project Study Group. *N Engl J Med* 2000; **342**: 921–9

34 John GC, Nduati RW, Mbori-Ngacha D *et al*. Genital shedding of human immunodeficiency virus type 1 DNA during pregnancy: association with immunosuppression, abnormal cervical or vaginal discharge, and severe vitamin A deficiency. *J Infect Dis* 1997; **175**: 57–62

35 Mostad SB, Jackson S, Overbaugh J *et al*. Cervical and vaginal shedding of human immunodeficiency virus type 1- infected cells throughout the menstrual cycle. *J Infect Dis* 1998; **178**: 983–91

36 Zhang H, Dornadula G, Beumont M *et al*. Human immunodeficiency virus type 1 in the semen of men receiving highly active antiretroviral therapy. *N Engl J Med* 1998; **339**: 1803–9

37 John GC, Rousseau C, Dong T *et al*. Maternal SDF1 3'A polymorphism is associated with increased perinatal human immunodeficiency virus type 1 transmission [In Process Citation]. *J Virol* 2000; **74**: 5736–9

38 Vernazza PL, Eron JJ, Fiscus SA, Cohen MS. Sexual transmission of HIV: infectiousness and prevention. *AIDS* 1999; **13**: 155–66

39 Soto-Ramirez LE, Renjifo B, McLane MF *et al*. HIV-1 Langerhans' cell tropism associated with heterosexual transmission of HIV [see comments]. *Science* 1996; **271**: 1291–3

40 Pope M, Frankel SS, Mascola JR *et al*. Human immunodeficiency virus type 1 strains of subtypes B and E replicate in cutaneous dendritic cell-T-cell mixtures without displaying

subtype-specific tropism. *J Virol* 1997; **71**: 8001–7

41 Whittle HC, Ariyoshi K, Rowland-Jones S. HIV-2 and T cell recognition. *Curr Opin Immunol* 1998; **10**: 382–7

42 Simonsen JN, Plummer FA, Ngugi EN *et al.* HIV infection among lower socioeconomic strata prostitutes in Nairobi. *AIDS* 1990; **4**: 139–44

43 Hayes RJ, Schulz KF, Plummer FA. The cofactor effect of genital ulcers on the per-exposure risk of HIV transmission in sub-Saharan Africa. *J Trop Med Hyg* 1995; **98**: 1–8

44 Halperin DT, Bailey RC. Male circumcision and HIV infection: 10 years and counting. *Lancet* 1999; **354**: 1813–5

45 Hussain LA, Lehner T. Comparative investigation of Langerhans' cells and potential receptors for HIV in oral, genitourinary and rectal epithelia. *Immunology* 1995; **85**: 475–84

46 Marx PA, Spira AI, Gettie A *et al.* Progesterone implants enhance SIV vaginal transmission and early virus load. *Nat Med* 1996; **2**: 1084–9

47 Smith SM, Baskin GB, Marx PA. Estrogen protects against vaginal transmission of simian immunodeficiency virus. *J Infect Dis* 2000; **182**: 708–15

48 Martin HL, Nyange PM, Richardson BA *et al.* Hormonal contraception, sexually transmitted diseases, and risk of heterosexual transmission of human immunodeficiency virus type 1. *J Infect Dis* 1998; **178**: 1053–9

49 Liu R, Paxton WA, Choe S *et al.* Homozygous defect in HIV-1 coreceptor accounts for resistance of some multiply-exposed individuals to HIV-1 infection. *Cell* 1996; **88**: 7–20

50 Samson M, Libert F, Doranz BJ *et al.* Resistance to HIV-1 infection in Caucasian individuals bearing mutant alleles of the CCR-5 chemokine receptor gene. *Nature* 1996; **382**: 722–5

51 O'Brien T, Winkler C, Dean M *et al.* HIV-1 infection in a man homozygous for CCR5Δ32. *Lancet* 1997; **349**: 1219

52 Biti R, French R, Young J, Bennetts B, Stewart G. HIV-1 infection in an individual homozygous for the CCR5 deletion allele. *Nat Med* 1997; **3**: 252–3

53 Balotta C, Bagnarelli P, Violin M *et al.* Homozygous delta 32 deletion of the CCR-5 chemokine receptor gene in an HIV-1-infected patient. *AIDS* 1997; **11**: F67–F71

54 Martinson JJ, Chapman NH, Rees DC, Liu Y-T, Clegg JB. Global distribution of the CCR5 gene 32 base-pair deletion. *Nat Genet* 1997; **16**: 100–3

55 Wu L, Paxton WA, Kassam N *et al.* CCR5 levels and expression pattern correlate with infectability by macrophage-tropic HIV-1 *in vitro*. *J Exp Med* 1997; **185**: 1681–92

56 Cocchi F, DeVico AL, Garzino DA, Arya SK, Gallo RC, Lusso P. Identification of RANTES, MIP-1 alpha, and MIP-1 beta as the major HIV-suppressive factors produced by CD8+ T cells. *Science* 1995; **270**: 1811–5

57 Paxton WA, Liu R, Kang S *et al.* Reduced HIV-1 infectability of CD4+ lymphocytes from exposed-uninfected individuals: association with low expression of CCR5 and high production of beta-chemokines. *Virology* 1998; **244**: 66–73

58 Quillent C, Oberlin E, Braun J *et al.* HIV-1-resistance phenotype conferred by combination of two separate inherited mutations of CCR5 gene. *Lancet* 1997; **351**: 14–8

59 Kostrikis LG, Neumann AU, Thomson B *et al.* A polymorphism in the regulatory region of the CC-chemokine receptor 5 gene influences perinatal transmission of human immunodeficiency virus type 1 to African-American infants. *J Virol* 1999; **73**: 10264–71

60 McDermott DH, Zimmerman PA, Guignard F, Kleeberger CA, Leitman SF, Murphy PM. CCR5 promoter polymorphism and HIV-1 disease progression. Multicenter AIDS Cohort Study (MACS). *Lancet* 1998; **352**: 866–70

61 MacDonald KS, Fowke KR, Kimani J *et al.* Influence of HLA supertypes on susceptibility and resistance to human immunodeficiency virus type 1 infection. *J Infect Dis* 2000; **181**: 1581–9

62 Winchester R, Chen Y, Rose S, Selby J, Borkowsky W. Major histocompatibility complex class II DR alleles DRB1*1501 and those encoding HLA-DR13 are preferentially associated with a diminution in maternally transmitted human immunodeficiency virus 1 infection in different ethnic groups: determination by an automated sequence-based typing method. *Proc Natl Acad Sci USA* 1995; **92**: 12374–8

63 Detels R, Mann D, Carrington M *et al.* Resistance to HIV-1 may be genetically mediated. *AIDS* 1996; **10**: 102–4

64 Ali S, Niang MA, N'Doye I et al. Secretor polymorphism and human immunodeficiency virus infection in Senegalese women. J Infect Dis 2000; 181: 737–9

65 Garred P, Madsen HO, Balslev U et al. Susceptibility to HIV infection and progression of AIDS in relation to variant alleles of mannose-binding lectin. Lancet 1997; 349: 236–40

66 Zhang C, Cui Y, Houston S, Chang LJ. Protective immunity to HIV-1 in SCID/beige mice reconstituted with peripheral blood lymphocytes of exposed but uninfected individuals. Proc Natl Acad Sci USA 1996; 93: 14720–5

67 Kaul R, Rowland-Jones SL. Methods of detection of HIV-specific CTL and their role in protection against HIV infection. In: Korber B, Brander C, Haynes BF et al. (eds) HIV Molecular Immunology Database. Los Alamos, NM: Los Alamos National Laboratory, Theoretical Biology and Biophysics, 1999; IV-35–44

68 Goh WC, Markee J, Akridge RE et al. Protection against human immunodeficiency virus type 1 infection in persons with repeated exposure: evidence for T cell immunity in the absence of inherited CCR5 coreceptor defects. J Infect Dis 1999; 179: 548–57

69 Clerici M, Shearer G. A Th1-> Th2 switch is a critical step in the aetiology of HIV infection. Immunol Today 1993; 14: 107–11

70 Clerici M, Sison AV, Berzofsky JA et al. Cellular immune factors associated with mother-to-infant transmission of HIV. AIDS 1993; 7: 1427–33

71 Clerici M, Levin JM, Kessler HA et al. HIV-specific T-helper activity in seronegative health care workers exposed to contaminated blood. JAMA 1994; 271: 42–6

72 Beretta A, Furci L, Burastero S et al. HIV-1-specific immunity in persistently seronegative individuals at high risk for HIV infection. Immunol Lett 1996; 51: 39–43

73 Furci L, Scarlatti G, Burastero S et al. Antigen-driven C-C chemokine-mediated HIV-1 suppression by CD4(+) T cells from exposed uninfected individuals expressing the wild-type CCR-5 allele. J Exp Med 1997; 186: 455–60

74 Wasik TJ, Bratosiewicz J, Wierzbicki A et al. Protective role of beta-chemokines associated with HIV-specific Th responses against perinatal HIV transmission. J Immunol 1999; 162: 4355–64

75 Kaul R, Plummer FA, Kimani J et al. HIV-1-specific mucosal CD8+ lymphocyte responses in the cervix of HIV-1-resistant prostitutes in Nairobi. J Immunol 2000; 164: 1602–11

76 Cheynier R, Langlade-Demoyen P, Marescot M-R et al. Cytotoxic T lymphocyte responses in the peripheral blood of children born to HIV-1-infected mothers. Eur J Immunol 1992; 22: 2211–7

77 Rowland-Jones SL, Nixon DF, Aldhous MC et al. HIV-specific CTL activity in an HIV-exposed but uninfected infant. Lancet 1993; 341: 860–1

78 Aldhous MC, Watret KC, Mok JY, Bird AG, Froebel KS. Cytotoxic T lymphocyte activity and CD8 subpopulations in children at risk of HIV infection. Clin Exp Immunol 1994; 97: 61–7

79 De Maria A, Cirillo C, Moretta L. Occurrence of HIV-specific CTL activity in apparently uninfected children born to HIV-1-infected mothers. J Infect Dis 1994; 170: 1296–9

80 Pinto LA, Sullivan J, Berzofsky JA et al. ENV-specific cytotoxic T lymphocyte responses in HIV seronegative health care workers occupationally exposed to HIV-contaminated body fluids. J Clin Invest 1995; 96: 867–76

81 Pinto LA, Covas MJ, Victorino RM. T-helper cross reactivity to viral recombinant proteins in HIV-2-infected patients [Published erratum appears in AIDS 1993; 7: following 1541]. AIDS 1993; 7: 1389–91

82 Langlade-Demoyen P, Ngo-Giang-Huong N, Ferchal F, Oksenhendler E. HIV nef-specific cytotoxic T lymphocytes in noninfected heterosexual contact of HIV-infected patients. J Clin Invest 1994; 93: 1293–7

83 Mazzoli S, Trabbatoni D, Lo Caputo S et al. HIV-specific mucosal and cellular immunity in HIV-seronegative partners of HIV-seropositive individuals. Nat Med 1997; 3: 1250–7

84 Bernard NF, Yannakis CM, Lee JS, Tsoukas CM. Human immunodeficiency virus (HIV)-specific cytotoxic T lymphocyte activity in HIV-exposed seronegative persons. J Infect Dis 1999; 179: 538–47

85 Bienzle D, MacDonald KS, Smaill FM et al. Factors contributing to the lack of human immunodeficiency virus type 1 (HIV-1) transmission in HIV-1-discordant partners [In Process Citation]. J Infect Dis 2000; 182: 123–32

86 Rowland-Jones SL, Sutton J, Ariyoshi K et al. HIV-specific cytotoxic T cells in HIV-exposed but uninfected Gambian women. Nat Med 1995; 1: 59–64

87 Rowland-Jones SL, Dong T, Fowke KR *et al.* Cytotoxic T cell responses to multiple conserved HIV epitopes in HIV-resistant prostitutes in Nairobi. *J Clin Invest* 1998; **102**: 1758–65

88 Hanke T, McMichael AJ. Design and construction of an experimental HIV-1 vaccine for a year 2000 clinical trial in Kenya. *Nat Med* 2000; **6**: 951–5

89 Zhang Z, Schuler T, Zupancic M *et al.* Sexual transmission and propagation of SIV and HIV in resting and activated CD4(+) T cells. *Science* 1999; **286**: 1353–7

90 Spira AI, Marx PA, Patterson BK *et al.* Cellular targets of infection and route of viral dissemination after an intravaginal inoculation of simian immunodeficiency virus into rhesus macaques. *J Exp Med* 1996; **183**: 215–25

91 Granelli-Piperno A, Finkel V, Delgado E, Steinman RM. Virus replication begins in dendritic cells during the transmission of HIV-1 from mature dendritic cells to T cells. *Curr Biol* 1999; **9**: 21–9

92 Giejtenbeek T, Kwon D, Torensma R *et al.* DC-SIGN, a dendritic cell-specific HIV-1-binding protein that enhances trans-infection of T-cells. *Cell* 2000; **100**: 587–97

93 Zhang LQ, MacKenzie P, Cleland A, Holmes EC, Leigh Brown AJ, Simmonds P. Selection for specific sequences in the external envelope protein of HIV-1 upon primary infection. *J Virol* 1993; **67**: 3345–56

94 Zhu T, Mo H, Wang N *et al.* Genotypic and phenotypic characterization of HIV-1 in patients with primary infection. *Science* 1993; **261**: 1179–81

95 Long EM, Martin Jr HL, Kreiss JK *et al.* Gender differences in HIV-1 diversity at time of infection. *Nat Med* 2000; **6**: 71–5

96 Cooper D, Gold J, Maclean P *et al.* Acute AIDS retrovirus infection. Definition of a clinical illness associated with seroconversion. *Lancet* 1985; **i**: 537–40

97 Vanhems P, Allard R, Cooper DA *et al.* Acute human immunodeficiency virus type 1 disease as a mononucleosis-like illness: is the diagnosis too restrictive? *Clin Infect Dis* 1997; **24**: 965–70

98 Schacker T, Collier AC, Hughes J, Shea T, Corey L. Clinical and epidemiological features of primary HIV infection. *Ann Intern Med* 1996; **125**: 257–64

99 Kahn JO, Walker BD. Acute human immunodeficiency virus type 1 infection. *N Engl J Med* 1998; **339**: 33–9

100 Vanhems P, Dassa C, Lambert J, *et al.* Comprehensive classification of symptoms and signs reported among 218 patients with acute HIV-1 infection. *J Acquir Immune Defic Syndr* 1999; **21**: 99–106

101 Lavreys L, Thompson ML, Martin Jr HL *et al.* Primary human immunodeficiency virus type 1 infection: clinical manifestations among women in Mombasa, Kenya. *Clin Infect Dis* 2000; **30**: 486–90

102 Vanhems P, Hughes J, Collier AC *et al.* Comparison of clinical features, CD4 and CD8 responses among patients with acute HIV-1 infection from Geneva, Seattle and Sydney. *AIDS* 2000; **14**: 375–81

103 Bollinger RC, Brookmeyer RS, Mehendale SM *et al.* Risk factors and clinical presentation of acute primary HIV infection in India. *JAMA* 1997; **278**: 2085–9

104 Pedersen C, Lindhardt BO, Jensen BL *et al.* Clinical course of primary HIV infection: consequences for subsequent course of infection. *BMJ* 1989; **299**: 154–7

105 Lindback S, Brostrom C, Karlssom A, Gaines H. Does symptomatic primary HIV-1 infection accelerate progression to CDC stage IV disease, CD4 count below 200 x 10⁶/ml, AIDS, and death from AIDS? *BMJ* 1994; **309**: 1535–7

106 Busch MP, Lee LL, Satten GA *et al.* Time course of detection of viral and serologic markers preceding human immunodeficiency virus type 1 seroconversion: implications for screening of blood and tissue donors. *Transfusion* 1995; **35**: 91–7

107 Daar ES, Little S, Pitt J *et al.* Diagnosis of primary HIV-1 infection. Los Angeles County Primary HIV Infection Recruitment Network. *Ann Intern Med* 2001; **134**: 25–9

108 Roth WK, Weber M, Seifried E. Feasibility and efficacy of routine PCR screening of blood donations for hepatitis C virus, hepatitis B virus, and HIV-1 in a blood-bank setting. *Lancet* 1999; **353**: 359–63

109 Daar ES, Moudgil T, Meyer RD, Ho DD. Transient high levels of viremia in patients with primary human immunodeficiency virus type 1 infection. *N Engl J Med* 1991; **324**: 961–4

110 Clark SJ, Saag MS, Decker WD *et al.* High titers of cytopathic virus in plasma of patients with symptomatic primary HIV-1 infection. *N Engl J Med* 1991; **324**: 954–60

111 Piatak M, Saag M, Yang L. High levels of HIV-1 in plasma during all stages of infection determined by competitive PCR. *Science* 1993; **259**: 1749–54

112 Pantaleo G, Graziosi C, Demarest JF *et al*. HIV infection is active and progressive in lymphoid tissue during the clinically latent stage of disease. *Nature* 1993; **362**: 355–8

113 Spiegel H, Herbst H, Niedobitek G, Foss HD, Stein H. Follicular dendritic cells are a major reservoir for human immunodeficiency virus type 1 in lymphoid tissues facilitating infection of CD4+ T-helper cells. *Am J Pathol* 1992; **140**: 15–22

114 Ariyoshi K, Harwood E, Chiengsong-Popov R, Weber J. Is clearance of HIV-1 viraemia at seroconversion mediated by neutralising antibodies ? *Lancet* 1992; **340**: 1257–8

115 Koup RA, Safrit JT, Cao Y *et al*. Temporal association of cellular immune responses with the initial control of viremia in primary human immunodeficiency virus type 1 syndrome. *J Virol* 1994; **68**: 4650–5

116 Koup RA, Ho DD. Shutting down HIV. *Nature* 1994; **370**: 416

117 Roos M, De Leeuw N, Claessen F *et al*. Viro-immunological studies in acute HIV-1 infection. *AIDS* 1994; **8**: 1533–8

118 Brugnoni D, Prati E, Malacarne F, Gorla R, Airo P, Cattaneo R. The primary response to HIV infection is characterised by an expansion of activated CD8+ CD28-cells. *AIDS* 1996; **10**: 104–6

119 Pantaleo G, Demarest JF, Soudeyns H *et al*. Major expansion of CD8+ T cells with a predominant Vb usage during the primary immune response to HIV. *Nature* 1994; **370**: 463–7

120 Borrow P, Lewicki H, Hahn BH, Shaw GM, Oldstone MB. Virus-specific CD8+ cytotoxic T-lymphocyte activity associated with control of viremia in primary human immunodeficiency virus type 1 infection. *J Virol* 1994; **68**: 6103–10

121 Lamhamedi-Cherradi S, Culmann-Penciolelli B, Guy B *et al*. Different patterns of HIV-1-specific cytotoxic T-lymphocyte activity after primary infection. *AIDS* 1995; **9**: 421–6

122 Wilson JD, Ogg GS, Allen RL *et al*. Direct visualization of HIV-1-specific cytotoxic T lymphocytes during primary infection. *AIDS* 2000; **14**: 225–33

123 Musey L, Hughes J, Schacker T, Shea T, Corey L, McElrath MJ. Cytotoxic-T-cell responses, viral load, and disease progression in early human immunodeficiency virus type 1 infection. *N Engl J Med* 1997; **337**: 1267–74

124 Pantaleo G, Demarest JF, Schacker T *et al*. The qualitative nature of the primary immune response to HIV infection is a prognosticator of disease progression independent of the initial level of plasma viremia. *Proc Natl Acad Sci USA* 1997; **94**: 254–8

125 Safrit JT, Koup RA. The immunology of primary HIV infection: which immune responses control HIV replication? *Curr Opin Immunol* 1995; **7**: 456–61

126 Price DA, Goulder PJ, Klenerman P *et al*. Positive selection of HIV-1 cytotoxic T lymphocyte escape variants during primary infection. *Proc Natl Acad Sci USA* 1997; **94**: 1890–5

127 Kelleher AD, Long C, Holmes EC *et al*. Clustered mutations in HIV-1 gag are consistently required for escape from HLA-B27-restricted cytotoxic T lymphocyte responses. *J Exp Med* 2001; **193**: 375–86

128 Allen TM, O'Connor DH, Jing P, *et al*. Tat-specific cytotoxic T lymphocytes select for SIV escape variants during resolution of primary viraemia. *Nature* 2000; **407**: 386–90

129 Gupta KK. Acute immunosuppression with HIV seroconversion. *N Engl J Med* 1993; **328**: 228–9

130 Vento S, Di PG, Garofano T, Concia E, Bassetti D. *Pneumocystis carinii* pneumonia during primary HIV-1 infection. *Lancet* 1993; **342**: 24–5

131 Zaunders JJ, Kaufmann GR, Cunningham PH *et al*. Increased turnover of CCR5+ and redistribution of CCR5- CD4 T lymphocytes during primary human immunodeficiency virus type 1 infection. *J Infect Dis* 2001; **183**: 736–43

132 Pedersen C, Dickmeiss E, Gaub J *et al*. T-cell subset alterations and lymphocyte responsiveness to mitogens and antigen during severe primary infection with HIV: a case series of seven consecutive HIV seroconverters. *AIDS* 1990; **4**: 523–6

133 Musey LK, Kreiger JN, Hughes JP, Schacker TW, Corey L, McElrath MJ. Early and persistent human immunodeficiency virus type 1 (HIV-1)-specific T helper dysfunction in blood and lymph nodes following acute HIV-1 infection. *J Infect Dis* 1999; **180**: 278–84

134 Gruters RA, Terpstra FG, De Goede RE *et al*. Immunological and virological markers in individuals progressing from seroconversion to AIDS. *AIDS* 1991; **5**: 837–44

135 Clerici M, Stocks NI, Zajac RA *et al*. Detection of three distinct patterns of T helper cell dysfunction in asymptomatic, human immunodeficiency virus-seropositive patients. Independence of CD4+ cell numbers and clinical staging. *J Clin Invest* 1989; **84**: 1892–9

136 Rosenberg ES, Billingsley JM, Caliendo A *et al*. Vigorous HIV-1-specific CD4+ T-cell responses associated with control of viraemia. *Science* 1997; **278**: 1447–50

137 Mellors JW, Kingsley LA, Rinaldo C *et al*. Quantitation of HIV-1 RNA in plasma predicts outcome after seroconversion. *Ann Intern Med* 1995; **122**: 573–79

138 Oxenius A, Price DA, Easterbrook PJ *et al*. Early highly active antiretroviral therapy for acute HIV-1 infection preserves immune function of CD8+ and CD4+ T lymphocytes. *Proc Natl Acad Sci USA* 2000; **97**: 3382–7

139 Levy JA. Caution: should we be treating HIV infection early? *Lancet* 1998; **352**: 982–3

140 Stranford SA, Ong JC, Martinez-Marino B *et al*. Reduction in CD8+ cell non-cytotoxic anti-HIV activity in individuals receiving highly active antiretroviral therapy during primary infection. *Proc Natl Acad Sci USA* 2001; **98**: 597–602

141 Rosenberg ES, Altfeld M, Poon SH *et al*. Immune control of HIV-1 after early treatment of acute infection. *Nature* 2000; **407**: 523–6

Interventions against sexually transmitted infections (STI) to prevent HIV infection

Philippe Mayaud and Duncan McCormick

London School of Hygiene and Tropical Medicine, London, UK

STIs have taken on a more important role with the advent of the HIV/AIDS epidemic, and there is good evidence that their control can reduce HIV transmission. The challenge is not just to develop new interventions, but to identify barriers to the effective implementation of existing tools, and to devise ways to overcome these barriers. This 'scaling-up' of effective strategies will require an international and a multisectoral approach. It will require the formation of new partnerships between the private and public sectors and between governments and the communities they represent.

Towards the end of the 15th century, a devastating epidemic of infectious syphilis swept Western Europe. Observers at that time quickly perceived the disease to be transmitted sexually, but this group of 'venereal diseases' was subsequently regarded as unproblematic until it was noted to be a severe problem among military personnel in the 19th and 20th centuries[1]. Interest in sexually transmitted infections (STIs) was further fuelled in the early 1980s by the advent of the HIV/AIDS epidemic and recognition of the role of STI in facilitating the sexual transmission of HIV[2]. Interest in STI control has reached a peak recently when it was shown that many interventions to control STIs can help reduce the spread of HIV. Furthermore, this can be achieved through the use of low technology in sustainable and cost-effective control programmes[3].

However, despite decades of control efforts, STIs still thrive today. There are problems in the effective implementation of control programmes because STIs are not just biological and medical problems, but also behavioural, social, political and economic problems – many facets that have not been adequately addressed in the past. This realisation is slowly translating into more comprehensive approaches to STI control involving several disciplines. Yet, there is growing evidence that the epidemiology of STIs and HIV is changing, and control efforts may be severely challenged once again.

Correspondence to:
Dr Philippe Mayaud,
Clinical Research Unit,
Department of Infectious
and Tropical Diseases,
London School of
Hygiene and Tropical
Medicine, Keppel Street,
London WC1E 7HT, UK

Public health importance of sexually transmitted infections

Sexually transmitted infections (STIs) constitute an important public health problem for the following reasons: (i) STIs are frequent with high prevalence and incidence; (ii) STIs can result in serious complications and sequelae; (iii) STIs have social and economic consequences; and (iv) a number of STIs have been identified as facilitating the spread of HIV.

Epidemiology of STIs

STIs are caused by over 30 pathogens, including bacteria, viruses, protozoal agents, fungal agents and ecto-parasites. The World Health Organization (WHO) estimates that approximately 340 million incident cases of the four main curable STIs (gonorrhoea, *Chlamydia* spp, syphilis and *Trichomonas vaginalis*) occur every year, with 85% in non-industrialised countries[4].

There are, however, substantial geographical variations in estimated prevalence and incidence. Sub-Saharan Africa, whilst accounting for 20% of the global STI estimates, has the highest prevalence and incidence rates. The overall yearly incidence rate of curable STIs in Africa is estimated at 254 per 1000 people in reproductive ages (15–49 years), but is only 77–91 per 1000 in industrialised countries[4]. The second highest rates are found in South and South-East Asia. This is not surprising given the large at-risk populations of young people in these countries, and – in the case of China – the recent opening of its borders to free trade, quickly followed by increases in prostitution and STI, which were once believed to have been controlled[5]. Similarly, in the early 1990s, major political and economic transitions took place in the Newly Independent States (NIS) of the former Soviet Union. Since that time, there have been unprecedented epidemics of syphilis and gonorrhoea with annual increases of 100–300%[6]. The reasons for the increase of STIs in many non-industrialised countries are multifactorial but relate to a great extent to the lack of access to effective and affordable STI services in many settings[7], or to the collapse of once relatively performant health systems in countries undergoing harsh economic and health reforms[6].

STIs impose an enormous burden of morbidity and mortality, both directly through their impact on reproductive and child health, and indirectly through their role in facilitating the sexual transmission of HIV infection. The greatest impact can be seen among women in whom severe complications include pelvic inflammatory disease, chronic pain, and adverse pregnancy outcomes (ectopic pregnancies, endometritis, spontaneous abortions, stillbirths and low birth weight). In both men and women, STIs play a major role in infertility. A growing number of malignancies are also attributed to STIs, notably cervical, anal and penile cancers as well as hepatocellular carcinoma. Congenital infections in the new-born include congenital syphilis, ophthalmia neonatorum and pneumonia.

The World Bank has estimated that STIs, excluding HIV, are the second commonest cause of healthy life years lost by women in the 15–44 year age group, responsible for some 17% of the total burden of disease in women of reproductive ages, outranked only by causes of maternal morbidity[8]. Yet it is only in recent years that STIs have been accorded any priority by national ministries of health or by the international community, mainly because of their potential interaction with HIV.

HIV–STI interactions

HIV and other STIs may interact with each other in the following ways (Fig. 1):

- HIV, by causing immunosuppression, can modify the natural history (duration), clinical presentation (severity), and response to treatment of certain STIs, notably other viral infections such as genital herpes simplex virus infection or human papillomavirus

- STIs, by causing ulceration or inflammation of the genital tract, may enhance the transmission of HIV by increasing infectiousness of HIV-positive individuals and/or the susceptibility of HIV-negative persons

Since the late 1980s, it had been noted that HIV-positive patients frequently gave a history of past STI or had serological evidence of past STI (*e.g.* increased prevalence of treponemal, chlamydial or herpes antibodies).

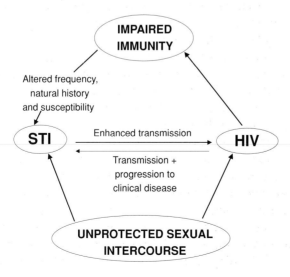

Fig. 1 Relationships between HIV and other STIs.

These studies suggested the existence of an 'epidemiological synergy' between HIV and other STIs[2]. However, one of the major hurdles in understanding this relationship was that HIV and other STIs share a common sexual transmissibility, driven by common sexual behaviours; thus, the observed association could be the result of a 'confounding' effect. This could only be overcome at the analytical stage through statistical methods for 'controlling' for the effect of behaviour, or in study design, by conducting prospective randomised-controlled intervention trials.

In a recent comprehensive review, Fleming and Wasserheit group the evidence that STIs facilitate the transmission of HIV into three categories[9]: (i) biological plausibility studies; (ii) HIV seroconversion studies; and (iii) randomised intervention studies.

Biological plausibility or mechanism studies

During sexual intercourse genital ulcers may bleed, leading to the increased risk of HIV transmission via the blood route. Studies of HIV infected people with genital ulcer disease (GUD) suggest that these ulcers may increase **infectiousness** as HIV virions have been detected in genital ulcer exudates among patients with chancroid or syphilis[10,11]. Similarly, HIV proviral DNA was found in herpes-associated GUD among men in Seattle[12]. Treatment or healing of GUD among HIV-seropositive individuals is accompanied by a decrease in HIV shedding[12,13]. Among HIV-seronegative individuals, GUD may increase **susceptibility** by disrupting mucosal integrity, by the recruitment and activation of HIV target cells, such as lymphocytes, and possibly by HIV taking advantage of CCR5 and chemokine receptors[14].

The effects of STI on excretion of HIV-1 in genital secretions have been investigated. There is evidence that among HSV-2 infected women, even in the absence of an ulcer, HSV-2 genital shedding is increased in HIV-seropositive individuals[15,16] and that both HIV-RNA and HSV-2 DNA shedding are increased in the presence of the other virus[16]. The biological basis for the 'promotion' of HIV infection is not entirely elucidated but it has been suggested that, in the presence of HSV, HIV can infect keratinocytes that lack CD4 receptors[17].

Non-ulcerative STIs such as gonococcal or chlamydial infections have also been shown to increase the frequency of HIV-DNA shedding in cervico-vaginal secretions among HIV-seropositive female sex workers in Ivory Coast[13], and Kenya[18]. A study among male patients in Malawi[19] observed an 8-fold increase in secretion of HIV-1 RNA in semen compared with a control group. The effect was marked for men having either gonorrhoea or *T. vaginalis* infections. In both men and women, successful treatment of patients with STI resulted in decreased frequency or quantity of HIV shedding[13,19].

Changes in the vaginal flora, such as seen in bacterial vaginosis, appear to be increasing the risk of HIV acquisition[20-22]. However, properly randomised intervention studies are still required to determine the real causal role of this frequent condition.

HIV seroconversion studies

Several studies have demonstrated that prior presence of an STI will enhance HIV acquisition. In Kenya, HIV-seronegative men attending a STI clinic with a chancroid ulcer were 4 times more likely than their counterparts without an ulcer to seroconvert in the few weeks of follow-up[23]. Other independent factors of HIV seroconversion included the lack of circumcision and a sexual contact with a sex worker. In a cohort study of Thai military conscripts, a significant 4-fold increase in the relative risk of HIV seroconversion was found among the men who were HSV seropositive at baseline, and a 2-fold significant increase among men who seroconverted for HSV in the intervening follow-up[24].

Randomised intervention studies

A large community-randomised controlled trial conducted in the Mwanza region of Tanzania showed that improved management of STIs in rural health centres and dispensaries, reduced the incidence of HIV infection by approximately 40% over a 2-year period[25] mediated by a decrease in the duration of symptomatic STIs[26]. This study has provided the clearest evidence to date of the impact of a feasible and cost-effective STI intervention in preventing HIV transmission.

It has now been realised that the prevention and care of STIs are interventions which improve the health status of the population and are also important strategies for the prevention of HIV transmission. Consequently, UNAIDS and WHO have recommended that high priority be given to the development of STI control programmes[4].

Approaches to STI control

Theoretical control models

STI control strategies have long been influenced by the 'transmission dynamics model' described by Anderson[27]. In this model, the transmission of a STI is expressed in terms of its basic reproductive number (R_0), *i.e.* the average number of new (or secondary) STI cases generated by an index (or primary) case in a defined population over a period of time. It has been demonstrated that R_0 is a function of the rate of partner change (c), the probability of transmission of the STI during sexual intercourse (β) and the duration of the infection (D)[27] – summarized in the formula $R_0 = \beta \times c \times D$. STI control programmes should, therefore, aim to reduce the basic reproductive rate by a combination of strategies, including behaviour

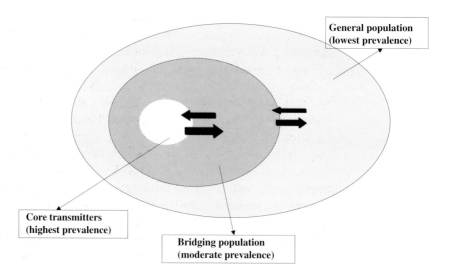

General population
(lowest prevalence)

Core transmitters
(highest prevalence)

Bridging population
(moderate prevalence)

Fig. 2 The structure of sexual networks (*reproduced with permission from:* Cates W & Dallabetta G, 1999[77]).

change aiming at decreasing the number of sexual partners, increased condom use and treatment of patients with STI. The latter component of STI control programmes aims to reduce the duration of infectivity of individuals with an STD.

This model has also highlighted the importance of groups of individuals who have much higher rates of sexual partnerships. These 'core groups' and their sexual partners – who may form 'bridge populations' between the core groups and the general populations (Fig. 2[77]) – have been shown to be epidemiologically important in driving the STI and HIV epidemics in many parts of the world[28].

Other models have been developed to conceptualise the strategies needed to control STI. The 'operational model' identifies the many different steps that patients with an STI pass through before they can they can be considered cured by health services (Fig. 3). At each step, a proportion of patients will drop out. By multiplying the percentages of patients taking each step, one obtains an estimate of the cure rate achieved by the health services of interest. This model shows how, in most non-industrialised countries, only a fraction of STI cases are successfully treated[29]. In this way,

Fig. 3 Operational model of the role of health services in STI case management (*reproduced with permission:* Laga M. 12th International AIDS Conference, Geneva 1998)

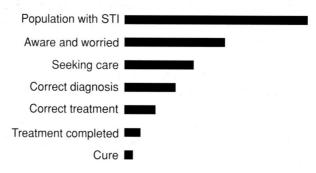

Population with STI
Aware and worried
Seeking care
Correct diagnosis
Correct treatment
Treatment completed
Cure

it clarifies the four main reasons for failure to control STIs: (i) failure to prevent unsafe sexual behaviour; (ii) failure of people with symptoms to access health services; (iii) failure to identify and treat patients with symptoms; and (iv) failure of health services to provide adequate treatment.

Each of these steps, in turn, suggests points for potential medical, health promotion, and service delivery interventions. Starting from the bottom of the model, broad options for STI control, therefore, include: (i) improving STI case management, including partner notification; (ii) improving treatment-seeking behaviour; (iii) case finding or screening for neglected or asymptomatic STIs; (iv) mass treatment of the general population and/or presumptive treatment of high-risk groups; and (v) primary prevention (information education and communication [IEC] strategies, condoms, microbicides, vaccines).

This paper will review the main strategies used under each of these approaches as a means to control STI, and prevent HIV.

STI interventions

STI case management

Early diagnosis and effective treatment of STIs is an essential component of STI control programmes. The traditional method for STI diagnosis has been through laboratory diagnosis of the aetiological agent. Whilst this is still the method of choice in many parts of the industrialised world, this approach is expensive both in terms of diagnostics, infrastructure, and maintenance. Additionally, it often results in delays in diagnosis and treatment. Moreover, most health centres and dispensaries in non-industrialised countries do not have access to reliable laboratory facilities. Consequently, clinicians either need to refer their patients to specialist centres, resulting in further delays, or they attempt to make a presumptive clinical diagnosis through the identification of particular clinical features related to various agents. This method has often proven inaccurate or incomplete[30].

To address the limitations of both aetiological and clinical diagnosis in the management of STIs, particularly for patients who attend the first level of primary health care, the WHO has developed and advocated the syndromic management approach. STI-associated syndromes are easily identifiable groups of symptoms and clinical findings on which the healthcare providers can base their presumptive diagnosis. Management is simplified by the use of clinical flowcharts, and allows time in the consultation to provide simple education messages, discuss partner notification and promote condoms. Antimicrobial therapy is provided at once to cover the majority of pathogens presumed responsible for that syndrome, in that specific geographical area[7].

Syndromic management is simple and lends itself to use in a variety of outlets such as STI clinics, primary healthcare (PHC) facilities, pharmacies, family planning/maternal and child health (FP/MCH) services and private practitioners clinics. The sensitivity and specificity of the approach for the diagnosis and management of urethral discharge syndrome and genital ulcer syndrome in various settings have been very satisfactory. Other advantages include cost-effectiveness, diagnosis and treatment at first visit and increased patient satisfaction[7].

There are two main limitations to syndromic management. Firstly, the cost of over-diagnosis and treatment of patients with no or only one infection. This includes the direct costs of the antimicrobials as well as the indirect costs in terms of adverse drug reactions, alteration in normal gut flora (*e.g.* shigella) and potential domestic violence. Over treatment is particularly a problem in areas of low STI prevalence. A study conducted in Matlab, Bangladesh, found that cervical infections were present in only 3 out of 320 women complaining of abnormal vaginal discharge while the prevalence of endogenous infection was 30%[31]. In this setting, the WHO algorithm had a sensitivity of 100% but a very low specificity (56%) while a locally-adapted speculum-based algorithm had sensitivity ranging between 0–59% depending on the pathogens to be identified with a specificity of 80% up to 97%. Clearly syndromic management in this setting did not deal adequately with the management of vaginal discharge and it was calculated that between 36% and 87% of costs would have been spent on uninfected women.

The second limitation is the poor sensitivity and specificity of the syndromic approach for the detection of cervical infections in women, even in settings with higher STI prevalence. The WHO has recommended a risk assessment score to be added to the vaginal discharge syndrome in order to increase the effectiveness of algorithms[7]. Evaluation of this approach has taken place in several countries, but has yielded disappointing results[7]: scores need to be setting-specific, with tremendous variations even within the same country; the performance of algorithms was not vastly improved; and, as in the case of the Matlab study, risk score was also found to be inadequate in societies where most women will not admit to extramarital or premarital sexual activity for threat of social sanctions[31].

Partner notification

Partner notification (PN) is a strategy consisting of contacting sexual partners of STI patients to offer them screening and treatment. PN aims to reduce asymptomatic disease in the community and shorten the average period of infectiousness. This, in turn, is expected to reduce disease transmission in the population[32]. However, while bacterial STIs can be identified and cured, thus breaking the chain of transmission, viral STIs such as HSV-2 and HIV have no cure and the rationale for PN is less obvious. In the context of syndromic management, it is even less clear which STI should be treated. The most practical approach has been to give the same treatment as for the index case, but this will clearly result in over-prescription of antibiotics. Very little work has been done to demonstrate the impact of PN on reducing the prevalence and incidence of STI in the population.

There has been more research to determine the best way to implement PN. There is strong evidence that simple PN forms given to the index patient ('patient referral') can be effective, and less labour intensive and costly than 'provider referral', where the services take responsibility of tracing contacts. Overall, it seems that PN is relatively ineffective in situations where there is low motivation of health providers, where sex with anonymous partners (*e.g.* sex workers) is common, where there is a high rate of sexual partner change and where resources are scarce and addresses unreliable[33]. Acceptability of PN depends upon confidentiality and availability of treatment[32], but strategies should take into account the sexual practices and ethnicity of the population as well as potential negative impacts such as violence against the index case (especially women).

Promotion of treatment seeking behaviour and the role of the private sector

A key step where many STI patients can be lost in the operational model is 'attendance to services'. Surveys of health-seeking behaviour in non-industrialised countries indicate that a substantial proportion of people with symptomatic STI seek treatment in the informal or private sector, from traditional healers, unqualified practitioners, street drug vendors, and from pharmacists and private practitioners and will only attend formal public health services after alternative treatments have failed[34]. Self-medication is also very popular in many settings, where up to 65% of men with symptoms of urethritis self treat[34-36].

Patients seek care in the private sector for many reasons. Public services often have restricted and inconvenient opening hours[35] while private services tend to tailor their opening times to suit their clients. Moreover, provider-to-client ratios vary greatly between sectors in many countries. For example in Lagos State, Nigeria, Green found a ratio of one traditional healer per 200 population, whereas in Mozambique, the physician to population ratio was 1:50,000[37]. In addition, private sector services are often seen as providing a more personalised and confidential service with less social and cultural distance between client and provider[34,35,37]. An additional barrier to public services utilisation is sometimes the cost of services, as was evidenced in Nairobi, Kenya: when user fees were introduced, a huge decrease in monthly attendances of the largest STI clinic in the city were recorded. Lifting of the fees a few months later resulted in increased attendances, although this never reached the same levels[38].

Quality of care in the private sector is difficult to assess due to the range of services offered and the difficulty in accessing practitioners. A study of private doctors in South Africa showed that fewer than one in ten patients received adequate doses of antibiotics and in 75% of cases an incorrect drug was prescribed[39]. In private practice there is a financial incentive which can affect the quality of care. In some cases, private practitioners may provide a sub-optimal dose of antibiotics in order that the client can afford treatment and in other cases, for example in China, practitioners may increase their income through over investigation and over prescription (Mabey D, personal communication).

There has been a number of interventions to improve private sector management of STIs. In Jamaica, seminars were provided for public and private physicians and nurses and post-training tests showed an increase in knowledge with regard to STI diagnosis, and most practitioners reported an increase in risk reduction counselling[40]. Similarly, training for pharmacists in Nepal showed an increase of 45% in the correct syndromic treatment of urethritis[41]. This figure dropped to 26% nine months after the training, indicating the need for continued training and supervision[42]. A study in Thailand using 'mystery shoppers' again showed improved treatment of STIs by drugstore staff after training[43].

Another strategy to increase effective treatment of STIs is the use of pre-packaged therapy (PPT) for syndromic treatment. A team in Uganda developed the 'Clear Seven' kit for patients with urethral discharge, which contains ciprofloxacin, doxycycline, condoms, partner referral cards and a clear instruction leaflet. The kit was socially marketed in clinics, pharmacies and retail drug shops. The study found that 'Clear Seven' users *versus* controls had significantly higher cure rates (84% *versus* 47%, $P > 0.001$), greater compliance (93% *versus* 87%) and increased condom use during treatment. Partner referral rates were similar for both groups[44]. Similar PPT kits have been used in Cameroon and South Africa with varying levels of acceptability by both health service staff and patients[45,46].

In general, the private sector should be viewed as a complement to, and not a replacement for, effective and accessible public services. Furthermore, the views of government health authorities and the medical community should be considered when attempting to stimulate effective collaboration between the sectors.

Screening and case finding

Case finding is the testing for STI in individuals seeking health care for reasons other than STI, and screening is defined as testing for STI in individuals not directly seeking health care (*e.g.* blood donors). Both strategies have an important role in the detection and treatment of asymptomatic STIs in the community. They should be principally directed towards ANC, FP and MCH clinic attendees as well as high-risk groups such as adolescents and sex workers.

Universal serological testing of ANC attendees for syphilis is recommended by WHO and is one of the most cost-effective health interventions available although programmes are poorly implemented in many countries[47]. Donors of blood, tissue and semen should be screened for at least syphilis, HIV and hepatitis B in order to protect recipients, and the potential exists for screening of populations such as military recruits and company employees. In all cases, careful attention should be paid to patient confidentiality, and if necessary counselling and treatment.

There is an urgent need for simple and cheap methods of identifying asymptomatic women with cervical infections in antenatal, family planning and maternal child health clinics. A simple sociodemographic risk score which identifies women at greater risk of infection has been tried but it has a poor sensitivity and predictive value[48,49].

Mass treatment

Mass treatment involves the single or periodic administration of effective drugs to a whole population in order to treat, reduce the reservoir, and prevent continued transmission of a specific infection. Mass treatment of STI has many potential advantages: asymptomatic patients are covered, no screening tests are needed, it can be combined with syndromic treatment services and may be highly cost-effective. However, there are concerns about the ethics of treating healthy subjects, adverse effects of treatment, development of drug resistance, logistical difficulties and expense. It has also been suggested that mass treatment may create a false sense of security and result in risk compensation behaviour.

Between 1994 and 1998, a community randomised trial was conducted in Rakai, Uganda, to test the hypothesis that repeated rounds of mass treatment for STI would reduce STI rates and HIV transmission[50]. The intervention comprised single dose oral treatment of all individuals with very effective antibiotics (azithromycin and ciprofloxacin) in the study areas and a single intramuscular penicillin injection for all patients with serological syphilis. Results showed significant reductions in the prevalence of some STIs, particularly among pregnant women in the intervention group. However, in contrast to the Mwanza study mentioned above, there was no effect on HIV incidence.

Reasons postulated for this paradoxical result include differences in the stage of the epidemic (mature epidemic in Rakai versus an earlier stage in Mwanza), differences in accessibility to STI services for patients with re-infection (continuous availability in Mwanza, intermittent in Rakai) and differences in the prevalences of treatable STI (higher proportion of GUD due to HSV-2 in Rakai than in Mwanza). It was concluded that the proportion of HIV infections attributable to the enhancing effect of STIs seems to decrease with the progression of the HIV epidemic[51]. The results of a third community randomised trial conducted in Masaka – adjacent district to Rakai, with the same epidemiological setting sharing the same epidemiological features but based on a similar intervention to the one used in Mwanza – are awaited with great anticipation.

It may be that single or multiple rounds of mass treatment combined with continuous availability of syndromic management could be an effective control strategy for many countries[52]. In the face of looming epidemics in Asia and elsewhere, this option needs to be fully explored. However, the comparative advantages of mass treatment and continuous provision of syndromic treatment should be determined through RCTs with STI services as standard provision in the control group[51].

Targeted periodic presumptive treatment

Targeted interventions are based on the concept of core groups, which play a key role in the epidemiology of HIV-1[28]. The 'epidemiological synergy' between STI and HIV is particularly important in core groups with a high incidence of STI and HIV. Moreover, Plummer showed in Kenya that progression to HIV disease is more rapid in prostitutes and it is likely that this rapid progression is related to concurrent STI infection[28]. This could have an important effect on accelerating the epidemic as frequent episodes of STI would accelerate the development of lowered immunity and increased HIV infectiousness while also increasing susceptibility to STIs.

Core groups are context specific and, when designing interventions, it is important to take account of the social and economic forces creating these groups and to balance disease control measures against the potential for victimisation. Interventions need to be designed in partnership with core group members they should be context specific and emphasise common goals and interests[53].

An example of a successful core group intervention took place in a South African mining community. The Lesedi project[54] provided STI treatment services including periodic presumptive treatment and prevention education to a core group of sex workers living around the mine. The study found that the intervention significantly reduced the prevalence of gonococcal and chlamydia infections (NG/CT: *Neisseria gonorrhoeae/Chlamydia trachomatis*) and GUD among women. Moreover symptomatic STIs were also reduced among the miners in the intervention area as compared to miners living further away[54]. The results of this study suggest that periodic presumptive treatment coupled with health education is a feasible approach to providing STI services to core groups.

Primary prevention

Primary prevention can be directed at changing the behaviour of individuals and these are particularly effective at reaching areas of need, especially when implemented in a clinical setting. These interventions often rely on the 'rational health model', which is based on the assumption that an individual has the power to make necessary changes. However, in many instances drugs/poverty/gender can diminish an individual's ability to act on his/her intentions[55]. Behavioural interventions are particularly important in adolescents as they have high rates of STI and are more susceptible to behaviour change intervention such as mutual monogamy, safer sexual practices and condom use. Many behavioural interventions for primary prevention of STI are similar to those for the prevention of HIV transmission. As these are discussed elsewhere in this volume, this paper will focus on those interventions specific to STIs.

Condoms

When used properly and consistently, condoms are one of the most effective methods of protection for individuals against STI. They are relatively cheap and free from side effects. They can be made readily available on a large scale through free distribution or social marketing – the promotion and use of marketing techniques to make products available at an affordable price.

However, in many countries only a small proportion of the sexually active population use condoms and those who do may do so irregularly and only with selected partners[56]. Barriers to consistent use of condoms include high price in some settings, low availability and inadequate social marketing but above all, lack of appeal to potential users. Women may also be forced into unprotected intercourse as a result of unequal power relations between men and women.

In Thailand, the 100% Condom Programme overcame many of these barriers and the programme has been linked to the decrease in the numbers of cases of STI and HIV[57]. However, similar declines in disease prevalence have been observed in Uganda where condom uptake is low[58]. It has been suggested that a large increase in condom use could fail to affect disease transmission at a population level due to a 'risk-compensation' mechanism[58]. This would imply that condom users switch from inherently safer strategies of partner selection and low rates of partner change, to a riskier strategy of maintaining higher rates of partner change plus reliance on intermittent condom use.

UNAIDS recommended best practice for condom programmes include campaigns to improve information, education and empowerment of individuals so that they can make informed decisions about condom use; ensuring easy access to high quality condoms; and conducting context specific research into behaviour and preferences as regards condom use[56].

Female controlled methods of STI prevention

STIs disproportionately affect women, and adolescent women are at increased risk of STI due to ignorance of appropriate preventative measures ,and unplanned or coercive sexual intercourse, where it may be difficult or impractical to negotiate safer sex. Female-controlled methods of protection against HIV and STIs are, therefore, taking on increased importance.

The female condom has important advantages such as efficacy, little reported disruption of sexual enjoyment, safety and in some areas increasing acceptance by women[59]. However, disadvantages include high cost, lack of visual and auditory appeal, difficulty of use, pre-planning of intercourse and mixed reactions among male partners. A randomised study conducted among sex workers in Thailand has demonstrated that women who were trained on using female condoms in addition to male condoms became more consistent users of either method and had, therefore, higher rates of protected intercourse, compared to women to whom only male condoms were promoted and provided[59].

Vaginal microbicides potentially offer a female-controlled means of protection from both infection and conception and have been under development since the early 1990s. Currently, there are about 36 compounds under development[60]. These compounds can have advantages over the female condom in that they can be developed with options for surreptitious use.

A detergent based chemical nonoxynol-9 (N-9) kills STI and HIV *in vitro* but while clinical trials suggest that the product provides some protection against gonococcus and chlamydia, results are disappointing for HIV[61]. There is also concern that repeated use of these compounds can disrupt the vaginal and rectal epithelium and actually make users more susceptible to pathogens[60]. This is a problem especially for female sex workers who would want to use it a lot.

New compounds are under development and evaluation. Studies using BufferGel (ReProtect) have shown positive spermicidal effects and also a decrease in symptoms of bacterial vaginosis[60] a condition which is highly prevalent in some areas and which increases susceptibility to HIV infection[20–22]. Other studies have shown that an antibody-based microbicide that persists in the vaginal tract for 2–3 days may be feasible. This would be useful for women who have multiple sexual contacts in a setting where it is difficult to re-apply a microbicide regularly. It is possible that anti-retroviral agents already approved for systemic treatment may be used intravaginally and in fact many researchers predict that 'intravaginal chemoprophylaxis' may require a combination of agents to be optimally effective.

Vaccines

Vaccines have enormous potential in the prevention and control of STIs and some are currently under development for *Neisseria gonorrhoeae*, *Chlamydia trachomatis*, herpes simplex virus, human papilloma virus and HIV. However, there are difficulties in making effective vaccines available for use by those in need.

Firstly, many STI agents do not evoke lasting immunity even subsequent to natural infection. Agents such as *N. gonorrhoeae* and HIV are constantly evolving and this makes it difficult to create a reliable and widely applicable vaccine. Secondly, there are problems with the logistics of vaccine delivery. A vaccine against hepatitis B has been available for about 20 years but most sexually active adults remain unprotected today. The practicalities of vaccination are well known through experiences with the EPI immunization programmes, but another important issue for STI vaccines is acceptability by the target population. Unique barriers to STI vaccine acceptance are likely to be encountered. For example, it could be argued that STI vaccination in adolescents would condone extramarital sex and, despite evidence to the contrary, such arguments are still used in opposition to sex education or condom distribution programmes at schools. Zimet suggests that issues around consent (parental and adolescent) are likely to be key and that substantial research will be required in order to guide programme design[62]. Thirdly, vaccination may influence sexual behaviour by promoting a feeling of invulnerability with a subsequent increase in risky behaviour.

Individual, community and targeted intervention strategies

An important consideration in STI control is to decide on strategies that target the individual, the community or special groups of individuals at higher risk of, or more vulnerable to, STIs within communities. Clearly, a number of strategies target the individual such as screening, case management and partner notification, whilst community strategies will include mostly primary prevention such as information, education and communication (IEC) campaigns, or vaccine programmes. In recent years, strategies to control STI through mass treatment programmes have been attempted.

Interventions targeted at individuals may fail to identify or influence behaviours of people at some level of risk but who do not identify themselves with the target group. On the other hand, although general population or community measures deliver a less intensive dose of intervention to each individual, it is distributed across a large population that includes many individuals at low risk. It has been suggested[53,55,63] that both types of intervention are appropriate at different points in the epidemic. At the start of an epidemic when individuals at risk are difficult to distinguish, general population interventions are appropriate. Targeting is indicated when sexual mixing patterns have been identified and later, when the epidemic moves into the general population and core groups have emerged, universal interventions are needed.

STI control programmes need a mix of individual and general population interventions. The challenge is how best to use and combine interventions and how to make sure policy and political support is conducive to help change the social or physical environment in which risk takes place. For example, restrictive policies about prostitution will hamper interventions targeting sex workers; sociocultural environments which promote homophobia or deny sexual health information to adolescents will prevent access of these vulnerable populations to appropriate sexual health services, or may encourage clandestine risk-taking. Economic empowerment of women can also be effective.

Challenges in STI control

Integration of STI prevention and care in reproductive health services

There is general consensus on the need to integrate STI services into reproductive health services. The rationale is that reproductive health programmes are already high profile and could attract additional funds necessary for STI treatment. In addition, integrated services could reach a wide female population.

It has been suggested that, at a minimum, STI/HIV risk assessment and prevention services should be provided in all MCH/FP clinics, and that integrated services should also include syphilis testing and treatment for all pregnant women attending antenatal services[47].

In economic terms it is thought that integration will optimise resources, reduce service delivery costs and patient transport costs as well as other opportunity costs relating to multiple health service visits[64]. However, there is little evidence that integration is in fact an effective public health measure[65]. A study of health systems in sub-Saharan Africa suggests that pre-existing vertical management and separate service delivery have hindered efforts to translate concepts into practice. For example, in Kenya the provision of drugs essential for STI treatment has remained separate from existing systems of procurement and in Ghana FP management has remained separate from other 'integrated' services. South Africa, on the other hand, has been more successful in developing an integrated and comprehensive service. This has been facilitated by South Africa's strong commitment, since 1994, to universal access to comprehensive primary healthcare (PHC). The South African approach has integrated all financial, human resources and logistical systems at provincial level, and the national programmes provide technical support to services through horizontal management systems at all levels. But the South African system is not trouble free. The provision of free comprehensive care has lead to increased demands on the health system and this has stretched the capacity of staff at health facilities as well as finances available for effective drugs. In addition, as elsewhere, an emphasis on clinical care has tended to be at the expense of health promotion services[65].

It is important to note that integration of STI services can miss one of the largest target groups – men. This is an important group as men, due to sexual behaviour and increased mobility, are at higher risk, initially, of contracting STI. However, once infected, the clinical management of men is simpler than for women. Investigators in Bangladesh found that there was a substantial unmet need for STI services for men and that, in addition, there was a demand for other reproductive and psychosexual services. It may, therefore, be appropriate to provide comprehensive reproductive health services to men as well as women and this may even prove to be an effective strategy for the control of STI[66].

The changing epidemiology of STI

Additional challenges to STI control include the capacity of pathogens to develop resistance to antimicrobials, and the emergence of some pathogens (HSV-2) or conditions (bacterial vaginosis) as novel significant causes of morbidity, including facilitation of HIV transmission.

Global antimicrobial resistance of *N. gonorrhoeae* and *Haemophilus ducreyi*

At present most regions of the world have a high prevalence of *N. gonorrhoeae* and *H. ducreyi* isolates resistant to common antibiotics such as penicillin, tetracyclin or cotrimoxazole[67]. Resistance is most common in areas of the world where effective treatment is unavailable or expensive and where diagnostic facilities are inadequate (Fig. 4). The high costs of effective agents such as azithromycin and ceftriaxone raise concerns that low or inadequate doses will be used and that this will facilitate the selection of resistance to these drugs also. Conversely, the decreasing costs of agents such as quinolones may precipitate their improper use and self-medication, also leading to increased resistance.

In order to provide effective treatment and prevent the transmission of resistant isolates, regimens need to be tailored to the prevalence of antimicrobial resistance in the locality. This in turn requires information on patterns of anti-microbial susceptibility. Many industrialised countries have

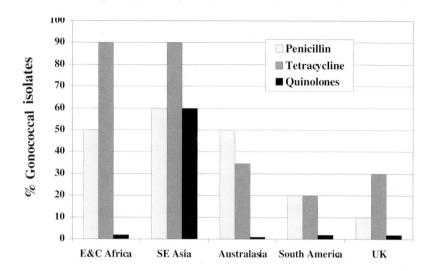

Fig. 4 Antimicrobial resistance of N. gonorrhoeae in selected countries in the 1990s [*Adapted from:* Ison CA, Dillon JR, Tapsall JW, 1998[67]].

programmes for *N. gonorrhoeae* surveillance, but continuous susceptibility data has been lacking in non-industrialised countries. This problem has been approached by the establishment of a global surveillance network – the gonococcal antimicrobial susceptibility programme (GASP). Co-ordinated by WHO, GASP aims to create a network of laboratories which will monitor susceptibility of gonococcal isolates and disseminate information on trends in susceptibility and resistance (Fig. 4). The network is only effectively working in the West Pacific and the Pan-American regions, but efforts are underway to promote the establishment of such networks in Africa.

Surveillance of *H. ducreyi* requires a viable culture of the organism. This is a barrier to effective surveillance as isolation of *H. ducreyi* is particularly difficult and often has a sensitivity of < 80%[67]. In addition, few centres have facilities for culture. Our knowledge of *H. ducreyi* resistance is limited to irregular sentinel surveillance data and hence the global prevalence of antibiotic resistant *H. ducreyi* is unknown[67].

The emergence of HSV-2 and the changing pattern of genital ulcer aetiologies
World-wide prevalence rates for infection with HSV-2 have been increasing over the last decades. In the US, recent seroprevalence studies indicate that 22–33% of the population is infected with HSV-2, representing a 33% increase over the past 20 years[68]. High seroprevalence rates of HSV-2 (40–70%) have been recorded in population-based studies in East and Southern Africa[69].

In countries where syphilis and chancroid are endemic, HSV-2 has traditionally been thought to be relatively less important as an aetiological agent of genital ulcer disease (GUD). This pattern is changing however[69]. Recent studies have found that, while GUD attributable to HSV-2 infection is increasing, *H. ducreyi* is decreasing in many areas. HSV-2 now typically

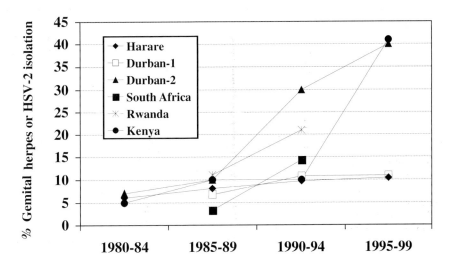

Fig. 5 Proportion of genital herpes or HSV-2 isolation over time among patients with genital ulcerative disease in selected sub-Saharan African settings. [*Adapted from:* O'Farrell B, 1999[69]]

represents 40–50% of detectable GUD aetiologies in some settings (Fig. 5). The implications of this increasing problem only begin to be fully appreciated. Given the fact that HSV-2 and HIV may have a synergistic effect, increased levels of HSV-2 in GUD will promote susceptibility to HIV or infectiousness of HIV-infected individuals, whilst HIV will contribute to the further spread of HSV-2 as well as the worsening of the natural course of GUD cases which will lead to many apparent failures of treatment. One consequence is that it may be important to revise the WHO guidelines for syndromic management of GUD[69] and possibly include anti-HSV treatment. Intervention trials evaluating the feasibility and impact of such treatment strategy, with an important outcome in terms of HIV shedding, are urgently required[16].

The role of vaginal and endogenous infections

Greater more attention has been accorded in recent years to bacterial vaginosis (BV) as a possible significant factor in women's sexual ill-health world-wide. BV is one of the most common causes of vaginal symptoms among women of reproductive ages and is associated with serious obstetric and gynaecological complication, including premature rupture of membranes, preterm birth and low birth weight infants, as well as pelvic inflammatory disease or endometritis following insertion of intra-uterine devices (IUD) or induced abortion[70]. Recent investigations in Thailand[20], Uganda[21] and Malawi[22] have reported associations between BV and HIV, suggesting a possible causal factor in HIV transmission.

Although the role of BV in women's health in non-industrialised countries has not been fully explored, it is potentially significant as suggested by high prevalence rates (20–50%) and the frequency of BV-associated morbidity in these regions. Moreover, even a moderate relative-risk may translate into a large population-attributable fraction of HIV infection.

It will be important to understand better the determinants of acquisition or maintenance of BV in women, including the role of hormonal factors, menstrual and sexual hygiene. The main obstacles to the control of BV are the difficulty of diagnosing the condition in primary health care clinics lacking microscopy and trained laboratory personnel, and the frequent relapse of the condition despite treatment. The challenges, therefore, will be to devise simpler and more effective methods to diagnose and treat BV and ways to implement and evaluate large-scale BV control programmes in non-industrialised countries[71].

Mobilising policy, priority setting and capacity building

The failure to control STIs in the past was not solely due to antibiotic resistance nor to any emergent or resurgent organisms, but simply through lack of political will to invest in control measures[72]. In order to mobilise policy, it is vital to identify the barriers that prevent research findings being translated into policy at country level[3]. One such barrier is a lack of appropriate models of service provision which facilitate the design of effective STI control programmes. Another is the lack of operational research into ways of adapting international research findings to the national context.

Many governments are reluctant to confront the STI and HIV epidemics and in many instances countries fail to prioritise activities in the face of severe financial and administrative constraints[73]. Spreading resources across programmes in many sectors risks stretching already scarce resources with negligible or even negative impact. An alternative approach for policy makers would be to implement a smaller, core set of interventions on a national scale and in this way provide a foundation for expansion of activities[73].

The operational model of STI control discussed above makes it clear that curative services alone contribute a small fraction to STI control efforts and will not solve the problem. It is essential, therefore, to build national capacity in areas that interact synergistically with case management to create an effective and sustainable approach to STI control. Training in all areas is essential and this needs to take place in a policy environment which enables managers to advocate for policy changes which can improve and sustain the national capacity to implement an effective STI control programme.

Future research orientations

In order to control STI better in the future, a number of important research questions will need to be answered, and a number of research strategies will need to be explored:

1   Operational research is required to establish the effectiveness of existing interventions and improve the implementation of these interventions in specific

contexts. For example, operational research to refine and adapt context specific syndromic management algorithms and to assess the cost-effectiveness of various STI case management approaches.

2 Randomised controlled trials (RCTs) are required to examine the comparative efficacy and cost-effectiveness of different partner notification strategies as well as research into cheap strategies for improving patient attendance.

3 There is an urgent need for the development and field-testing of simple rapid diagnostic tests for *N. gonorrhoeae* and *C. trachomatis* so that asymptomatic infections can be detected and treated. Research is required to rationalise available and future diagnostic techniques in order to guide choices as to who should be tested.

4 The development of vaccines and vaginal microbicides is especially urgent for the incurable viral STIs (HPV, HSV-2, HIV). Both the World Bank and UNAIDS have stated that their organisations are making a strong commitment to purchase and distribute effective microbicides when they become available.

5 There is a need for RCTs to assess the effectiveness of primary prevention and behavioural interventions, particularly among vulnerable populations such as adolescents, using STI and HIV incidence as outcome measures. One such trial is currently underway in Mwanza, Tanzania, but more are needed in different cultural and epidemiological settings.

6 Capacity building is an important pre-requisite to enable research in non-industrialised countries and this needs to be developed along with functioning support structures, access to information and positive feed-back – in the form of publications, grants and policy change[74].

7 In 1999, the World Bank indicated that the international community has the responsibility for ensuring the production of global public goods[75]. However, funding for research and the development of new technology may be a problem when private firms do not have sufficient incentives to develop the technology – the main beneficiaries live in impoverished countries that cannot afford to pay. It is, therefore, a priority to promote public-private partnerships to develop medical products, and to conduct research into how this may best be achieved.

Conclusions

STIs have taken on a more important role with the advent of the HIV/AIDS epidemic, and there is good evidence that their control can reduce HIV transmission. Although many cost-effective tools such as condoms, effective drugs and the syndromic approach to case management are already in existence (Table 1), there is an urgent need for research into more interventions such as vaginal microbicides, vaccines and behaviour change.

Table 1 Public health package for STI control: the key elements

Promotion of safer sexual behaviour and primary prevention
Condom programmes
Promotion of appropriate health care seeking behaviour
Integration of STI care into basic healthcare services
Comprehensive and syndromic STI case management
Specific services for populations at high risk
Control of congenital syphilis and neonatal conjunctivitis
Development of female-controlled methods (microbicides, female condoms)

Table 2 Challenges for effective STI control

Inappropriate STI services
    diagnostic tests, drugs, condoms
    training, attitudes, staff numbers
    involving public and private providers
Strategies for women, lack of integrated services
Strategies for adolescents, linked with education
Lack of male responsibility, gender inequalities
Societal norms ('shame'), education, information
Structural issues and capacity
Political/policy will, neglect
Economics, poverty, instability, migration

However, even where existing tools are available, there are barriers to the effective utilisation of these tools (Table 2). These barriers include unavailability or unsuitability of STI services, cultural factors in sexual and health-care seeking behaviour, difficulties in the provision of essential drugs, a lack of political will to develop appropriate policies, and financial support for STI control programmes.

The challenge, therefore, is not just to develop new interventions, but to identify barriers to the effective implementation of existing tools, and to devise ways to overcome these barriers. This 'scaling-up' of effective strategies will require an international and a multisectoral approach. It will require the formation of new partnerships between the private and public sectors and between governments and the communities they represent[76].

References

1   Brandt AM, Jones AS. Historical perspectives in sexually transmitted diseases: challenges for prevention and control. In: Holmes KK, Sparling PF, Mardh PA *et al.* (eds) *Sexually Transmitted Diseases*, 3rd edn. New York: McGraw-Hill, 1999; 15–21
2   Wasserheit JN. Epidemiologic synergy: interrelationships between human immunodeficiency virus infection and other sexually transmitted diseases. *Sex Transm Dis* 1992; **19**: 61–77
3   Mayaud P, Hawkes S, Mabey D. Advances in control of sexually transmitted diseases in developing countries. *Lancet* 1998; **35** (**Suppl III**): 29–32

4   Gerbase AC, Rowley JT, Mertens TE. Global epidemiology of sexually transmitted diseases. *Lancet* 1998; **351 (Suppl III)**: 2–4

5   Cohen MS, Henderson GE, Aiello P *et al*. Successful eradication of sexually transmitted diseases in the People's Republic of China: implications for the 21st century. *J Infect Dis* 1996; **174 (Suppl II)**: S223–9

6   Riedner G, Dehne KL, Gromyko A. Recent declines in reported syphilis rates in eastern Europe and central Asia: are the epidemics over? *Sex Transm Infect* 2000; **76**: 363–5

7   Dallabetta GA, Gerbase AC, Holmes KK. Problems, solutions, and challenges in syndromic management of sexually transmitted diseases. *Sex Transm Infect* 1998; **74 (Suppl 1)**: S1–11

8   World Bank. *World Development Report 1993: Investing in Health*. New York: Oxford University Press, 1993

9   Fleming DT, Wasserheit JN. From epidemiological synergy to public health policy and practice: the contribution of other sexually transmitted diseases to sexual transmission of HIV infection. *Sex Transm Infect* 1999; **75**: 3–17

10   Kreiss JK, Coombs R, Plummer FA *et al*. Isolation of human immunodeficiency virus from genital ulcers in Nairobi prostitutes. *J Infect Dis* 1989; **160**: 380–4

11   Plummer FA, Simonsen JN, Cameron DW *et al*. Cofactors in male-female sexual transmission of HIV-1. *J Infect Dis* 1991; **68**: 639–54

12   Schacker T, Ryncarz AJ, Goddard J, Diem K, Shaughnessy M, Corey L. Frequent recovery of HIV-1 from genital herpes simplex virus lesions. *JAMA* 1998; **280**: 61–6

13   Ghys P, Fransen K, Diallo MO *et al*. The association between cervico-vaginal HIV-1 shedding and STIs, immunosuppression, and serum HIV-1 load in female sex workers in Abidjan, Cote d'Ivoire. *AIDS* 1997; **11**: F85–93

14   Cohen MS. Sexually transmitted diseases enhance HIV transmission: no longer a hypothesis. *Lancet* 1998; **351 (Suppl III)**: SIII5–7

15   Mostad SB, Kreiss JK, Ryncarz AJ *et al*. Cervical shedding of herpes simplex virus in human immunodeficiency virus-infected women: effects of hormonal contraception, pregnancy and vitamin A deficiency. *J Infect Dis* 2000; **181**: 58–63

16   Mbopi-Keou FX, Gresenguet G, Mayaud P *et al*. Interactions between herpes simplex virus type 2 and human immunodeficiency virus type 1 infection in African women: opportunities for intervention. *J Infect Dis* 2000; **182**: 1090–6

17   Heng MCY, Heng SY, Allen SG. Co-infection and synergy of human immunodeficiency virus-1 and herpes simplex virus-1. *Lancet* 1994; **343**: 255–8

18   Mostad SB, Overbaugh J, DeVange DM *et al*. Hormonal contraception, vitamin A deficiency, and other risk factors for shedding of HIV-1 infected cells from the cervix and vagina. *Lancet* 1997; **350**: 922–7

19   Cohen MS, Hoffman IF, Royce RA *et al*. Reduction of concentration of HIV-1 in semen after treatment of urethritis: implications for prevention of sexual transmission of HIV-1. *Lancet* 1997; **349**: 1868–73

20   Cohen CR, Duerr A, Pruithithada N *et al*. Bacterial vaginosis and HIV seroprevalence among female commercial sex workers in Chiang Mai, Thailand. *AIDS* 1995; **9**: 1093–7

21   Sewankambo N, Gray RH, Wawer MJ *et al*. HIV-1 infection associated with abnormal vaginal flora morphology and bacterial vaginosis. *Lancet* 1997; **350**: 546–9

22   Taha TE, Hoover DR, Dallabetta GA *et al*. Bacterial vaginosis and disturbances of vaginal flora: association with increased acquisition of HIV. *AIDS* 1998; **12**: 1699–706

23   Cameron DW, Simonsen JN, D'Costa LJ *et al*. Female to male transmission of human immunodeficiency virus type 1: risk factors for seroconversion in men. *Lancet* 1989; **ii**: 403–7

24   Nopkesorn T, Mock PA, Mastro TD *et al*. HIV-1 subtype E incidence and sexually transmitted diseases in a cohort of military conscripts in northern Thailand. *J Acquir Immune Defic Syndr Hum Retrovirol* 1998; **18**: 372–9

25   Grosskurth H, Mosha F, Todd J *et al*. Impact of improved treatment of sexually transmitted diseases on HIV infection in rural Tanzania: randomised controlled trial. *Lancet* 1995; **346**: 530–6

26   Mayaud P, Mosha F, Todd J *et al*. Improved treatment services significantly reduce the prevalence of sexually transmitted diseases in rural Tanzania: results of a randomised controlled trial. *AIDS* 1997; **11**: 1873–80

27   Anderson RM. Transmission dynamics of sexually transmitted infections. In: Holmes KK, Sparling

PF, Mardh M-A *et al.* (eds) *Sexually Transmitted Diseases*, 3rd edn. New York: McGraw-Hill, 1999; 25–37

28 Plummer FA, Nagelkerke NJD, Moses S, Ndinya-Achola JO, Bwayo J, Ngugi E. The importance of core groups in the epidemiology and control of HIV-1 infection. *AIDS* 1991; 5 (**Suppl 1**): S169–76

29 Adler M, Foster S, Grosskurth H, Richens J, Slavin H. *Sexual Health & Care: Sexually Transmitted Infections. Guidelines for Prevention and Treatment*, 2nd edn. DFID, Health & Population Occasional Paper. London: Department for International Development, 1998

30 Adler MW. Sexually transmitted diseases control in developing countries. *Genitourin Med* 1996; 72: 83–8

31 Hawkes S, Morison L, Foster S *et al.* Reproductive-tract infections in women in low-income, low-prevalence situations: assessment of syndromic management in Matlab, Bangladesh. *Lancet* 1999; 354: 1776–81

32 Cowan FM, French R, Johnson AM. The role and effectiveness of partner notification in STI control: a review. *Genitourin Med* 1996; 72: 247–52

33 Potterat JJ. Contact tracing's price is not its value. *Sex Transm Dis* 1997; 24: 519–21

34 Crabbe F, Carsauw H, Buve A, Laga M, Tchupo J-P, Trebucq A. Why do men with urethritis in Cameroon prefer to seek care in the informal health sector? *Genitourin Med* 1996; 72: 220–2

35 Van der Geest S. Self-care and the informal sale of drugs in South Cameroon. *Social Sci Med* 1987; 25: 293–305

36 Khamboonruang C, Beyer C, Natpratan C *et al.* Human immunodeficiency virus infection and self-treatment for sexually transmitted diseases among northern Thai men. *Sex Transm Dis* 1996; 23: 264–9

37 Green EC. *AIDS and STDs in Africa, Bridging the Gap between Traditional Healing and Modern Medicine*. Bolder: Westview, 1994

38 Moses S, Manji F, Bradley JE *et al.* Impact of user fees on attendance at a referral centre for sexually transmitted diseases in Kenya. *Lancet* 1992; 340: 463–6

39 Connolly AM, Wilkinson D, Harrison A, Lurie M, Abdool Karim SS. Inadequate treatment for sexually transmitted diseases in the South African private health sector. *Int J STD AIDS* 1999; 10: 324–7

40 Green M, Hoffman IF, Brathwaite A *et al.* Improving sexually transmitted diseases management in the private sector: the Jamaica experience. *AIDS* 1998; 12 (**Suppl II**): 67–72

41 Casey M, Richards RME. A training programme for drug retailers in Nepal. *Pharmacy Int* 1994; 5: 114–6

42 Tuladhar SM, Mills S, Acharya S *et al.* The role of pharmacists in HIV/STD prevention: evaluation of and STD syndromic management intervention in Nepal. *AIDS* 1998; 12 (**Suppl 2**): 81–7

43 Mendoza AM, Chinvarasopak W. Mobilising pharmacists for STD control. *AIDScaptions* 1996; 111, No 1

44 Kambugu FSK, Jacobs B, Lwanga A *et al.* Evaluation of a socially marketed pre-packaged treatment kit for men with urethral discharge in Uganda. *XIIIth International AIDS Conference*, Durban, July 2000, Abstract ThOrC765

45 Crabbe F, Tchupo J-P, Manchester T *et al.* Prepackaged therapy for urethritis: the 'MSTOP' experience in Cameroon. *Sex Transm Infect* 1998, 74: 249–52

46 Wilkinson D, Harrison A, Lurie M, Abdool Karim SS. STD syndrome packets: improving syndromic management of sexually transmitted diseases in developing countries. *Sex Transm Dis* 1999; 26: 152–6

47 Temmerman M, Hira S, Laga M. STDs and pregnancy. In: Dallabetta G, Laga M, Lamptey P. (eds) *Control of Sexually Transmitted Diseases. A Handbook for the Design and Management of Programs*. Arlington, VA, USA: AIDSCAP/FHI/USAID, 1996; 169–86

48 Thomas T, Choudhri S, Kariuki C, Moses S. Identifying cervical infection among pregnant women in Nairobi, Kenya: limitations of risk-assessment and symptom-based approaches. *Genitourin Med* 1996; 72: 334–8

49 Mayaud P, Uledi E, Cornelissen J *et al.* Risk scores to detect cervical infections in urban antenatal clinic attenders in Mwanza, Tanzania. *Sex Transm Inf* 1998; 74 (**Suppl 1**): S139–46

50 Wawer MJ, Sewankambo NK, Serwadda D *et al.* Control of sexually transmitted diseases for AIDS prevention in Uganda: a randomised community trial. Rakai Project Study Group. *Lancet* 1999; 353: 525–35

51 Grosskurth, H, Gray R, Hayes R, Mabey D, Wawer M. Control of sexually transmitted diseases for HIV-1 prevention: understanding the implications of the Mwanza and Rakai trials. *Lancet* 2000; **355**: 1981–7

52 Korenromp EL, Van Vliet C, Grosskurth H *et al*. Model based evaluation of single round mass treatment of sexually transmitted diseases for HIV control in a rural African population. *AIDS* 2000; **14**: 573–93

53 Sumatytojo E, Carey JW, Doll LS, Gayle H. Target and general population interventions for HIV prevention: towards a comprehensive approach. *AIDS* 1997; **11**: 1201–9

54 Steen R, Dallabetta G. The use of epidemiological mass treatment and syndrome management for sexually transmitted disease control. *Sex Transm Dis* 1999; **26**: S12–20

55 O'Reilly KR, Piot P. International perspectives on individual and community approaches to the prevention of sexually transmitted disease and human immunodeficiency virus infection. *J Infect Dis* 1996; **174**: S214–22

56 UNAIDS. *The male condom*. Technical update. Geneva: UNAIDS, August 2000

57 Nelson KE, Celentano DD, Eiumtrakul S *et al*. Changes in sexual behavior and a decline in HIV infection among young men in Thailand. *N Engl J Med* 1996; **335**: 297–303

58 Richens J, Imrie J, Copas A. Condoms and seat belts: the parallels and the lessons. *Lancet* 2000; **355**: 400–3

59 UNAIDS. *The female condom and AIDS. UNAIDS point of view/UNAIDS Best Practice Collection.* Geneva: UNAIDS, April 2000

60 Stephenson J. Microbicides: ideas flourish, money to follow? *JAMA* 2000; **283**: 1811–2

61 Rosenthal SL, Cohen SS, Stanberry LR. Topical microbicides: current status and research considerations for adolescents. *Sex Transm Dis* 1998; **25**: 368–77

62 Zimet GD, Mays RM, Fortenberry JD. Vaccines against sexually transmitted infections: promise and problems of the magic bullets for prevention and control. *Sex Transm Dis* 2000; **27**: 49–52

63 Aral SO, Holmes KK, Padian NS, Cates W. Overview: individual and population approaches to the epidemiology and prevention of sexually transmitted diseases and human immunodeficiency virus infection. *J Infect Dis* 1996; **174 (Suppl 2)**: 127–3

64 Mayhew S. Integrating MCH/FP and STD/HIV services current debates and future directions. *Health Policy Planning* 1996; **11**: 339–53

65 Lush L, Cleland J, Walt G, Mayhew S. Integrating reproductive health: myth and ideology. *Bull World Health Organ* 1999; **77**: 771–7

66 Hawkes S. Why include men? Establishing sexual health clinics for men in rural Bangladesh. *Health Policy Planning* 1998; **13**: 1210–30

67 Ison CA, Dillon JR, Tapsall JW. The epidemiology of global antibiotic resistance among *Neisseria gonorrhoea* and *Haemophilus ducreyi*. *Lancet* 1998; **381 (Suppl III)**: SIII.8–11

68 Fleming DT, McQuillan GM, Johnson RE *et al*. Herpes simplex type-2 in the United States, 1976 to 1994. *N Engl J Med* 1997; **337**: 1105–11

69 O'Farrell B. Increasing prevalence of genital herpes in developing countries: implications for heterosexual HIV transmission and STI control programmes. *Sex Transm Infect* 1999; **75**: 377–84

70 Hillier S, Holmes KK. Bacterial vaginosis. In: Holmes KK, Sparling PF, Mardh, PA *et al*. (eds) *Sexually Transmitted Diseases*. New York: McGraw-Hill, 1999; 563–86

71 Mayaud P. Tackling bacterial vaginosis and HIV in developing countries. *Lancet* 1997; **350**: 530–1

72 Weber J. HIV and sexually transmitted diseases. *Br Med Bull* 1998; **54**: 717–29

73 Ainsworth M, Teokul W. Breaking the silence: setting realistic priorities for AIDS control in less-developed countries. *Lancet* 2000; World AIDS series: WA35–40

74 Editorial. Enabling research in developing countries. *Lancet* 2000; **356**: 1043

75 World Bank. *Confronting AIDS: Public Priorities in a Global Epidemic*, revised edn. New York: Oxford University Press, 1999

76 Watts C, Kumaranayake L. Thinking big: scaling-up HIV-1 interventions in sub-Saharan Africa. *Lancet* 1999; **354**: 1492

77 Cates W, Dallabetta G. The staying power of sexually transmitted diseases. *Lancet* 1999: **354**(Suppl December): SIV62

78 Laga M. 12th International AIDS Conference, Geneva 1998

Behavioural interventions to prevent HIV infection: rapid evolution, increasing rigour, moderate success

C Bonell* and **J Imrie†**

*Social Science Research Unit, Institute of Education, University of London, London, UK and †Department of Sexually Transmitted Diseases, Royal Free and University College Medical School, University College London, London, UK

Behavioural interventions aim to alter behaviours that make individuals more vulnerable to becoming infected or infecting others with HIV. Research in this field has developed rapidly in recent years. Increased rigour in the design and conduct of evaluations and moderate successes in bringing about behaviour change in target populations are the key achievements so far. This paper reflects on these developments, addresses recent innovations and highlights likely areas for future work. Discussion focuses on maximising the potential effectiveness of new interventions, methodological issues relating to evaluation and implementation of interventions into practice. The paper concludes there is evidence that interventions deemed effective under evaluation conditions can be implemented in HIV prevention services and that this is the next major challenge. The immediate goal should be consolidation of the learning that has occurred, particularly efforts to maintain theoretical and evaluative rigour whilst encouraging increased collaborative partnerships between researchers, service providers and affected communities.

The lack of an effective HIV vaccine means prevention through behaviour change is the most important available strategy to reduce new infections. It is well established that behaviour rather than identity determines risk of HIV infection and certain social groups are more vulnerable to infection than others. Effective HIV prevention programmes need to include interventions that target identified groups at increased risk, as well as the general population, with the balance between these being determined by current epidemiology and future projections[1,2].

Behavioural interventions aim to reduce behaviours that make individuals more vulnerable to becoming infected, or infecting others, with HIV. These interventions have generally aimed to increase use of condoms or reduce numbers of partners[3–6]. More recently, 'negotiated safety' interventions have sought to promote condom protected sex

*Correspondence to:
John Imrie, Department
of Sexually Transmitted
Diseases, Mortimer
Market Centre, Mortimer
Market, off Capper
Street, London
WC1E 6AU, UK*

between individuals of different HIV sero-status, acknowledging that partners who know themselves to be of the same status may have unprotected sex, but have suggested this is only an adequate risk reduction strategy if both partners agree to have no unprotected sex with others[7]. Sexual behaviour is not a static phenomenon, but is influenced by many factors, including characteristics of the individual as well as their social and economic context. Thus, while the aim of behavioural interventions is **relatively** simple, the circumstances in which they operate often necessitates their being complex and multi-dimensional. To date, there has been a huge diversity of interventions, employing methods that variously focus on the individual (*e.g.* counselling), the community (*e.g.* community development) and society (*e.g.* changes in legislation and public policy).

Research into behavioural interventions for HIV prevention has rapidly developed in the course of the last ten or so years. This development is characterized by increasing rigour and moderate success. This paper reflects on developments, addressing recent innovations and highlighting some important areas for future work. The paper is structured around: maximizing the potential effectiveness of new interventions; evaluating interventions; and implementing interventions more widely. The discussion is largely confined to interventions targeting the prevention of HIV, and other poor sexual health outcomes such as sexually transmitted infections (STIs) and unwanted pregnancies in industrialised countries. Although non-industrialised and middle-income countries are hardest hit by the HIV epidemic, the reality of behavioural intervention research so far is that it has been disproportionately situated in the richer countries. This is, however, slowly changing, and there is an emerging literature concerned with behavioural interventions in resource-poor countries.

Maximising the likely effectiveness of interventions

Use of theory

There is widespread agreement that the use of theory is central to developing effective behavioural interventions[8–10]. Theory in this context refers to either a formal theory of individual or social behaviour (see below), or evidence regarding the social or individual constraints that either promote or inhibit behaviour change[10]. Nearly all behavioural interventions for HIV prevention can broadly be classified as complex interventions – that is they consist of separate elements that are combined in order for the intervention to function as intended and to deliver the desired outcome[9,10]. People may respond differently to singular components and what constitutes the 'active ingredient' may be different for each person. One of the great attractions of theoretical approaches is they can serve as an explicit framework to enable a thorough consideration of what factors must be addressed to bring about the desired behaviour change, and how. At the same time, this framework will guide evaluators' identification of process and outcome measures to be examined.

So far, there is little in the way of clear guidance on deciding which theory is most appropriate, or how best to apply it. Examining the results of reported research is rarely helpful. Reported intervention studies seldom provide explanations for the choice of theory. Equally, they rarely describe how a chosen theory guided development of the intervention or choice of outcome measures[11]. Furthermore, evidence to support the specific application of many theories is limited and of varying quality. Application of the theory of the social construction of sexuality, for example, has little basis in research[12]. The application of other theories, such as the theory of planned behaviour, has been extensively investigated[13,14]. Most of these studies have used observational designs; there have been remarkably few attempts to test the theories experimentally[11].

Health promotion theory

Health promotion theory, unlike the other theories discussed below, does not attempt to determine how various factors affect health outcome, but rather it attempts to categorise and prescribe health promotion approaches[15]. Nevertheless, it is often central in determining what factors interventions target and identifying the most appropriate modalities of delivery. Caplan categorises health promotion in terms of two dimensions[16]. The first dimension focuses on whether health promotion aims to affect the individual's actions or to modify the environment (material or social) within which they live. For example, HIV prevention programmes might, on the one hand, try to improve gay men's sexual assertiveness, or on the other, try to encourage the development of a less homophobic society. Caplan's[16] second dimension focuses on the extent to which health promotion is driven by the priorities articulated by affected individuals and communities, or by those of 'experts'.

Health promotion theory is often prescriptive, encouraging interventions that focus on the societal determinants of health, and activities developed and delivered in partnership with affected communities, to redress a perceived existing bias towards individualistic and 'top-down' interventions. This prescriptive element is stressed in documents such as the World Health Organization's *Global Strategy of Health for All by the Year 2000*[17]. In practice, however, most health promotion, including that addressing HIV infection, remains individual-focused and expert-driven[18]. To date, some interventions have sought the involvement of affected communities[19], and a few have addressed the environmental determinants of risk[3,20]. Recognition of the need for this collaborative approach, particularly in dealing with the most vulnerable groups, is slowly being reflected in the literature[3,4].

Social psychological theories

The growing commitment to using theory in intervention development stems partly from the evidence that nearly all sexual health and HIV prevention programmes that have demonstrated some impact on sexual risk behaviour have drawn on social psychological models[6,8,9,11]. These theories relate behaviour to individual cognitions (*i.e.* thoughts, attitudes or beliefs). If these cognitions can be modified, and there is a demonstrable corresponding shift in behaviour, then there is good reason to target these cognitions in behavioural interventions.

There are a number of different models; these have mostly evolved from the Health Belief Model[21]. Only one of these, the AIDS Risk Reduction Model, has been specifically designed to address behavioural change in relation to HIV[22]. The rest have been borrowed from other areas of behavioural research and adapted to meet the needs of HIV prevention. There is substantial overlap between the various theories with regard to the cognitions on which they focus. The theories do, however, differ from one another in a number of ways, including their range of application, formal structure, and complexity. Table 1 summarises the main cognitions that these models focus on, theories with which they are associated, and examples from the recent literature of interventions employing them.

A critique that has emerged in the literature is that social psychological models often overlook the situational factors that might shape sexual behaviour, such as the effects of recreational drugs, and negotiation with one's sexual partner[23]. Others have argued that the more sophisticated models do take into account how situational factors might impact at the individual level[24]. Theoretically-based behavioural interventions should be able to overcome any such difficulties by employing modelling and qualitative testing prior to application[10].

Sociological theories

Sociological theories also offer considerable potential for guiding the design of behavioural interventions. These theories relate the actions of individuals to the societies in which they live. Unfortunately, one weakness of some potentially useful sociological theories is that there is as yet little empirical support for their application in interventions. One example is the social construction of sexual identity[12]. This theory suggests that sexual identities develop in the course of social interaction with same-sex peers during adolescence, generally being based on prior, non-sexual gender identities. Where conventional gender roles predominate, interactionists suggest that young women view sexual activity as a service to men, while

Table 1 Overview of the main social psychological theories used in behavioural interventions for HIV prevention with examples of evaluated behavioural interventions

Model or theory	Psychological and behavioural determinants	Examples of target thoughts, attitudes or beliefs	Examples of evaluated theory-based interventions
Health belief model	Perceived susceptibility Perceived seriousness of illness Belief in the effectiveness of proposed behaviour Perceived benefit of adopting behaviour Barriers to behaviour adoption Cues to action	*Am I really at risk of HIV?* *Getting HIV would mean health issues would dominate all aspects of my life* *Proper use of condoms reduces the chance of HIV being passed on to me* *Using condoms all the time, I could avoid HIV* *I don't like the feel of wearing a condom* *How many of my friends have HIV and are ill?*	Intervention with female sex workers[58]. Series of 3 sessions that aimed to increase knowledge about HIV and sexually transmitted infections, increased perceived susceptibility to HIV and improve skills related to condom use and condom negotiation with partners. Another intervention using outreach workers targeted clients of the sex workers and the sex workers' pimps and focused on similar points.
Theory of planned behaviour	Attitudes Perceived norms Behaviour intentions	*Sex is just as enjoyable if we use condoms as without condoms* *My friends all use condoms and would expect me to as well* *I intend to make my sexual behaviour less risky by using condoms all the time*	Clinic-based trial of counselling approaches[55]. Compared 3 strategies. Enhances counselling (i.e. more sessions) focused on addressing misconceptions about behaviour, developing individualised risk reduction strategies by improving behavioural intentions and skills training to improve self-efficacy.
Social cognitive theory	Expected outcomes Self-efficacy	*Using condoms all the time, I could avoid HIV* *I know I can get my partner to use condoms*	Inner-city African American adolescents[59]. Black male adolescents randomly assigned to receive an AIDS risk reduction intervention aimed at increasing AIDS-related knowledge and address problematic attitudes toward high risk sexual behaviour.
Stages of change	Pre-contemplation Contemplation Preparation Action Maintenance	*People like me don't need to use condoms* *Using condoms can reduce the chances of getting HIV* *I want to reduce my chances of getting HIV* *I am only going to have sex if we use condoms* *Always using condoms is worthwhile because it reduces my chances of getting HIV*	Clinic-based intervention with gay men[31]. Single session (7 h) small-group workshop. Exercises addressed relevance of personal goals, setting goals, assessing motivations for behaviour change, coping strategies, body image and self-esteem, condom skills and lifestyle balance.
AIDS risk reduction model (ARRM)	Self-labelling Commitment Taking action Maintenance	*I didn't think so before, but I know what I do puts me at risk of HIV infection* *My sex life can be enjoyable if I use condoms I can do it. Condoms are easily available and I know that people will help me* *This was a good decision that I'm going to keep to it*	Intervention with minority women[17]. Three small-group sessions of 3–4 h meeting weekly over 3 weeks. Each session helped women to recognise personal susceptibility, identify ways of reducing risk, building commitment to change behaviours and developing necessary skills to do so (e.g. condom negotiation).

young men see it as a form of personal achievement, and homosexual activity is viewed as antithetical to conventional gender self-identity[12]. Behavioural interventions informed by this theory can encourage people to explore how their understanding of sexuality has been formed predominantly through interaction with their peers, influenced by wider society, so that negative views of one's identity, or stereotypical behaviour can be challenged.

One sociological theory[4] for which there is some empirical evidence in relation to HIV prevention is the theory of 'diffusion of innovations'. This theory describes how material or cultural innovations come to be adopted by communities. Through analysis of the take-up of innovations in different fields, Rogers identified factors that influence the rate of adoption[25]. These include: the characteristics of the social system; the innovation itself; and the characteristics of early and later adopters. According to this theory, early adopters might influence key opinion leaders who in effect become peer-educators within their communities[25]. One limitation is that the theory assumes innovations remain unchanged as a result of their diffusion[25]. While this might be true of physical products, it is easy to imagine that cultural products, such as health promotion messages, might become modified and even distorted in the process of diffusion. This model has been used to inform several carefully evaluated peer-education programmes, including at least two targeting gay men[4,26]. The contrasting findings of these two studies are discussed below.

Sociological analyses also have much to offer behavioural intervention research in explaining socio-economic and cultural factors that can contribute to a population's vulnerability to infection[27,28]. Such theorizing has been an important influence in the targeting of HIV prevention interventions, and in the focus on social and personal empowerment[3,5,27,29].

Use of formative research

Theories can offer general guidance concerning factors addressed by interventions, but there are other aspects they cannot inform. For example, social psychological theory cannot provide guidance on the ideal number and schedule of intervention sessions. Additional research is required to determine which factors need most attention with a specific audience and setting[5,27]. 'Formative research', often in the form of qualitative inquiry, should occur prior to the development of an intervention. Such research can be analogous to phase I development of interventions in clinical medicine, but also has the added benefit of allowing exploration of acceptability, appropriateness and feasibility of the modes of deployment of an intervention[10].

Despite growing recognition of the important contribution of formative research prior to deployment and evaluation of an intervention, findings from this important research phase are often not widely disseminated in the published literature[11]. Shain *et al* report on the formative research they conducted prior to the development and evaluation of an HIV prevention intervention[5,27]. Their 18 month study involved 25 focus groups and 102 in-depth interviews with both men and women to collect background information on values and beliefs, behaviours, strategies to motivate behavioural change and barriers to change as well as the logistics of intervention[27]. They also specify how the background behaviours and beliefs identified, were directly addressed through the intervention[27]. Subsequently, the researchers demonstrated links between the adoption of risk reduction strategies that targeted these behaviours and a decrease in the acquisition of sexually transmitted infections[30]. Funders have recognised the value of these research processes[6,10]. In future, they will need to demonstrate their commitment to funding formative research processes, which in reality are not optional bolt-ons, but central to the development of successful interventions[10].

Evaluating interventions

Rigorous evaluation of effectiveness

While there is little disagreement about the importance of evaluating behavioural interventions, there is still on-going controversy about the most appropriate evaluation methodologies. Evaluation is important to ensure implementation of effective interventions in appropriate settings with appropriate target groups; to stop ineffective or harmful interventions being further deployed[26,31,32]; and to determine the cost-effectiveness of interventions[33]. In order to conclude that an intervention is effective, we need to establish a significant association between positive outcomes and exposure to the intervention in question. This requires minimising the possibility that such an association reflects the effects of some unacknow-ledged factor (*i.e.* confounding), or underlying differences between those who received the intervention and those who do not (*i.e.* bias).

Many, including ourselves, would argue that experimental evaluations, and randomised controlled trials (RCTs) in particular, provide the best means to achieve these objectives. In an uncontrolled study, if an evaluator detects an improvement in the outcome measures compared with baseline measures this might reflect the effects of the intervention or of some other time-related confounding factor (*e.g.* secular trends). However, by comparing the outcomes of the intervention group with those of an equivalent control group, the researcher can take account of this confounding and thus make an assessment of the effects of the intervention itself.

Random allocation, and to a lesser extent matching, appear to offer the best means of ensuring that intervention and control groups resemble each other in terms of factors, for example, age and sexual behaviour that, if they varied between the two groups, could affect outcomes and so bias results. Randomisation should distribute both the known and unknown factors that influence outcomes equally between the groups[34]. It is thus an elegantly simple device for taking account of the multiplicity of social influences on outcomes studied in research[35]. The problem with matching is that it requires knowing about all the relevant factors that can influence outcome, and this is unlikely to be the case. For this reason, RCTs are generally regarded as the most rigorous evaluation design[36].

Increased rigour is a key development in recent behavioural intervention research. The quality of evidence obtained from an evaluation is now likely to be assessed on more than merely random allocation to intervention and control groups. Assessment requires the reporting of baseline characteristics of the intervention and control groups, the mode of randomization, attrition rates in each group at each follow-up, all of the outcomes of both these groups, and sample size calculations in relation to outcomes[11,34].

Acceptance of RCTs in the field of behavioural interventions for HIV prevention is still by no means unanimous[37,38]. Critics have suggested that allocation (random or otherwise) of participants to interventions and control groups is impossible in certain interventions. This, they argue is particularly so in interventions where those from affected communities participate in planning and delivery[37,39]; interventions delivered *via* community networks and structures[40]; and interventions addressing the socio-economic or legislative environment[39]. There are, however, examples of quasi-experimental evaluations of interventions in all these categories, including a group-work intervention developed collaboratively with local voluntary agencies[3]; peer-education sexual health promotion interventions employing community networks[4,41]; and interventions targeting societal determinants of risk among adolescents[20,42].

Another criticism of RCTs of sexual health promotion is that contamination between intervention and control groups will prevent adequate control of confounding[37,43]. In other words, there is more chance that health promotion messages, as opposed to clinical interventions, will come to influence control as well as intervention-group participants. One methodological development that seeks to counter problems of contamination is cluster RCTs. In these, whole sites rather than individuals, are allocated to intervention or control, the belief being that intervention and control site participants are then less likely to interact. Examples of clusters used in experimental evaluations of sexual health promotion include: gyms[26] and cities[41]. However, the possibility exists that an intervention aimed at an intervention cluster could still affect a control cluster, for example because residents of an 'intervention' city travel to a 'control' city, and have sex or otherwise interact with its residents. There is, however, evidence that well-designed studies can avoid problems of contamination between intervention and control clusters by employing clusters whose residents do not intermingle[41] or by statistically controlling for the effects of contamination[44].

These counter-arguments regarding allocation and contamination are not meant to suggest that allocation and contamination difficulties never impede or prevent the use of experimental evaluations in the field of sexual health promotion. Certain interventions, especially those addressing socio-economic and legislative determinants of behaviour, may be difficult or impossible to trial[28,34,42]. Allocation to control and intervention groups may be impossible for practical or ethical reasons. It would have been highly problematic, for example, to evaluate the HIV prevention effect of removing discrimination in the age of consent for male homosexual intercourse by doing so in some UK 'clusters', but not others. Where experimental evaluations genuinely are impossible, other methods, despite providing less clear evidence on effectiveness, must suffice.

Choice of outcome measures

To demonstrate with confidence the effectiveness of behavioural interventions, evaluators need to use outcome measures that reflect the objectives of the intervention and the aims of key stakeholders, including the affected communities. This makes the choice of outcome measures complex. For example, if the aim of an intervention is to reduce sexual risk taking behaviours among young heterosexual women, the choice of outcome measures is not necessarily clear. Should evaluators focus only on measures of behaviour (either the proportion or the actual number of episodes of sex that are deemed to be less risky)? Do indicators of morbidity and other negative sexual health outcomes (e.g. unplanned pregnancy) offer a better measure? The answer is rarely clear-cut and will depend partly on the behaviour of the target population and partly on the aims of the intervention[11,34]. The most appropriate outcomes will therefore be specific to the intervention and the evaluation design, but should always be identified as such at the outset[11,34].

In HIV prevention research, the incidence of new HIV infections in intervention and control groups offers the most valid measure of effect of interventions. However, this has almost never been possible in evaluations of single interventions in industrialised country settings because of low incidence. Nevertheless, other biological outcomes may be suitable proxy indicators of reduced risk[11]. These might, for example, include incident sexually transmitted infections[11]. However, the relationship between sexual behaviour and sexually transmitted infections is not direct or simple[11,45,46]. Studies have shown that specific sexual behaviours cannot predict reductions in infections[32,45,46].

Biological measures can have their own validity problems, concerning definition and ascertainment. Definitions of sexually transmitted infections that are too broad can include infections acquired through less risky sex (*e.g.* oral sex). Ascertainment of cumulative diagnosed infections by record review at the end of an evaluation will yield more endpoints, but miss asymptomatic infections[11,32]. Ascertainment of infections by screening at a given time post-intervention has the advantage of including asymptomatic infections, but requires large numbers to detect differences between trial groups[47]. Bias in measurement of cumulative diagnosed infections is more likely if the intervention changes the probability that individuals will attend clinics. Another potential bias is that of missing infections diagnosed at other clinics[32]. Within the context of an RCT, intervention group participants may be more likely than controls to 'hide' an infection acquired during the study from researchers by having it treated elsewhere[11].

The emphasis on biological endpoints here is not intended to undermine the importance of behavioural measures. However, empirical research has questioned the validity and the accuracy of self-reported sexual behaviour[11,32,48,49]. Use of new technologies, such as computer-assisted self-interview (CASI), instead of traditional face-to-face interviews, are an important methodological advance that may go some way toward addressing the underlining problem[50]. However, unblinded randomised evaluations of behavioural interventions will continue to be vulnerable to biased self-reporting. Even with careful explanation of equipoise, it is difficult to exclude the possibility that people who know they are receiving a certain intervention will feel obliged to under-report risk behaviours more than people who know they are in a control group. Stephenson *et al*'s review of rigorous behavioural intervention trials found that all reported some improvement in one or more self-reported behavioural outcomes, but only two interventions reported declines in sexually transmitted infection rates[11]. It cannot, therefore, be assumed that interventions having a beneficial effect on reported sexual behaviour will have a similar effect on sexually acquired infections[11,32].

The question of which measures constitute the most appropriate outcomes in a given evaluation is unlikely to be resolved quickly, and continued research into the complex epidemiological relationship between behaviours and sexually transmitted infections is needed[45,46,48]. However, as suggested at the outset, the key is that outcomes should be realistic and reflect the aims of the intervention. Where a complex intervention aims to address various determinants of risk in order to reduce

HIV transmission, it is perfectly reasonable to measure biological outcomes. Failure to measure biological measures means that, as evaluators, we will have no means to know whether ultimately we have affected them[11]. However, more modest interventions, such as educational projects, may not in isolation hope to influence biological end-points and so including biological outcome measures might be unrealistic.

A number of behavioural interventions have been reported as effective in increasing rates of condom use, reducing numbers of partners and reducing incidence of STIs within a population[3-5,51]. However, the outcomes of 'negotiated safety' interventions remain unevaluated. While the effects of these interventions have not been as dramatic as the reported effects of STI treatment programmes in reducing HIV infection[52], behavioural and STI treatment approaches to HIV prevention are complementary.

Process evaluation

All outcome evaluations, whether they employ control groups or not, should be conducted alongside process evaluations so that effective interventions can be carefully described, the processes by which an intervention exerts effects (or fails to do so) can be explored, and the context within which an intervention will and will not be effective can be examined[53]. A recent example of such a study is a controlled trial of peer education for gay men in London, which had no apparent impact on HIV risk behaviours[26]. Because the study had an integral process evaluation, the researchers were able to identify possible explanations for intervention 'failure', such as the unacceptability of the intervention to the peer educators who were asked to provide the it[26].

Implementing effective behavioural interventions in HIV prevention practice

The overarching goal of behavioural intervention research is to ensure interventions, particularly those for which there is good evidence of effectiveness, are implemented widely in HIV prevention services. A number of interventions have been identified as 'effective' and ready for implementation[6], yet service providers have been slow to take up these interventions and incorporate them into their services[54]. This is an area where we feel there is likely to be intensified interest in the future[55]. This section examines some of the obstacles to widespread implementation of evidence-based interventions and some of the potential responses.

One of the principal obstacles to wider implementation of interventions may be the degree to which they are targeted and developed for a specific audience[5]. As discussed above, theories used to develop interventions may not be directly transferred from one cultural setting to another. Kelly et al's application of the theory of diffusion of innovations with gay men in the US was demonstrably effective in reducing risk-taking behaviour, while Elford et al's application in the UK was not[4,26]. A recent review of the most rigorously evaluated interventions concluded that an explicit understanding of behaviours, beliefs and risk perceptions seems to be key to developing successful interventions and that the generalisability of interventions may be determined by contextual specificities indicated in the formative research stage[11]. If true, this suggests that an intervention shown to be effective with one target group, cannot be applied with another, or in different setting, with the same anticipated benefit without some new formative research to assess its appropriateness and viability. One strategy that avoids this is to develop interventions, informed by theory and formative research, and to conduct their subsequent evaluation, across diverse populations and in different geographical and possibly, cultural settings[47,51,56]. However, evaluations on this scale are costly, require major personnel resources and are rarely financially or practically feasible for a single intervention.

A second obstacle, critics of randomised trials argue, is that the generalisability of interventions evaluated using trials is especially questionable because of the unusual level of control and care exercised by those conducting the evaluation[37]. Rather than supporting arguments against trials, this suggests that, in order to maximise the likely generalisability of an intervention, similar development processes should be used for interventions that will undergo a trial evaluation as for those that would not. In other words, we should involve affected communities as well as the intended providers of behavioural interventions in the planning and undertaking of intervention studies from the outset[55]. The involvement of affected communities and providers in the development and evaluation of interventions is not inimical either to the use of theory in developing interventions or the employment of rigorous methods of evaluation[53].

Finally, at the level of technology transfer, there are structural obstacles to the implementation of evidence-based interventions. Somlai et al's findings from a survey of community-based prevention organisations in the US showed that few offered workshops on risk self-appraisal and risk-reduction skills even though there was evidence to suggest these approaches were effective with some groups[57]. In the US, a number of programmes are now in place to support and enhance technology transfer between researchers and prevention providers[6,55]. There is also a very small but growing literature that provides the descriptions and evidence for the effectiveness of such work at the level of the HIV prevention providers[55,58].

Conclusions

Development, evaluation and implementation of behavioural interventions has progressed rapidly in the last decade or so. Yet most critical reviews conclude that such interventions have only been modestly successful in reducing HIV transmission risk[11]. However, this should not be a cause for despondency. The necessary rapidity of such developments, generally with limited funding, means that evidence of success should be celebrated. Moreover, the evidence that with appropriate support interventions demonstrated effective under evaluation conditions can be implemented into HIV prevention services suggests that there is real potential for success. What is now required is a consolidation of all the learning that has occurred, and in particular an effort to maintain and further develop theoretical and evaluative rigour, whilst encouraging a participative ethos and multidimensional focus within HIV prevention behavioural interventions.

Acknowledgements

We would like to thank colleagues in the Department of Sexually Transmitted Diseases and the Social Science Research Unit for helpful comments on preliminary drafts of this paper. Our thoughts on psychological and sociological theory have been informed and stimulated by those of Dr Daniel Wight of the MRC Social and Public Health Sciences Unit, Glasgow University, Scotland.

References

1 Anderson R. Prevention works. Plenary paper presented at the *XIIIth International AIDS Conference*, Durban, South Africa. 9–14 July 2000

2 Wasserheit JN, Aral SO. Dynamic topology of sexually transmitted disease epidemics: implications for prevention strategies. *J Infect Dis* 1996; **174** (**Suppl 2**): S201–13

3 Kegeles SM, Hays RB, Coates TJ. The Mpowerment project: a community-level HIV prevention intervention for young gay men. *Am J Public Health* 1996; **86**: 1129–36

4 Kelly JA, Murphy D, Sikkema K *et al*. Outcomes of a randomized controlled community-level HIV prevention intervention: effects on behaviour amongst at-risk gay men in small US cities. *Lancet* 1997; **350**: 1500–5

5 Shain RN, Piper JM, Newton ER *et al*. A randomised, controlled trial of a behavioral intervention to prevent sexually transmitted disease among minority women. *N Engl J Med* 1999; **340**: 93–100

6 CDC. *HIV/AIDS Prevention Research Synthesis Project, Compendium of HIV Prevention Interventions with Evidence of Effectiveness*. Atlanta, GA: Centers for Disease Control and Prevention, 1999

7 Dowsett G. *Practising Desire: Homosexual Sex in the Era of AIDS*. Stanford, CA: Stanford University, 1996

8   NIH. *Interventions to Prevent HIV Risk Behaviors.* NIH Consensus Statement Online 1997 Feb 11–13 [cited 2001, June, 5]; 15(2): 1-41.
    http://odp.od.nih.gov/consensus/cons/104/104_statement.htm

9   King R. *Sexual Behavioural Change for HIV: Where Have Theories Taken Us?* Geneva: UNAIDS, 1999

10 Campbell M, Fitzpatrick R, Haines A *et al.* Framework for design and evaluation of complex interventions to improve health. *BMJ* 2000; **321**: 694–6

11 Stephenson J, Imrie J, Sutton S. Rigourous trials of sexual behaviour interventions in STI/HIV prevention: what can we learn from them? *AIDS* 2000; **14 (Suppl 3)**: S115–24

12 Gagnon JH, Simon W. *Sexual Conduct: The Social Sources of Human Sexuality.* London: Hutchinson, 1974

13 Ajzen I. The theory of planned behavior. *Organizational Behavior Hum Decision Processes* 1991; **50**: 179–211

14 Sutton S. Using the theories of reasoned action and planned behaviour to develop health behaviour interventions: Problems and assumption. In: Rutter DR, Quine L. (eds) *Changing Health Behaviour: Research and Practice with Social Cognition Models.* Buckingham: Open University Press, 2001 (In press)

15 Rawson D. The growth of health promotion theory and its rational reconstruction: lessons from the philosophy of science. In: Bunton R, MacDonald G. (eds) *Health Promotion: Disciplines and Diversity.* London: Routledge, 1992; 202–24

16 Caplan R. The importance of social theory for health promotion: from discussion to reflexivity. *Health Promotion Int* 1993; **8**: 147–57

17 World Health Organization. *Global Strategy of Health for All by the Year 2000.* Copenhagen: WHO Regional Office for Europe, 1981

18 Parish R. Health promotion: rhetoric and reality. In: Bunton R, Nettleton S, Burrows R. (eds) *The Sociology of Health Promotion.* London: Routledge, 1995; 13–23

19 Altman D. Expertise, legitimacy and the centrality of community. In: Aggleton P, Davies P, Hart G. (eds) *AIDS: Facing the Second Decade.* London: Falmer, 1993; 1–12

20 Olsen RJ, Farkas G. Employment opportunity can decrease adolescent childbearing within the underclass. *Eval Program Planning* 1991; **14**: 27–34

21 Becker MH. The health belief model and personal health behaviour. *Health Educ Monographs* 1974; **2**: 324–508

22 Catania JA, Kegeles SM, Coates TJ. Towards an understanding of risk behavior: an AIDS risk reduction model (ARRM). *Health Educ Q* 1991; **17**: 53–72

23 Davies P. Acts, sessions and individuals: a model for analyzing sexual behaviour. In: Boulton M. (ed) *Challenge and Innovation. Methodological Advances in Social Research on HIV/AIDS.* London: Taylor & Francis, 1994; 57–68

24 Abraham C, Sherran P. Modelling and modifying young heterosexuals' HIV-preventive behaviour; a review of theories, findings and educational implications. *Patient Educ Counsel* 1994; **23**: 173–86

25 Rogers EM. *The Diffusion of Innovations.* New York, NY: Free Press, 1983

26 Elford J, Bolding G, Sherr L. Peer education has no significant impact on HIV risk behaviours among gay men in London. *AIDS* 2000; **15**: 535–8

27 Ramos R, Shain R, Johnson L. 'Men I mess with don't have anything to do with AIDS': using ethno-theory to understand sexual risk perception. *Sociol Q* 1995; **36**: 483–504

28 Parker RG, Easton D, Klein CH. Structural barriers and facilitators in HIV prevention: a review of international literature. *AIDS* 2000; **14 (Suppl 1)**: S22–32

29 Homans H, Aggleton P. Health education, HIV infection and AIDS. In: Aggleton P, Homans H. (eds) *Social Aspects of AIDS.* Lewes: Falmer, 1988; 154–76

30 Shain RN, Perdue S, Piper JM *et al.* Sexual risk reduction behaviors amenable to intervention: The importance of context. *Conference Proceedings, 13th Meeting of the International Society for Sexually Transmitted Disease Research,* 11–14 July 1999. Denver CO, USA. Abstract 001

31 Christopher FS, Roosa MW. An evaluation of adolescent pregnancy prevention program: is 'just say no' enough? *Fam Relat* 1990; **39**: 68–72

32 Imrie J, Stephenson JM, Cowan FM *et al.* A cognitive behavioural intervention to reduce sexually transmitted infections among gay men: randomised trial. *BMJ* 2001; **322**: 1451–6

33 Holtgrave DR, Kelly JA. Preventing HIV/AIDS among high risk urban women: the cost effectiveness of behavioral group intervention. *Am J Public Health* 1996; **86**: 1442–5

34 Stephenson J, Imrie J. Why do we need randomised controlled trials to assess behavioural interventions? *BMJ* 1998; **316**: 611–3

35 Oakley A. Who's afraid of the randomised controlled trial? In: Roberts H. (ed) *Women's Health Counts*. London: Routledge, 1990; 167–94

36 Chalmers I, Enkin M, Keirse MJNC. *Effective Care in Pregnancy and Childbirth*. Oxford: Oxford University, 1990

37 Kippax S, van de Ven P. An epidemic of orthodoxy? Design and methodology in the evaluation of the effectiveness of HIV health promotion. *Crit Public Health* 1998; **8**: 371–86

38 van de Ven P, Aggleton P. What constitutes evidence in HIV/AIDS education? *Health Educ Res* 1999; **14**: 461–71

39 Nutbeam D. Oakley's case for using randomised controlled trials is misleading. *BMJ* 1999; **318**: 944–5

40 Downie RS, Tannahill C, Tannahill A. *Health Promotion: Models and Values*. Oxford: Oxford University, 1996

41 Williamson LM, Hart GJ, Flowers P, Frankis JS, Der GJ. The gay men's task force: the impact of peer-education on the sexual health behaviour of gay men in Glasgow. *Sex Transm Infect* 2001; In press

42 Rotheram-Borus MJ. Expanding the range of interventions to reduce HIV among adolescents. *AIDS* 2000; **14 (Suppl 1)**: S33–40

43 Webb D. *Measuring Effectiveness in Health Promotion*. Southampton: University of Southampton, 1997

44 Torgerson DJ. Contamination in trials: is cluster randomisation the answer? *BMJ* 2001; **322**: 355–7

45 Peterman TA, Lin LS, Newman DR *et al*. Does measured behavior reflect STD risk? An analysis of data from a randomized controlled behavioral intervention study. *Sex Transm Dis* 2000; **27**: 446–51

46 Fishbein M, Jarvis B. Failure to find a behavioral surrogate for STD incidence – what does it really mean? *Sex Transm Dis* 2000; **27**: 452–5

47 National Institute of Mental Health Multisite HIV Prevention Trial Group. The NIMH multisite HIV prevention trial: reducing HIV sexual risk behaviour. *Science* 1998; **280**: 1889–94

48 Aral SO, Peterman TA. Do we know the effectiveness of behavioural interventions? *Lancet* 1998; **351 (Suppl 3)**: 33–6

49 Zenilman JM, Weisman CS, Rompalo AM *et al*. Condom use to prevent incident STDs: the validity of self-reported condom use. *Sex Transm Dis* 1995; **22**: 15–21

50 McQueen D, Campostrini S. Monitoring behavioural change in the population: a continuous data collection approach. In: Boulton M. (ed) *Challenge & Innovation. Methodological Advances in Social Research on HIV/AIDS*. London, Taylor & Francis, 1994; 39–56

51 Kamb ML, Fishbein M, Douglas JM *et al*. Efficacy of risk-reduction counselling to prevent human immunodeficiency virus and sexually transmitted diseases: a randomized control trial. *JAMA* 1998; **280**: 1161–7

52 Hayes R, Nicholl A, Grosskurth H *et al*. A community trial of the impact of improved sexually transmitted disease treatment on the HIV epidemic in rural Tanzania. *AIDS* 1995; **9**: 1–26

53 Peersman G, Harden A, Oliver S. *Effectiveness of Health Promotion Interventions in the Workplace: A Review*. London: Health Education Authority, 1998

54 DiFrancesico W, Kelly JA, Otto-Salaj L *et al*. Factors influencing attitudes with AIDS service organizations toward the use of research-based HIV prevention interventions. *AIDS Educ Prev* 1999; **11**: 72–86

55 Anon. Turning HIV prevention research into practice (special supplement). *AIDS Educ Prev* 2000; **12 (Suppl A)**: 1–145

56 CDC AIDS Community Demonstration Projects Research Group. Community-level HIV intervention in five cities: final outcome data from the CDC AIDS Community Demonstration Projects. *Am J Public Health* 1999; **89**: 336–45

57 Somlai AM, Kelly JA, Otto-Salaj L et al. Current HIV prevention activities for women and gay men among 77 ASOs. *J Public Health Manage Pract* 1999; **5**: 23–33

58 Kelly JA, Somlai AM, DiFranceisco W *et al*. Bridging the gap between the science and service of HIV prevention: transferring effective research-based HIV prevention interventions to community AIDS service providers. *Am J Public Health* 2000; **90**: 1082–8

59 Ford K, Wirawan D, Fajans P *et al*. Behavioral interventions for reduction of sexually transmitted disease/HIV transmission among female commercial sex workers and clients in Bali, Indonesia. *AIDS* 1996; **10**: 213–22

60 Jemmott JB, Jemmott LS, Fong GT. Reductions in HIV risk-associated sexual behaviors among black male adolescents: effects of an AIDS prevention intervention. *Am J Public Health* 1992; **82**: 372–7

HIV care in non-industrialised countries

Charles F Gilks

Division of Tropical Medicine, Liverpool School of Tropical Medicine, Liverpool, UK

The HIV/AIDS epidemic is now most rapidly expanding in the non-industrialised world. As more and more poor people fall sick and die prematurely, the issue of care for the HIV-infected person living in a resource-poor country is of paramount importance. Rational and comprehensive care packages need to be based on proper understanding of the natural history of infection and accurate measurement of the HIV/AIDS disease burden. In the early stages of infection, disease progression is the same in non-industrialised nations as it is in industrialised countries. Once virulent diseases start, survival is short largely because of limited access to inadequate health care. Therefore, early HIV-related disease, as well as AIDS, are targets for care. Needs are diverse but can be considered as more of the same (*e.g.* to cope with additional cases of TB generated by HIV) and those new services such as voluntary counselling and testing and palliative care. Budgets are limited everywhere, but prioritisation can be promoted through drawing up a hierarchy of care needs. Specific HIV/AIDS services and the provision of anti-retroviral therapy come after basic services are implemented. Affordable ways to use disease-modifying drugs need to be pursued that are relevant to non-industrialised countries and which do not promote AIDS exceptionalism.

Human immunodeficiency virus (HIV) infection has now been recorded in every region of the world. With high-quality disease surveillance, the end-stage clinical manifestations of infection characteristic of acquired immunodeficiency syndrome (AIDS) were first noticed in a rich industrialised country. However, two decades after it was first described, it is abundantly clear that the main brunt of the epidemic is falling on resource-poor countries particularly in sub-Saharan Africa[1].

This has been a mixed blessing for non-industrialised nations. Undoubtedly, far more resources have been devoted to studying the virus and the spectrum of infectious and other diseases associated with a waning immune system than would have been the case if HIV had been an exclusively tropical problem. When an effective preventive vaccine is eventually manufactured, all will benefit. However, much of the new knowledge and many of the new products generated are geared to resource-rich nations and, therefore, usually have little relevance to resource-poor regions. This is particularly so with recent developments in

Correspondence to:
Prof. Charles F Gilks,
Division of Tropical
Medicine, Liverpool
School of Tropical
Medicine,
Pembroke Place,
Liverpool L3 5QA, UK

the care of the HIV-infected person – dependent on high-technology approaches to diagnosing and managing clinical disease, and ready access to highly active anti-retroviral therapy that is almost universally accessible in the West[2].

With all that has been published and written about HIV/AIDS care, it may seem strange to say that in non-industrialised countries the first problem is a relative dearth of knowledge about the spectrum of HIV-related disease, how to diagnose and treat in a resource-poor setting. It is also an undoubted problem that very little has been done to describe rational and appropriate approaches to care in communities where at best most sick people only have access to the bare minimum of clinical services[3]. And whilst there is now clear awareness of the global inequity in the differential access to anti-retroviral therapy (ART) according to the financial status of the patient's homeland, and much has been written and said about drugs, HIV care in the non-industrialised world is not just about lack of drug[4].

Natural history of HIV/AIDS relevant to care

High background morbidity, not rapid early disease progression

One feature distinguishes the natural history of HIV in non-industrialised countries from that described in rich industrialised societies – dealing with the consequences of progressive ill-health and immunosuppression on a background of poverty and lack of resources. The environment for most poor people is unhygienic and unhealthy, characterised by high exposure to ordinary, as well as opportunistic, pathogens. With such exposure, it is well recognised that infants in the tropics suffer far higher rates of acute respiratory infections, tuberculosis and diarrhoeal disease than in the West.

Adults are also similarly exposed. Knowing that HIV infection predisposes to specific bacterial and mycobacterial infections in the West, it will come as no surprise that, in the slums and shanties of the non-industrialised world, tuberculosis, pneumococcal disease and non-typhi salmonellosis are all leading clinical problems[5]. As these pathogens are all virulent and quite capable of causing disease in the immuno-competent adult as well as child, it again will come as no surprise that such HIV-related problems cause significant morbidity in the early stages of disease progression[6]. Survival following these early events may also be relatively good. Thus one carefully conducted cohort study in Uganda noted a median survival in excess of 4.1 years following pulmonary tuberculosis and 3.36 years following acute bacterial infection[7].

Another consequence of high exposure to virulent pathogens is that early manifestations of HIV may develop quite soon after sero-conversion. These features are incorporated in the WHO staging system[8] and if time to the different stages is considered (*e.g.* from seroconversion to stage 2 median 29 months; and to stage 3, 46 months[7]) transition time can be interpreted as rapid disease progression. This particularly happens in cohorts where individuals are known to be HIV-positive, and where staging data may be backed up by limited clinical investigation of morbid events – because clinical manifestations are often over-fitted into AIDS diagnoses[9]. Furthermore, several stage 2 (weight loss, minor mucocutaneous manifestations) and stage 3 events (marked weight loss, unexplained prolonged fever) are common in HIV-uninfected community controls when included, and these events occur at relatively high frequencies irrespective of HIV status[7]. When staging is carefully conducted and matched with CD4 counts, it is clear that survival times for patients in the early stages of HIV do not indicate rapid progression[7,10].

Several groups propose that the higher background rates of endemic disease (in particular helminth infections, tuberculosis, sexually transmitted infections and, in many areas, malaria) generate 'immune activation' which drives rapid progression. Whilst this may be demonstrated *in vitro* in both HIV-infected and uninfected Africans (in and out of Africa)[11], it is difficult to reconcile this with lack of evidence of this occurring in the early stages of HIV. Whilst viral loads may go up with acute malaria, this may only be transient and associated with acute febrile episodes; the outcome this may have on progression is likely to be limited[12]. The most likely candidate disease significantly to disturb the immune system is tuberculosis. Even here whilst individual studies may show worse survival with TB, the control groups may not be strictly comparable[13]; a comprehensive recent review found little evidence epidemiologically of a significant interaction[14]. In African patients in the UK, there is no difference in survival with tuberculosis – indeed survival is better if TB is the first AIDS-indicator disease[15].

Poor survival with clinical AIDS

Poverty also influences disease presentation and quality of care. With few resources at hand, health seeking behaviour may be significantly compromised with delay resulting in late clinical presentation, and this is likely to increase mortality even in readily treatable conditions. It is extremely hard to quantify this in any fashion. Household studies would need to be very large, and identifying morbidity in any ethical study requires that the event is properly managed and treated. An indirect measure of this is the much higher rates of mortality for community-acquired pneumonia in predominantly young adults in Kenya of 10%[16]; in the UK comparable age-adjusted rates would be only 1–2%.

Whatever impact late presentation may have, it is compounded by inadequate healthcare services in which the facilities may be very basic and the quality of care provided highly compromised. The supply of essential drugs cannot always be maintained and simple diagnostic tests and radiology may not be available because of lack of supplies or machine faults. Trained staff may not be on hand to deliver even a limited basic package of care, either because they are not paid a living wage and need second jobs, or because HIV/AIDS is itself taking a toll on clinical staff. There are sadly no data to suggest in the non-industrialised world that healthcare staff are using superior knowledge about HIV to reduce their own risks of infection. There is little primary medical care and continuity of care in the community on discharge can rarely be organised.

These issues are likely to be critical with more severe ill-health and immunosuppression. There are far more data from Africa on mortality with an AIDS-defining illness, or when a patient develops stage 4 illness. All studies suggest that survival is far shorter than in the West[17]. In a rural Ugandan cohort, median survival with stage 4 clinical AIDS was 9 months[18]. In an urban Ugandan cohort, median survival with a CD4 count less than 200 was 9 months, whereas survival in an urban US cohort before the introduction of highly active anti-retroviral therapy median survival was 19–20 months[10]. Whether this is all just inadequate health care, or whether inadequately treated virulent infections significantly up-regulate viral replication, drop CD4 counts and hasten death is not clear.

Clearly some patients do present with profound immuno-suppression[19], but it is unclear how long they have been in this state, whether it is recent and a consequence of viral activation, or long-standing. In some patients with virulent infections, low CD4 counts rise on therapy[6]. It must also be remembered that these data do not indicate rapid progression to the point of development of AIDS, only impaired survival with AIDS. Unfortunately, many authors look just at time-to-death and conclude that rapid disease progression throughout the course of HIV infection must be taking place[20], assuming that all death occurs at a similar point in the disease process[21].

Rarity of the classical Western opportunistic infections

With high early morbidity and mortality in non-industrialised countries, it is to be expected that fewer people will survive long enough to develop profound immunosuppression or will survive long in such a state. Thus even with the ubiquitous exposure to opportunistic infections (OIs) in the environment, the rate of developing such conditions will be far lower in resource-poor countries for people who are poor and use government facilities. It is important to point out that the more affluent users of private hospitals are likely to experience a more typical western pattern of OIs, but these groups are in all non-industrialised countries just a small minority.

Pneumocystis pneumonia occurs but is consistently identified only in small numbers of patients who are from highly selected populations and bronchoscoped[22], or at autopsy[23]. Whilst *Mycobacterium avium* infection does occur in Kenya, it is estimated to occur in only about 1% of HIV/AIDS patients admitted to hospital[24]. Autopsy data suggest, in some areas at least, that toxoplasma lesions may be common[23], but clinical studies suggest far fewer patients actually present with encephalitis; it seems that many of these lesions may be clinically silent, contributing little to clinical outcome. Geography may play some role here with potentially different rates of toxoplasm exposure, although in Kenya where rates of clinical disease are very low, the majority of adults have toxoplasma antibodies[25]. The most important true opportunists seem to be fungal, with *Cryptococcus neoformans* a problem across the tropics[26] and *Penicillium marnefii* restricted to South-East Asia[27].

Epidemiology of the HIV/AIDS disease burden

The size of the HIV/AIDS disease burden

Surveillance for HIV infection is now well established in most non-industrialised countries, with surveys of at-risk or sentinel groups regularly conducted. However, one epidemiological issue has not received appropriate attention, the burden of HIV/AIDS disease. Incredibly, in the second decade of the epidemic, no non-industrialised country has yet generated figures that document comprehensively the actual volume of HIV/AIDS disease presenting to the health services for care. Disease surveillance is at best haphazard, often relying just on the reporting of 'clinical AIDS' cases. This omits early HIV-related disease, as much presents without stigmata of underlying HIV infection.

Such an approach is based on western experience, where AIDS dominates clinical care but has little relevance where early non-AIDS disease is at least as important[21]. Only with tuberculosis is regular serological surveillance carried out and this is still far too haphazard in most countries. Most care is delivered in health centres and community clinics, yet almost no disease surveillance has been carried out at this

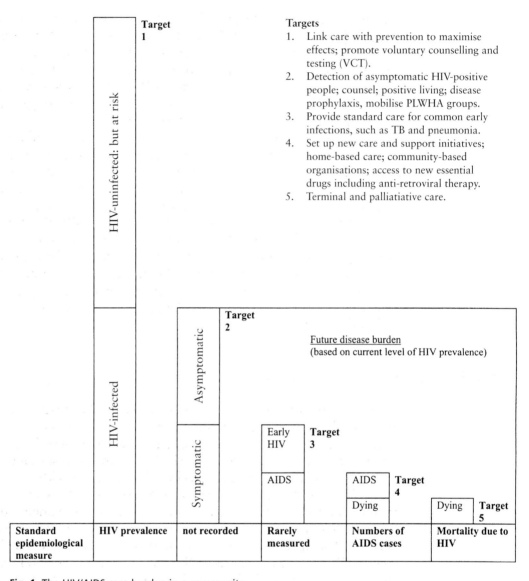

Fig. 1 The HIV/AIDS care burden in a community.

Targets within the figure:

Targets
1. Link care with prevention to maximise effects; promote voluntary counselling and testing (VCT).
2. Detection of asymptomatic HIV-positive people; counsel; positive living; disease prophylaxis, mobilise PLWHA groups.
3. Provide standard care for common early infections, such as TB and pneumonia.
4. Set up new care and support initiatives; home-based care; community-based organisations; access to new essential drugs including anti-retroviral therapy.
5. Terminal and palliatiative care.

level. Without knowing how much HIV/AIDS disease is presenting, where and at what stage of disease progression, it is impossible to describe adequately the care burden of any community (Fig. 1).

The HIV epidemic is dynamic and rapidly evolving across the non-industrialised world. Some countries may at last be showing stability or reductions in HIV prevalence[1]. However, this has not yet had time to translate into stability in disease burden, where the number of people falling sick and needing significant healthcare equals the number of people dying. In all non-industrialised countries, far more people are starting to fall sick with HIV/AIDS and steady state may be decades away. The consequences of this on the health system will be profound, but have hardly been touched upon. Clearly the demand for care will escalate for the foreseeable future; and because current disease surveillance focusing just on clinical AIDS is far too crude and inexact to generate any meaningful information or to capture changes evolving over time, active surveillance must be set up[28].

All HIV-related disease is 'new' in the sense that it would not have developed without the HIV epidemic. In high-prevalence countries this additional, new burden of disease presenting for care may be very large and growing, and may have a significant impact on healthcare services themselves. This is because the existing, pre-AIDS disease burden has not diminished in any way as the epidemic of HIV/AIDS disease has taken off. Few high-prevalence countries have been able to increase health spend in anticipation of this additional burden of disease; indeed, some health budgets have actually diminished in real terms. Another problem with inadequate disease surveillance is that it is quite unclear how such unprecedented shifts in the burden of disease have been met by health services.

The evolving and ever-growing disease burden

We have conducted two longitudinal studies in hospitals facing large HIV care burdens – one serving a rural district, Hlabisa in KwaZulu Natal, the other a government facility in an urban centre, Nairobi. The earliest evidence of the impact of HIV is the rapid and sustained rise in TB cases. In Hlabisa, the TB workload had doubled within 3 years of HIV being identified in the district in 1990; by 1997, 57% of all TB was attributable to HIV with an HIV prevalence in new patients of 67% (when a condition like HIV is common in the background population, it must be assumed that some patients with TB are coincidentally infected)[29]. In contrast, clinical AIDS cases were relatively rare in 1997 indicating the relatively long period the later stage diseases take to develop and perhaps that significant proportion of people die before developing clinical AIDS.

In Nairobi, the trends with time are equally revealing. Over a decade (1988–1997), the number of HIV-infected patients admitted per day to one hospital increased steadily from 4.3 to 13.9. There was a consistent pattern of disease over the study period, with bacteraemia and myco-bacteraemia predominating, and there was no evidence of the classic western opportunistic infections emerging as the AIDS epidemic has matured[30]. HIV prevalence in patients hospitalised in Nairobi doubled from 19% in 1988/1989 to 39% in 1992. Initial trends suggested that the sick HIV/AIDS cases were crowding out the HIV-uninfected patients and that mortality rates were rising, effects that had been widely predicted[31]. However, in 1997, admissions increased irrespective of HIV status, so the HIV prevalence stabilised at 40% whilst hospital bed occupancy nearly doubled from 105% to 190%. Far fewer patients with clinical AIDS were admitted over the decade (39% of HIV-positive patients initially falling to 24% in 1997) probably because of changes in health-seeking behaviour. Carers seem less likely to bring in potential AIDS sufferers because of perceived stigmatisation or lack of confidence that much can be achieved. With a changing spectrum of early versus late disease/AIDS over the time period, in-patient mortality actually significantly fell – from 36% to 23% – despite the rise in bed occupancy[32]. These counter-intuitive results may be unique to Nairobi, or a common feature in non-industrialised countries. It is very frustrating to note that there are no other comparable data bases to refer to. If these responses are common, then they have important implications for care particularly if patients with end-stage disease remain in the community.

Planning and implementing a comprehensive care policy

Comprehensive care across the continuum

HIV/AIDS is a spectral disease that progresses through several more or less distinct stages. This is important when considering what care needs to be provided, because this clearly relates to the different stages of disease (Fig. 2). This is not so obvious if there is limited perception of the importance of early disease; or if it is invisible because there is no surveillance system in place to record it[21]. On the other hand, it is emphasised by discussing the need to provide 'comprehensive care across the continuum', a phrase first coined by van Praag when in the WHO.

An overt focus on clinical AIDS has tended to obscure the earlier, more treatable part of the disease process, minimised the true impact that is being felt in hospitals and perhaps health centres and constrained the development of comprehensive care policies. Care is not synonymous with home-based care and trying to deliver services just for patients with AIDS is an incomplete response. Focusing on AIDS alone, re-inforces the negative, that we have little control over this disease, and can do very little good – rather than the positive, that much early disease is successfully treated and that even with basic drugs and facilities something can always be done. It is bad for the patient and his or her carer who need to be encouraged and educated into realising that they can do something for themselves by early presentation of symptoms – especially in TB but with other acute problems too. It is also very bad for staff motivation and morale and although poorly documented both recruitment and staff retention are becoming major problems for health services in high-prevalence countries.

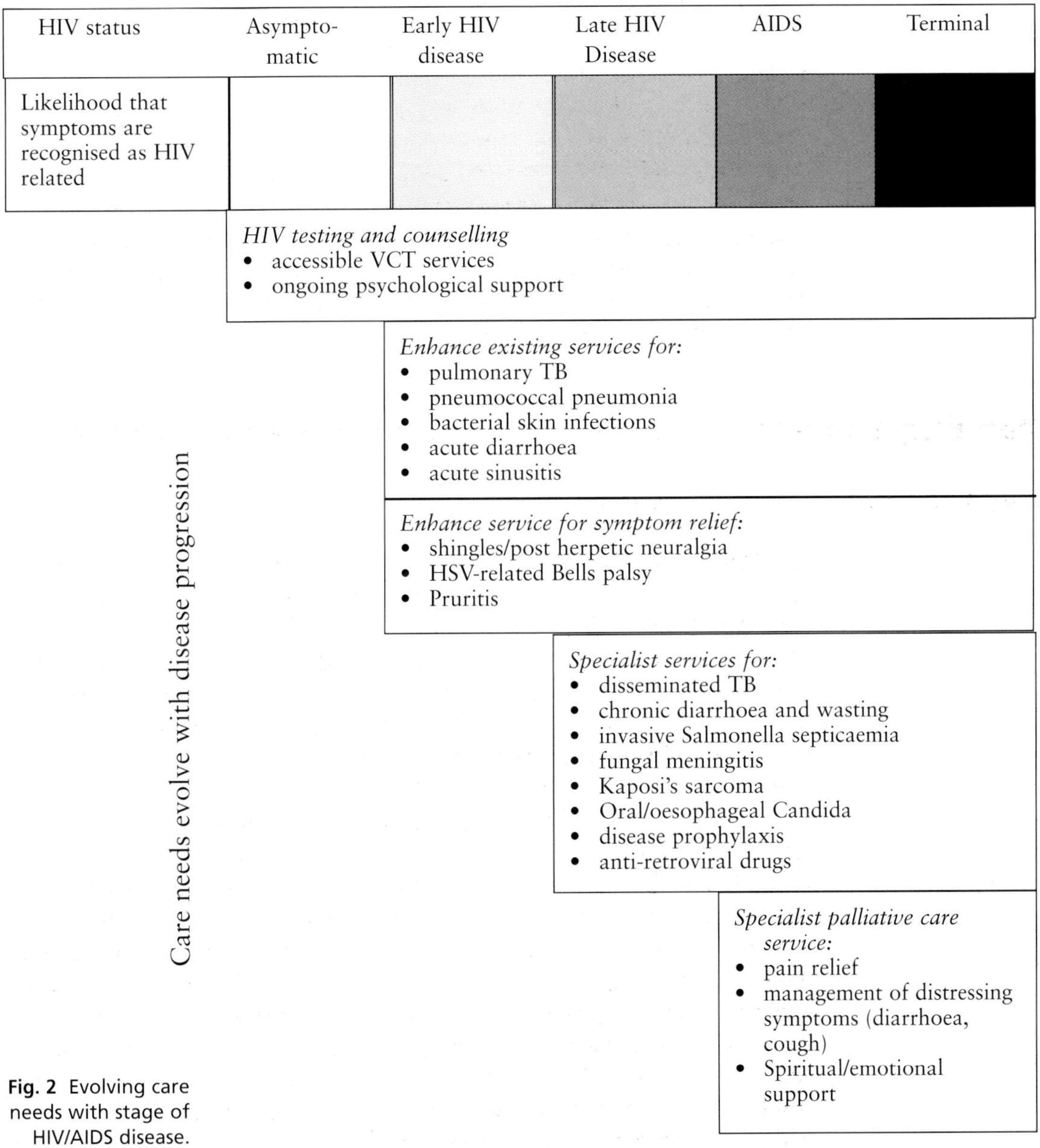

HIV status	Asympto-matic	Early HIV disease	Late HIV Disease	AIDS	Terminal
Likelihood that symptoms are recognised as HIV related					

HIV testing and counselling
- accessible VCT services
- ongoing psychological support

Enhance existing services for:
- pulmonary TB
- pneumococcal pneumonia
- bacterial skin infections
- acute diarrhoea
- acute sinusitis

Enhance service for symptom relief:
- shingles/post herpetic neuralgia
- HSV-related Bells palsy
- Pruritis

Specialist services for:
- disseminated TB
- chronic diarrhoea and wasting
- invasive Salmonella septicaemia
- fungal meningitis
- Kaposi's sarcoma
- Oral/oesophageal Candida
- disease prophylaxis
- anti-retroviral drugs

Specialist palliative care service:
- pain relief
- management of distressing symptoms (diarrhoea, cough)
- Spiritual/emotional support

Care needs evolve with disease progression

Fig. 2 Evolving care needs with stage of HIV/AIDS disease.

New services to set up

Planning a response involves identifying what new services or interventions are needed that were either not widely promoted or did not exist prior to the HIV/AIDS epidemic. The most important of these are counselling services which have a pivotal role in HIV/AIDS care[33]. Voluntary counselling and testing (VCT) is the entry point to care – without a person knowing his or her positive HIV status, it is obvious that specific care services cannot be effectively utilised. Because of the stigmatisation and discrimination around the diagnosis, it is universally accepted that there are special constraints around making a diagnosis of HIV infection that do not exist with other infectious or terminal conditions. This involves discussing the possibility of the diagnosis, then if the patient or client so wishes, informing the person of the test result. The process is voluntary and implies consent to the test procedure. This is a new concept which has come with HIV in non-industrialised as in industrialised countries. It has meant putting in place a new cadre of staff trained in counselling and implementing a new service. It is also a service which links the entry-point to care effectively with HIV prevention[34,35]. One may hope that with more people knowing their HIV status that the demand for effective care services downstream may then grow, as in the West people living with HIV/AIDS have been very effective advocates for this. One important point to note in linking care with prevention is that in non-industrialised countries, the credibility of AIDS programmes will increasingly be judged by the quality of care they offer[36].

At the other end of the disease process is the need for palliative care services[37]. Whilst death is not new, the HIV/AIDS epidemic has focused attention on the needs of the dying[3]. Prior to HIV, death usually came at the extremes of life and the economically active adults (usually the women or mother) provided the necessary care and support. There was relatively little call for specialised terminal care. Unfortunately, all this has changed with the HIV epidemic as it is precisely this group who are falling sick and dying; whilst some people die relatively quickly with overwhelming infection, many have chronic and debilitating end-stage disease. The traditional social safety net in most non-industrialised countries is the extended family. This is being overwhelmed by the death of so many breadwinners and heads of household and cannot cope.

More of the same

The early disease burden comprises virulent infections such as TB, pneumonia and Gram-negative sepsis, which may present with fairly typical clinical features but at much higher rates. Blood-stream invasion is common[38]. These diseases usually respond well to standard therapy[3,17].

Indeed impressive improvements can be achieved in survival without high-technology inputs or non-essential drugs[30]. With TB, the delivery of standard therapy with DOTS is a major advance. Thus the problem in managing these patients is not that the diseases are new and require new facilities and drugs, but simply that there is extra volume to treat. It must be emphasised that HIV-uninfected people get TB, pneumonia and invasive bacterial infections, albeit at lower rates than those with underlying HIV infection. It is important to concentrate on care services that will serve all – both for equity, and because those negative will increasingly be expected to care for their sick relatives in the community.

This is recognised very well for tuberculosis control, perhaps because TB is vertically organised and there is an effective global TB unit in WHO. Certainly the most important HIV-associated disease from a care perspective as well as public health perspective is TB. However, most TB control is delivered outside hospital, and delivering 'more of the same' needs also to take into account clinical problems that present to the general medical services. Whilst in Nairobi it is not invariably the case that these services will collapse[32], without somehow being strengthened and supported the staff will suffer great stress and morale and motivation will inevitably suffer.

Research relevant to non-industrialised countries

Clinical and operational research has a vital role to play in planning rational care policies for a new epidemic. Unfortunately, most research on HIV/AIDS disease is conducted in resource-rich countries and is of very little relevance to non-industrialised countries. Sufficient data exist to be clear that there is a different spectrum of disease in poor communities; that virulent bacterial and mycobacterial infections predominate, and will respond to standard treatment. One remaining issue is whether such morbidity can be prevented.

A number of studies have shown that preventive treatment (chemoprophylaxis) given for 3–12 months protects against TB in adults infected with HIV, at least in the short-to-medium term. Protection is greatest in subjects who are ppd-skin test positive[39]. This intervention requires all patients to be carefully screened for active TB to prevent inadvertent monotherapy. Co-trimoxazole chemoprophylaxis offers protection against morbidity, and in patients with tuberculosis against mortality, in a region with low community levels of drug resistance, largely by preventing pneumonia, bacterial infections and malaria[40,41]. In most non-industrialised countries co-trimoxazole resistance is widespread and it is not clear how effective chemoprophylaxis will be in such areas. The problems with any intervention which requires regular pill-taking is ensuring adequate adherence and in a resource poor environment may limit the widespread implementation of primary prevention. Unfortunately, pneumococcal polysaccharide vaccination, a single injection deliverable without any adherence issues, has recently proved to be ineffective and may even be harmful in African adults infected with HIV[42]. More research is required in appropriate primary disease prophylaxis.

A hierarchy of care

Prioritising care needs

Non-industrialised countries are invariably short of financial resources and cannot afford to implement all of these initiatives included in a comprehensive and rational care package. There is a clear need to prioritise the more critical from those less vital, which depends on what infrastructure already is in place. With this in mind it is possible to construct a hierarchy of care services (Table 1)[43].

Such a practical approach may appear to be inimical, and indeed some AIDS activists dispute the validity and morality of such an approach – specialist services including ART must be made available now, as it is in the West. Others feel that this is grounded in reality and that, whilst it is important to press for more resources just for HIV/AIDS, in the real world there are competing needs in public health and disease care and priorities have to be selected. It would seem sensible only to advocate widespread specialist services when other more basic services for HIV/AIDS patients can be assured.

Access to anti-retroviral therapy

To many activists in the West, the main issue about HIV/AIDS care is even more focused on the huge inequity in access to ART in the non-industrialised world, now bearing the main brunt of the HIV epidemic. Somehow mechanisms must be found to provide drugs so that the single global standard of care for HIV/AIDS, that practised in the West, can be adopted. This ignores the huge investment necessary in the capacity to use such drugs properly (training, laboratory monitoring, drug distribution); and runs the risk of being inequitable itself, as so many resources are devoted to HIV/AIDS. What about malaria, tuberculosis and the other diseases of poverty the majority HIV-uninfected also suffer from. AIDS exceptionalism of this magnitude runs the very real risk of generating a major backlash and cannot be sustainable[44].

Table 1 A hierarchy of different care levels for resource-poor countries

Care level	Services	Comments
The essential minimum *To be able to deliver any form of HIV/AIDS care and support, a certain minimum level of specific services needs to be provided.*	• Universally accessible HIV testing. • Support and counselling for the person with HIV/AIDS. • Information and education which includes clear prognosis and advice on care and support issues. • Access to PWHIV/AIDS groups.	• Most countries in Africa have started implementing these basic minimum essential services. • Once implemented, providing basic HIV/AIDS education and information, and training staff in counselling and support skills, is relatively cheap and sustainable.
Basic care delivery within the existing healthcare services *Most HIV/AIDS clinical care in Africa is delivered by the existing health services, which are under increasing pressure as demand grows. Extra capacity must be developed; if not services will deteriorate or collapse and the whole community will suffer.*	• Restructured tuberculosis control services with the capacity to cope with rising demand. • Restructured hospital services with the capacity to cope with rising and changing case-load in equitable fashion (HIV/AIDS and non-HIV equally considered). • Improved primary healthcare services (health centres, clinics and dispensaries) to include specific HIV/AIDS care packages. • More resources for terminal care.	• DOTS is being introduced and will improve the capacity for TB control to be delivered. • Where confidence exists in hospital care, crowding out of patients and reduced quality of services are becoming evident. No solutions are yet identified. • Often spare capacity in clinics and health centres; little yet done to develop existing potential or improve referral patterns.
Introducing specific HIV/AIDS clinical services *It will usually be appropriate to set up specific (new) HIV/AIDS clinical services only if basic level services are in place, and the existing health services are delivering effective basic care.*	• The purchase and provision of drugs for opportunistic infections that are not on essential drugs list. • Establishment of technology to diagnose and manage common opportunistic infections. • Provision of clinics and centres from where primary/secondary prophylaxis can be delivered.	• To pay for such services, more money has to be voted to the health sector or redistributed within existing health budget. • For many African countries, the initial stumbling block has been the treatment of fungal infection • Equity and access issues complex and largely unresolved.
Providing disease-modifying anti-retroviral therapy *At present this is very expensive to implement; it is likely to be more cost-effective to increase life-span in Africa by reducing the incidence and improving outcome of specific HIV/AIDS infections, particularly TB.*	• The purchase and provision of anti-retroviral drugs in keeping with current consensus guidelines. • Establishment of technology to manage HIV/AIDS patients on anti-retroviral therapy. • Expansion of existing HIV/AIDS treatment clinics to accommodate anti-retroviral therapy.	• Massive investment necessary to finance such a new initiative, and sustain it once implemented. • If poorly implemented, threat of drug-resistance is major concern. • Equity and access issues complex and largely unexplored.

What is needed is to integrate AIDS care into mainstream care and to improve globally access to care. Resources for healthcare need to be increased in an equitable fashion. Within such a system, the issue with ART is how these can be incorporated in a way that is sustainable and affordable. The research question is how best to use powerful, but expensive, ART in ways appropriate to a resource-poor environment. Recognising that these drugs can be used in a variety of ways in addition to the 'standard of care' in the West is vital. If that is accepted, then it is possible to seek ways that ART can be used for short-term benefit which either governments can subsidise, or individuals can choose to buy. Erecting one standard of care, life-long triple therapy, means that such approaches are by definition sub-standard. But it then erects impossible barriers for governments to fund, or individuals to purchase. Pragmatism suggests that we need to explore ways to use ART for short-term benefit to increase access. Then at least some of the therapeutic advances made over the last decade would impact on non-industrialised countries.

References

1 UNAIDS/WHO. AIDS Epidemic Update: December 1999. Geneva: WHO, 1999
2 Carpenter CCJ, Cooper DJ, Fischl MA et al. Antiretroviral therapy in adults: updated recommendations of the International AIDS Society – USA panel. JAMA 2000; **283**: 381–90
3 Gilks CF, Floyd K, Haran D, Kemp J, Squire B, Wilkinson D. *Care and Support for People with HIV/AIDS in Resource-poor Settings. Health and Population* Occasional Paper in Sexual and Reproductive Health, Department for International Development. London:DFID June 1997.
4 Gilks CF, Katabira E, de Cock KM. The challenge of providing effective care for HIV/AIDS in Africa. AIDS 1997; **11 (Suppl B)**: S99–106
5 Gilks CF. Acute bacterial infections and HIV disease. Br Med Bull 1998; **54**: 383–93
6 Gilks CF, Ojoo SA, Ojoo JC et al. Invasive pneumococcal disease in a cohort of pre-dominantly HIV-1 infected female sex workers in Nairobi, Kenya. Lancet 1996; **347**: 718–24
7 Morgan D, Ross A, Malamba S, Whitworth J. Early manifestations of HIV-1 infection in Uganda. AIDS 1998; **12**: 591–6
8 WHO. Interim proposal for a WHO staging system for HIV infection and disease. Wkly Epidemiol Rec 1990; **65**: 221–8
9 Anzala OA, Nagelkerke NJD, Bwayo JJ et al. Rapid progression to disease in African sex workers with HIV-1 infection. J Infect Dis 1995; **171**: 686–9
10 French N, Mujugira A, Nakiyingi J, Mulder D, Janoff EN, Gilks CF. Immunological and clinical staging in HIV-1-infected Ugandan adults are comparable and provide no evidence of rapid progression but poor survival with advanced disease. J AIDS 1999; **22**: 509–16
11 Rizzardini G, Trabattoni D, Saresella M et al. Immune activation in HIV-infected African individuals. AIDS 1998; **12**: 2387–96
12 Hoffman IF, Jere CS, Taylor TE *et al.* The effect of *Plasmodium falciparum* malaria on HIV-1 RNA blood plasma concentration. *AIDS* 1999; **13**: 487–94
13 Whalen CC, Nsubuga P, Okwera A *et al.* Impact of pulmonary tuberculosis on survival of HIV-infected adults: a prospective epidemiologic study in Uganda. *AIDS* 2000; **14**: 1219–28
14 Del Amo J, Malin A, Pozniak A, de Cock KM. Does tuberculosis accelerate the progression of HIV disease? Evidence from basic science and epidemiology. *AIDS* 1999; **13**: 1151–8

15 Del Amo J, Petruckevitch A, Phillips A *et al*. Disease progression and survival in HIV-1-infected Africans in London. *AIDS* 1998; **12**: 1203–9

16 Scott JAG, Hall AJ, Muyodi C *et al*. Aetiology, outcome and risk factors for mortality among adults with acute pneumonia in Kenya. *Lancet* 2000; **355**: 1225–30

17 Grant AD, Djomand G, de Cock K. Natural history and spectrum of disease in adults with HIV/AIDS in Africa. *AIDS* 1997; **11 (Suppl B)**: S43–54

18 Morgan D, Maude GH, Malamba SS *et al*. HIV-1 disease progression and AIDS-defining disorders in rural Uganda. *Lancet* 1997; **350**: 245–50

19 Grant D, Djomand G, Smets P *et al*. Profound immunosuppression across the spectrum of opportunistic disease amongst hospitalized HIV-infected adults in Abidjan, Cote d'Ivoire. *AIDS* 1997; **11**: 1357–64

20 Deschamps M, Fitzgerald DW, Pape JW, Johnson WD. HIV infection in Haiti: natural history and disease progression. *AIDS* 2000; **14**: 2515–21

21 Gilks CF. The clinical challenge of the HIV epidemic in the developing world. *Lancet* 1993; **342**: 1037–9

22 Kamanfu G, Mlika-Cabanne N, Girard P-G *et al*. Pulmonary complications of HIV infection in Bujumbura, Burundi. *Am Rev Respir Dis* 1993; **147**: 658–63

23 Lucas SB, Hounnou A, Peacock C *et al*. The mortality and pathology of HIV infection in a West African city. *AIDS* 1993; **7**: 1569–79

24 Gilks CF, Brindle RJ, Mwachari C *et al*. Disseminated *Mycobacterium avium* infection among HIV-infected patients in Kenya. *J Acquir Immune Def Syndr* 1995; **8**: 195–8

25 Brindle R, Holliman R, Gilks C, Waiyaki P. Toxoplasma antibodies in HIV-positive patients from Nairobi. *Trans R Soc Trop Med Hyg* 1991; **85**: 750–1

26 Heyderman RS, Gangaidzo IT, Hakim JG *et al*. Cryptococcal meningitis in human immunodeficiency virus-infected patients in Harare, Zimbabwe. *Clin Infect Dis* 1998; **26**: 284–9

27 Supparatpinyo K, Khamwan C, Baosoung V, Nelson KE, Sirisanthana T. Disseminated *Penicillium marneffei* infection in Southeast Asia. *Lancet* 1994; **344**: 110–3

28 Gilks CF. Improving HIV/AIDS disease surveillance in low-income countries [Editorial comment]. *AIDS* 1997; **11**: 1881–2

29 Floyd K, Reid RA, Wilkinson D, Gilks CF. Admission trends in a rural South African hospital during the early years of the HIV epidemic. *JAMA* 1999; **282**: 1087–91

30 Arthur G, Nduba VN, Kariyuki S, Kimari J, Bhatt S, Gilks CF. Trends in blood-stream infections for HIV-infected adults admitted to hospital in Nairobi, Kenya over the last decade. *Clin Infect Dis* 2001; In press

31 Gilks CF, Floyd K, Otieno LS, Adam AM, Bhatt SM, Warrell DA. Some effects of a rising case-load of adult HIV-related disease on a hospital in Nairobi. *J Acquir Immune Defic Syndr* 1998; **18**: 234–40

32 Arthur G, Bhatt SM, Muhindi D, Achia J, Kariuki S, Gilks CF. The changing impact of HIV/AIDS on Kenyatta National Hospital, Nairobi from 1988/9 through 1992 to 1997. *AIDS* 2000; **14**: 1625–31

33 Global Programme on AIDS. *Counselling for HIV/AIDS: A Key to Caring*. Geneva: WHO/GPA/TCO/HCS/95.15, 1995

34 The voluntary HIV-1 Counselling and Testing Efficacy Study Group. Efficacy of voluntary HIV-1 counselling and testing in individuals and couples in Kenya, Tanzania and Trinidad: a randomised trial. *Lancet* 2000; **356**: 103–12

35 Sweat M, Gregorich S, Sangiwa G *et al*. Cost-effectiveness of voluntary HIV-1 counselling and testing in reducing sexual transmission of HIV-1 in Kenya and Tanzania. *Lancet* 2000; **356**: 11–21

36 World Health Organization. *The Global AIDS Strategy: WHO AIDS Series Number 11*. Geneva: WHO, 1992

37 Wood CGA, Whittet S, Bradbeer CS. ABC of palliative care. HIV infection and AIDS. *BMJ* 1997; **315**: 1433–6

38 Archibald LK, Mcdonald LC, Rheanpumikankit S *et al*. Fever and HIV infection as sentinels for emerging mycobacterial and fungal bloodstream infections in hospitalized patients > 15 years old, Bangkok. *J Infect Dis* 1999; **180**: 87–92

39 Wilkinson D, Squire SB, Garner P. Effect of preventive treatment for tuberculosis in adults infected with HIV: systematic review of randomised placebo controlled trials. *BMJ* 1998; **317**: 625–9

40 Anglaret X, Chene G, Attia A *et al.* Early chemoprophylaxis with trimethoprim-sulphamethoxazole for HIV-1-infected adults in Abidjan, Cote d'Ivoire: a randomised trial. *Lancet* 1999; **353**: 1463–8

41 Wiktor SZ, Sassan-Morokro M, Grand AD *et al.* Efficacy of trimethoprim-sulphamethoxazole prophylaxis to decrease morbidity and mortality in HIV-1-infected patients with tuberculosis in Abidjan, Cote d'Ivoire: a randomised controlled trial. *Lancet* 1999; **353**: 1469–75

42 French N, Nakiyingi J, Carpenter LM *et al.* 23-valent pneumococcal polysaccharide vaccine in HIV-1-infected Ugandan adults: double-blind, randomised and placebo controlled trial. *Lancet* 2000; **355**: 2106–11

43 Gilks CF, Katabira E, de Cock KM. The challenge of providing effective care for HIV/AIDS in Africa. *AIDS* 1997; **11 (Suppl B)**: S99–106

44 Casarett DJ, Lantos JD. Have we treated AIDS too well? Rationing and the future of AIDS exceptionalism. *Ann Intern Med* 1998; **128**: 756–9

Immune interventions

John Wilkinson and Frances Gotch

Department of Immunology, Imperial College of Science, Technology and Medicine, Chelsea and Westminster Hospital, London, UK

A better understanding of the immune response to HIV and the deleterious effect that HIV infection may have on the immune system in general, allows us to consider how best to restore protective immune responses to HIV and other opportunistic pathogens in the immunocompromised host. In this chapter, we summarise areas of current innovation and provide an update of the current state of knowledge concerning interventions which could result in the immuno-compromised state being reversed. We describe the kinds of immune responses, which are thought to be useful in combating both the human immuno-deficiency virus and other pathogenic organisms, and methods which are being considered to stimulate such responses. Lessons which may be learned from other disease states, which lead to immunodeficiency and methods for measuring successful outcome of treatment will be described.

The HIV-infected immune system

Correspondence to: Dr John Wilkinson, Department of Immunology, Imperial College of Science, Technology and Medicine, Chelsea and Westminster Hospital, 369 Fulham Road, London SW10 9NH, UK

The immune system is capable of mounting very strong attacks on invading pathogens and is able to eliminate many of them completely. Cellular immune responses are a critical part of the host's defence against viral infections with CD8[+] T-lymphocytes forming a primary component. Evidence for strong CD8[+] antiviral pressure can be appreciated by the number and variety of strategies which viruses have evolved to avoid apoptosis and CTL recognition, thus prolonging the life of the virally-infected cell and enabling viral replication and dissemination (reviewed by Meinl *et al*[1]). The importance of CD4[+] T cell responses should also not be underestimated, providing 'help' both to T- and B-cells. Since the original description of CD4[+] and CD8[+] T-lymphocytes as 'helper' cytokine-producing cells and 'lytic' CTLs, respectively, the two have not remained mutually exclusive with CD4[+] T-lymphocytes demonstrating cytotoxic activity and CD8[+] T-lymphocytes exhibiting potent cytokine and chemokine-producing activity.

The overall *in vivo* effect of HIV-1 infection and its interaction with the body's natural response mechanism is of severe damage to the immune system, destroying the means by which the body responds and defends itself against infections. Infection with HIV produces a wide range of qualitative and quantitative immunological changes, the most prominent being the changes that affect the CD4[+] T-lymphocytes. In normal physiology, the CD4[+] T-lymphocyte provides regulatory factors that enhance the function of many other cell types. It is widely believed that many of the defects in function in these other cells seen during HIV infection are linked to changes in CD4[+] T-lymphocyte number and function.

Studies of HIV-specific immunity soon after primary infection show early induction of both CD4[+] and CD8[+] cell-mediated immunity. However, in most cases, these immune responses achieve only weak control of viral replication. The mechanisms by which HIV escapes immune control include both immunological and viral factors. The major determinant of the rate of disease progression is the balance between the evolutionary pressures upon HIV from the immune system at large, and the success of the virus population in adapting to these pressures. HIV undergoes a continual process of evolution reflected in the viral load and the CD4[+] T-lymphocyte count of the individual and in the changes evident in the genotype of the viruses present. During primary infection, viruses utilising the CCR5 co-receptor are likely to predominate. Virus strains able to use the CXCR4 chemokine receptor may predominate with time and are associated with a switch from NSI to SI phenotype and hence a much greater quantitative loss in CD4[+] T-lymphocytes. This constant evolution helps HIV stay one step ahead of the immune system, which is primed to respond to the previous generation of virus.

CD4[+] T-lymphocytes

The first cells infected by HIV are likely to be the activated CD4[+] T-lymphocytes in the lymphoid tissue, and tissue macrophages that are in a differentiated state. CD4[+] T-lymphocytes either express CD45RA[+], a cell surface marker which defines the subset of antigen naive cells, or CD45RO[+], which characterises the memory cell subset. Naive cells originate typically from the thymus and remain in a resting state until they encounter foreign antigen. When antigen and co-stimulatory signals are presented by antigen presenting cells, naive cells become activated and switch to the memory phenotype displaying an effector function and with the ability to respond quickly to antigen. Initial exposure to HIV results in the rapid recruitment of activated memory CD4[+] T-lymphocytes, which, being the primary targets for HIV infection, are preferentially depleted while in advanced stages of the disease the proportion of naive cells also declines.

Besides the progressive fall in the numbers of peripheral blood CD4[+] T-lymphocytes in HIV-infected individuals, immunological abnormalities in T-helper cell function occur early in HIV infection, even before the CD4[+]

T-lymphocyte numbers diminish. Reduced proliferative capacity and diminished IL-2 production by peripheral blood mononuclear cells in response to stimulation is one of the hallmarks of HIV disease and these functions decrease progressively with disease. CD4[+] T cell responses to HIV-specific antigens are difficult to detect even early in the disease process with responses to recall antigens lost as disease progresses and finally a loss of response to mitogens becoming apparent.

CD4[+] T-lymphocytes in HIV-infected individuals, which recognise antigen in association with class II MHC molecules on the antigen presenting cell, have demonstrated responses to a variety of HIV proteins (*env*, *gag* and *pol*) in early-stage disease. Further, the association between certain MHC HLA class II haplotypes and HIV disease progression suggests a positive role for the host's immune system in determining clinical outcome (reviewed by Westby *et al*[2]).

Human CD4[+] T-lymphocytes can be separated into Th1 and Th2 subsets, secreting cytokines that may play an immunoregulatory role in HIV infection by defining the lymphokine and thus the effector cell profile which can possibly affect progression to AIDS (reviewed by Clerici and Shearer[3]). Derived from a common precursor (Th0-type) cell capable of expressing a broad range of different cytokines, generally Th1 cells differentially secrete IL-2, IFN-γ, TGF-β and IL-12, whilst Th2 cells secrete IL-4, IL-5, IL-6 and IL-10. Studies by Clerici and Shearer[3] have suggested that specific humoral immune responses are determined by the cytokines they produce, with a switch during HIV disease progression from Th1 (increasing cellular immunity) to Th2 (enhancing antibody production) type cytokine production. The interaction of the Th1 and Th2 cell subsets is competitive, with over-expression of cytokines by one cell type suppressing the activity of the other, such that the predominance of Th2 cells could be responsible for the decrease in Th1 activity, thus leading to the switch (Fig. 1).

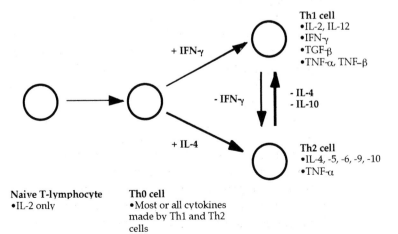

Fig. 1 Model for the differentiation of CD4[+] T-lymphocytes with regard to cytokine expression (adapted from Clerici and Shearer[3]).

Naive T-lymphocyte
•IL-2 only

Th0 cell
•Most or all cytokines made by Th1 and Th2 cells

+ IFN-γ

- IFN-γ

+ IL-4

Th1 cell
•IL-2, IL-12
•IFN-γ
•TGF-β
•TNF-α, TNF-β

- IL-4
- IL-10

Th2 cell
•IL-4, -5, -6, -9, -10
•TNF-α

CD8+ effector cells

The contribution of CD8+ T-lymphocytes towards cellular immunity has been highlighted in two recent studies which eliminated CD8+ T-lymphocytes from SIV-infected rhesus monkeys during primary or chronic infection[4,5]. CD8+ depletion during primary infection resulted in uncontrolled viraemia with a subsequent inability to generate neutralising antibody responses and rapid progression to disease. Elimination of CD8+ cells during chronic infection resulted in a rapid and marked increase in viraemia that was suppressed with the re-appearance of SIV-specific CD8+ T cells. Similarly, CD8+ T-lymphocytes have been shown to play an important role in controlling HIV infection, either by a direct killing effect on HIV infected cells and/or by the secretion of soluble antiviral factors which suppress HIV replication.

Within the T-lymphocyte compartment, naive (cells which have not encountered antigen), effector (cells with specialised functions such as cytotoxic and suppressor activity) and memory T-lymphocytes can be identified. Memory cells, the progeny of CTLs that escape activation-induced cell death[6], are an important component of the immune system, responding efficiently to recall antigens, demonstrating less stringent requirements for activation and secreting a broader range of cytokines. Phenotypically, naive, effector and memory cells differ in the expression of several surface antigens, including CD29, LFA-1 and CD45RO, although these markers may just reflect cellular activation. However, in the murine model, various groups have demonstrated that the lymph node homing receptor CD62L is strongly down regulated on CTL compared to naive cells, with memory cells demonstrating heterogeneous expression.

One of the hallmarks of HIV-infection is the dynamic expansion and activation of CD8+ T-lymphocytes. During primary HIV infection (PHI), the CD8+ cell compartment can increase remarkably in number; a 10-fold expansion was observed in one individual with acute HIV infection who declined anti-retroviral therapy (ART)[7]. Nearly 90% of these CD8+ T cells expressed markers of immune activation at seroconversion. An effect of such enormous expansion and activation may be that HIV-specific CD8+ T-lymphocytes are eventually deleted through a process of clonal exhaustion.

CD8+ cytotoxic T-lymphocytes

CD8+ CTL recognise virus-infected cells upon presentation of an 8–10 amino acid peptide epitope by the infected target cell and may be directed against both structural (*gag*, *pol* and *env*) and regulatory (*tat*, *rev* and *nef*) proteins of HIV. Classically, this response is HLA-restricted and requires cell-to-cell contact and appears as early as 5 days following seroconversion, as demonstrated in the SIV model of acute infection. Additionally, the reduction in viraemia in acute HIV infection is associated with the onset of a virus-specific, class I HLA-restricted, CD8[+] CTL response, which is similar to that which has been observed in acute virus infections in mice (reviewed by Gotch and Hardy[8]).

Precursors of HIV-specific CTL have been detected prior to the appearance of neutralising antibodies, suggesting that HIV-specific cell-mediated immune responses play a major role in down-regulating HIV viraemia following seroconversion. These cells are probably responsible for the destruction of the virus expressing cells, reducing the pool of HIV-producing cells, and leading to the decrease in HIV viraemia at seroconversion. Various studies have demonstrated that in early HIV-1 infection, the induction of memory CTLs, particularly those specific for *env*, help control viral replication, with this activity associated with slower declines in CD4[+] T-lymphocyte counts.

CTLs remain in relatively high numbers during the asymptomatic period of HIV infection, but their numbers decline with progression to disease. Direct measurements (using the complementarity-determining region 3 of the T-cell antigen receptor as molecular markers for individual CTL clones) have indicated that the level of CD8[+] CTL effectors is around 1% of all PBMC in the chronic phase of HIV disease[9], with antigen-specific CTLs representing > 25% of the total number of circulating CD8[+] T-lymphocytes during the acute phase[10]. Long-term survivors demonstrate high precursor frequencies of CTL (Table 1) and there is evidence that CTL may have a protective role in exposed but uninfected individuals.

In longitudinal studies, variant HIV species encoding mutated CTL epitopes in regions critical for MHC binding (particularly *gag*, but *nef*, *tat* and *pol* also) may emerge during the course of infection, with progression to AIDS occurring when new strains of virus are produced

Table 1 Salient features associated with long-term survivors

Preservation of the lymph node architecture

Demonstrate a lower viral load, by approximately one log

May express a heterozygote CCR5Δ32 mutation of the co-receptor gene

Associated with a deletion in *nef* in the infecting viral species

May demonstrate infection with relatively non-virulent strains of HIV-1 (often M-tropic)

Possess high levels of neutralising antibodies to the virus in their blood

PBMC continue to demonstrate Th1-type CD4[+] T-lymphocytes

Demonstrate high precursor frequencies of CTL

Both the cytotoxic and suppressing ability of the CD8[+] cells is maintained

Modified from Barker *et al*[53] and Gea-Banacloche *et al*[54].

that cannot be controlled by the generation of CTL with new specificities. Increasing viral diversity in itself does not correlate with CD4[+] T-lymphocyte loss and progression to AIDS; in fact, rapid CD4[+] T-lymphocyte decline has been associated with relatively homogenous viral populations. However, just prior to, or coincident with, a rapid decline in CD4[+] T-cell numbers, basic amino acid substitutions clustered within and downstream of the gp120 V3 domain can be detected, suggesting that the virus continually accumulates changes in its amino acid sequences well into the time of marked CD4[+] T cell decline[11].

CD8[+] suppressor cells

The inability to recover virus from asymptomatic HIV-infected individuals unless CD8[+] T-lymphocytes were first removed led to the discovery of CD8[+] suppressor responses. When the CD8[+] effector cells were added back to the assay, virus replication was again suppressed in a dose-dependent manner. Many studies have confirmed the presence of CD8[+] anti-HIV suppressor activity (CASA) and similar results have been reported in SIV- and HIV-infected non-human primates. CASA demonstrates a broad spectrum of activity against target cells infected with either cytopathic or non-cytopathic strains of HIV-1, HIV-2, and SIV, with autologous CD8[+] T-lymphocytes demonstrating stronger CASA than allogeneic cells. CASA is not HLA-restricted, does not involve cell killing, and is mediated through a novel soluble factor(s), termed CD8[+] antiviral factor (CAF).

The degree of CASA and levels of CAF correlate with the patient's clinical state, with CD8[+] T-lymphocytes from asymptomatic individuals exhibiting the strongest CASA, followed by CD8[+] T-lymphocytes from symptomatic patients and then AIDS patients who demonstrate the least activity, although, an overlap in the relative anti-HIV suppressor activity exhibited by CD8[+] T cells from these cohorts has been reported. In addition, CASA in lymphoid tissue has also been observed to correlate with the clinical state of the individual. CASA in the peripheral blood has been detected before neutralising antibodies to HIV, suggesting a positive role for this cellular immune response in controlling viral replication soon after HIV infection (reviewed by Levy et al[12]).

Immunosuppression and opportunistic infections

In most patients, chronic HIV infection results in a generalised progressive impairment of cell-mediated immune responses and, as a result, a failure to control the replication of opportunistic pathogens such as cytomegalovirus (CMV), human papilloma virus (HPV), human herpes virus 8 (HHV8), *Cryptosporidium* and *Microsporidium*. Opportunistic infections are the clinical manifestations of uncontrolled replication of opportunistic pathogens which usually exist as latent subclinical infections.

Long-term survival

Although only a relatively small number of patients fall into this category, the reasons for long-term survival could provide insights into possible therapeutic approaches to HIV. Definitions of long-term survival vary; generally, individuals living with HIV infection for more than 8 years (median duration) with no symptoms and a CD4+ T-lymphocyte count above 500 cells/ml are considered long-term survivors. Some consistent features of their infection are outlined in Table 1.

Understanding the immune factors that maintain this natural suppressive response, which may also partly account for the resistance to infection in exposed but uninfected individuals and increased longevity in some HIV-infected individuals, are important when the development of safe and effective immune interventions such as therapeutic or prophylactic vaccines are considered. The stimulation of the cell-mediated immune response with a therapeutic vaccine may be a key factor in the restoration of the immune system following anti-retroviral therapy (ART), where the immune system may be persuaded to assist in the control of continued HIV replication once the viral load has been rendered undetectable. It is important to note that whilst ART may reduce viral load to undetectable levels, viral replication continues within the host. Additionally, with such a high incidence of AIDS in the non-industrialised world, the development of a preventive vaccine that results in vigorous HIV-specific cellular immune responses may be one option for an effective long-term solution to the control of the AIDS pandemic.

Anti-retroviral therapy (ART)

The efficacies of current anti-retroviral agents and treatment strategies cannot be simply assessed by quantitation of CD4+ T-lymphocytes (a surrogate marker for overall immune function), as alterations in their number does not explain all the effects of therapeutic intervention; but must be assessed by their ability to reconstitute the immune system on a wider scale. There are currently no measures of HIV-specific immunity routinely available in clinical practice. Assays to determine HIV-specific immune function, including neutralising antibody responses, CTL assays and assays for CD4[+] T cell function are only available in the research laboratory, but may be essential for the clinical monitoring of current ART which incorporates immune based therapies.

Following PHI, the level of viraemia at 4–12 months (the 'set-point') correlates with disease progression. Treatment initiated at higher CD4[+] T-lymphocyte and lower HIV-1 RNA levels, has been associated with greater and more durable immune responses, leading to the possibility of preventing the dissemination of HIV, the preservation of the immune function and the increased likelihood of restoring important components of the HIV-specific immune response[13] and responses to other important opportunistic pathogens, such as CMV, HSV and HHV8, which have been diminished or lost. In addition, early treatment during PHI, and even at seroconversion, may prevent the stable reservoir of integrated proviral HIV DNA, present in resting CD4[+] T-lymphocytes both in the peripheral blood and lymph nodes, which persists through ART[14,15].

Highly active anti-retroviral therapy (HAART)

Encouraging results have been observed with a number of combination drug regimens containing various potent antiviral agents which target the HIV enzymes (i) reverse transcriptase, associated with HIV replication, and/or (ii) the protease enzymes, essential for the maturation of the HIV virion. Plasma HIV-1 RNA levels in the peripheral blood in treated patients may be below those seen in long-term survivors. Many studies link the durability of response to HAART with the magnitude of the initial response, with greater initial therapy-induced HIV RNA decreases strongly associated with the reduced risk of progression to AIDS or death (reviewed by DeGruttola *et al*[16]). The advent of combination therapy has led to the partial control of HIV-1 replication *in vivo*, demonstrated by a decline in AIDS incidence and mortality in the Western world. In addition, HAART has helped revolutionise our understanding of HIV-1 viral kinetics in infected individuals and has given us an opportunity to observe changes in the immune system.

Immune reconstitution with HAART

The decrease in the incidence of mortality and opportunistic diseases observed since the introduction of HAART is compelling clinical evidence of improvements in immune function specific for or 'directed at' HIV and for opportunistic pathogens. HAART is associated with decreases in viral burden, which are paralleled by increases in CD4[+] T-lymphocyte counts and improvements in T-cell function, even in individuals with advanced stages of HIV-1 disease. The extent of immune restoration that can be achieved may be determined by the state of the immune system, in particular by the number of naive T-lymphocytes, prior to the commencement of HAART[17].

Despite the significant increases in CD4[+] T-lymphocyte numbers with HAART, only a small proportion of individuals demonstrate increases which approach the normal range following 2 years of therapy. In the majority of cases, these increases in T-lymphocytes rarely reach normal levels, and immune reconstitution does not necessarily follow long-term HIV-1 suppression with HAART[18]. However, Furrer and co-workers have reported that even a partial restoration of the immune system may protect some individuals against opportunistic infections[19].

In one of the first studies to assess immune reconstitution, Kelleher and co-workers[20] noted significant increases in both naive and memory CD4[+] T-lymphocytes, as well as increased lymphocyte proliferation responses to mitogen, recall antigens and HIV-1-specific proteins in HIV-1 infected individuals treated with ritonavir®. Similarly, Autran and co-workers reported the appearance of memory CD4[+] T-lymphocytes during the first 4 months of HAART, followed by increased numbers of functional naive CD4[+] T-lymphocytes by 12 months[17].

In addition to increases in CD4[+] T-lymphocytes, increases in CD8[+] T-lymphocytes are observed with ART, both demonstrating a biphasic response to HAART[21]. Memory CD8[+] T-lymphocytes expand rapidly within weeks resulting in an overall increase in total CD8[+] number, but decline again in the subsequent months. The proportion of naive CD8[+] T-lymphocytes increases slowly maintaining the number of total CD8[+] T-lymphocytes at an almost constant level[17,20,21].

Infection with HIV-1 leads to the extensive activation of T-lymphocytes resulting in anergy and increased apoptosis. With HIV-1 disease progression the proportion of activated T-lymphocytes increases, which correlates to increases in plasma HIV RNA levels. Initiation of HAART has been reported to rapidly reduce the number of activated CD4[+] and CD8[+] T-lymphocytes as measured by the expression of CD38 and HLA-DR cell surface antigens[17,20,22].

In addition to increasing the proliferative responses of CD4[+] T-lymphocytes to recall antigens and/or to mitogens[17,20,23,24], HAART has resulted in the detection of new DTH responses to recall antigens in a third of those individuals tested[24]. Proliferative T-lymphocyte responses improve slowly as demonstrated in studies of up to 1.5 years' duration; however, normal levels were still not attained[23]. Individuals with a significant improvement in lymphocyte proliferative responses demonstrated a more sustained suppression of plasma HIV RNA, greater CD4[+] increases and an early increase of memory and naive CD4[+] T-lymphocytes[25]. In support of early treatment of individuals with HAART, improved HIV-specific T-helper responses were observed in individuals treated early[23,26,27], but not in those with chronic more advanced HIV-1 disease[17,24].

Despite 12 months of HAART, achieving undetectable viral loads, HIV-1 specific $CD4^+$ T cell proliferative responses were not restored in early HIV-1 disease[23,26,27]. In some individuals with HAART-associated undetectable viraemia, there is an apparent loss of HIV-1-specific CTL[28], a loss of CASA[29] and a decline of HIV-1 specific cytotoxic $CD4^+$ T-lymphocytes[30] probably as a result of reduced HIV antigen levels. Different therapeutic approaches may, therefore, be required to restore fully HIV-1-specific T cell responses lost during early infection. Additional vaccination strategies may be needed to maintain the HIV-1 specific immune response in subjects receiving HAART.

Structured treatment interruptions

Following encouraging reports in PHI treated patients[26], a number of groups are studying the effects of transient interruptions of ART in patients with well-controlled viraemia (<50 copies). Such studies are being performed in an attempt to boost HIV-specific immune responses using the viral rebounds that result from treatment interruption as a form of 'auto-immunisation'. Early success with this approach has been documented by Walker and colleagues, who demonstrated a significant increase in virus-specific CTL responses and a broadening to include more targeted epitopes in patients with PHI following each successive structured treatment interruptions[13]. However, for the majority of individuals, discontinuation of HAART in patients with chronic infection usually results in an increase in the level of viraemia which rapidly (within 4 weeks) returns to pre-HAART levels[31]. The fact that the levels of viraemia usually return to initial levels, and not below, suggest that prolonged effective suppression of virus in these individuals may not result in a significant improvement of the HIV-specific immune response. In addition, interruption of HAART in chronically infected individuals results in a rapid decline of $CD4^+$ T-cells[32] and structured treatment interruptions may lead to the replenishment of viral reservoirs[33] with the immunological benefits from this approach possibly short-lived[34].

The effect of HAART on opportunistic infections

Immune reconstitution, in terms of an increase in T-cell function, can be evidenced clinically by the resolution of opportunistic infections with ART. When HIV replication is controlled, in terms of undetectable viral loads as a result of HAART, a reduction in the incidence of diseases

Table 2 Summary of the objectives of immune based strategies

To maintain and/or potentiate the existence of:

       HIV-specific immune responses

       non-specific immune responses

       immune responses to opportunistic infections

To induce *de novo* HIV-specific immune responses

To restore pre-existing HIV-specific immune responses which have been lost with disease progression

To enable long-term survivor status in the absence of ART

To decrease latent/proviral reservoirs

To eliminate the infected host of virus

Modified from Pantaleo[38].

caused by opportunistic pathogens has been observed[19,35]. Pathogen-specific immune responses are restored with HAART leading to the resolution of CMV retinitis, HIV-related TB, HPV related cervical disease, Kaposi's sarcoma, cryptosporidiosis and microsporidiosis in many treated patients. A reduction in CMV and HHV8 DNA in the blood of treated patients suggests that replication of these opportunistic pathogens also decline with HAART. This sudden increase in immune function may ironically result in localised inflammation to opportunistic pathogens or 'immune restoration disease' (reviewed by French[36]).

Immune-based therapies

It has become apparent that ART alone will not be able to contain fully HIV replication or eradicate virus in most chronically infected individuals. Current estimations suggest that to eradicate the reservoir of infected memory T-cells may take up to 60 years of continuous control of HIV replication with ART[37]. Therefore, the key to long-term control of HIV replication is likely to be the restoration of the immune system, especially HIV-specific immunity which is lost soon after infection with HIV, in individuals with chronic infection, and to preserve immune competence in those with acute infection. Novel therapeutic approaches are, therefore, required for the treatment of HIV.

Objectives of immune-based strategies have been defined by Pantaleo[38] and are summarised in Table 2. A number of immune-based strategies have been investigated in several clinical trials and, with the exception of IL-2 therapy and granulocyte-macrophage colony-stimulating factor (GM-CSF), there has been no clear evidence of clinical benefit or improvement in virological and immunological parameters (reviewed by Emery and Lane[39]).

IL-2 therapy

IL-2, a cytokine secreted by activated T-cells that regulates lymphoid proliferation and maturation, decreases with HIV disease progression. Various studies with IL-2 as an immune based therapy for HIV have demonstrated increases in CD4[+] T cell number, but no significant changes in viral load[39,40]. However, whether the observed increases in CD4[+] T-cell number translate into increased immunocompetence remains unclear. Immune recovery may be enhanced by co-administration of IL-2 with HAART, improving both CD4[+] T-cell number and function. The ESPRIT and SILCAAT trials, looking at IL-2 administration in different cohorts of patients, aim to evaluate immune recovery. Preliminary data suggest IL-2 administration with HAART results in greater increases in CD4[+] T cell numbers than IL-2 alone[41].

IL-2 may stimulate viral replication in latent viral reservoirs, activating the CD4[+] T cells and 'flushing out' the virus. In the presence of HAART, the virions should not be able to infect new CD4[+] target cells. In a recent study evaluating the frequency of latently infected CD4[+] T-cells in patients receiving HAART, with or without IL-2, individuals receiving IL-2 demonstrated a significantly lower number of CD4[+] T cells containing replication-competent HIV than the patients receiving HAART alone[42]. However, discontinuation of HAART in this group led to an increase in viraemia, suggesting that the latent reservoir had not been abolished.

GM-CSF therapy

Significant increases in CD4[+] T cell counts have been observed when the cytokine GM-CSF is administered to patients with advanced HIV infection. In addition, significantly fewer changes in ART were necessary and the incidence of an opportunistic infection or death was significantly lower in the GM-CSF group compared to the placebo control. GM-CSF was also shown to augment phagocytosis of *Mycobacterium avium* complex (MAC) by HIV-infected macrophages *in vitro*[43]. In late stage patients receiving HAART, the addition of GM-CSF and IL-2 appeared more effective in inducing both HIV-specific and non-specific proliferative responses[44], highlighting the positive role of such immunomodulators in the treatment of HIV.

CD8[+] T-cell re-infusion

The expansion *in vitro* and re-infusion of HIV-specific CTLs may provide an alternative effective therapeutic approach. Preliminary studies, expanding and re-infusing bulk CD8⁺ T-lymphocytes in the presence or absence of IL-2 demonstrated no changes to CD4⁺ or CD8⁺ T-lymphocyte numbers, nor was there any reduction in HIV viral load. Recent studies have demonstrated the short-term survival of transferred CTL clones. In a study raising and re-infusing *gag* and *pol* CTL clones, and monitoring their fate *in vivo* with the use of a class I tetramer stain, Tan and colleagues observed a rapid rate of apoptosis of the infused cells with over 90% undergoing activation-induced cell death within 48 h[45].

Therapeutic vaccines

For a therapeutic vaccine to be effective it should induce HIV-1 specific immune responses that have been previously absent. With the reduction in HIV antigen as a result of HAART, HIV-specific immune responses such as T-cell proliferative responses and CD8⁺ CTL and CASA decline. The aim of a therapeutic vaccine is, therefore, to remind the immune system what the viral pathogen 'looks like' and elicit an immune response accordingly. The possibility of slowing progression to AIDS by therapeutic immunisation with an HIV vaccine is one such approach currently receiving interest in the literature[46].

Early trials of therapeutic vaccination yielded disappointing results, but because these vaccines were administered in the pre-HAART era, it is not surprising that the trials failed to show a clinical benefit. Present studies are concentrating on vaccinating with an HIV-1 antigen concurrent with ART, and studies are being conducted as to when such treatment should take place. Results from two randomised trials comparing four envelope vaccine candidates in HIV-infected patients have shown that patients with higher CD4⁺ T-cell counts and lower viral loads may benefit the most from this approach. In addition, a great diversity in immune response between the four vaccination groups was observed, suggesting there is strain specificity to the antigen used[47].

The HIV-1 Immunogen (Remune®) is a gp120-depleted inactivated HIV-1 antigen, which has been evaluated in HIV-infected adults since 1987. Remune® has resulted in increased DTH responses, anti-HIV p24 responses, lymphocyte proliferative responses and increased intensity of antibody bands by Western blot analysis (reviewed by Gotch *et al*[48]). Patients treated with Remune® have recently been shown to elicit a strong CD4⁺ T helper cell proliferative response to their own virus as well as demonstrating strong cross-reactive immune response to HIV-1 subtypes B, E and C. Additionally, Remune® was associated with increased levels of perforin and MIP-1β, markers of CD8⁺ T-cell activity, and phenotyping of the proliferating cells that were induced by Remune® has revealed that it is predominantly the CD4⁺ and CD8⁺

memory phenotypes that are induced by the HIV-1 antigen[49]. However, a recent publication[50] 'failed to demonstrate that the addition of HIV-1 Immunogen to ART conferred any effect on HIV progression-free survival relative to that achievable by ART alone'.

Several studies of recombinant gp160 (VaxSyn®) as a therapeutic vaccine have been performed. No advantage in patients receiving VaxSyn®, in terms of CD4+ counts, viral load, time to initiation of ART, incidence of opportunistic infections or death, was observed compared to placebo controls (reviewed by Gotch *et al*[48]). However, prior to the era of HAART, immunotherapy of patients with recombinant gp160 vaccine demonstrated an increase in T-cell proliferative responses despite suboptimal viral control[51]. Such studies will lead to further investigations of new treatment strategies using HAART to produce complete viral suppression in combination with vaccination and/or cytokines, to regenerate the kinds of anti-HIV responses that have been associated with long-term survivors.

Conclusions

With more than 30 million people world-wide living with HIV disease, over 90% of whom will not have access to HAART, a prophylactic vaccine to prevent increasing numbers of people becoming infected remains a priority. The ultimate therapeutic goal is that in the era of HAART where the HIV viral load can be reduced to minimal levels, immune responses generated by therapeutic vaccines will eventually be able to control viral replication in the absence of ART[13,52].

It has become clear that viral eradication can not be achieved with the anti-retroviral agents that are currently available. The future of AIDS treatment lies with immune-based therapies that will restore the host immune system into one that is competent, fully functional and able to deliver the appropriate immune response. Studying those individuals who manage to control activation of the latent cell pool and remain with low or undetectable viral loads (long-term survivors) has provided insights into the immune response required for the long-term control of HIV infection. Such insights together with our increasing understanding of the role of the cellular immune system provide a realistic basis for immune-based intervention.

Acknowledgements

We would like to thank Nesrina Imami for helpful criticism of this manuscript. JW is funded by MRC grant #G9825083. FG is supported by funding from MRC, Wellcome Trust, NIH and EU.

References

1   Meinl E, Fickenscher H, Thome M, Tschopp J, Fleckenstein B. Anti-apoptotic strategies of lymphotropic viruses. *Immunol Today* 1998; **19**: 474–9

2   Westby M, Manca F, Dalgleish A. The role of host immune responses in determining the outcome of HIV infection. *Immunol Today* 1996; **17**: 120–6

3   Clerici M, Shearer G. TH-1→TH2 switch is a critical step in the etiology of HIV infection. *Immunol Today* 1993; **14**: 107–11

4   Jin X, Bauer DE, Tuttleton SE *et al.* Dramatic rise in plasma viremia after CD8(+) T-cell depletion in simian immunodeficiency virus-infected macaques. *J Exp Med* 1999; **189**: 991–8

5   Schmitz JE, Kuroda MJ, Santra S *et al.* Control of viremia in simian immunodeficiency virus infection by CD8+ lymphocytes. *Science* 1999; **283**: 857–60

6   Opferman JT, Ober BT, Ashton-Rickardt PG. Linear differentiation of cytotoxic effectors into memory T lymphocytes. *Science* 1999; **283**: 1745–8

7   Ferbas J, Daar ES, Grovit FK *et al.* Rapid evolution of human immunodeficiency virus strains with increased replicative capacity during the seronegative window of primary infection. *J Virol* 1996; **70**: 7285–9

8   Gotch F, Hardy G. The immune system: our best antiretroviral. *Curr Opin Infect Dis* 2000; **13**: 13–7

9   Moss P, Rowland-Jones S, Frodsham P *et al.* Persistent high frequency of human immunodeficiency virus-specific cytotoxic T cells in peripheral blood of infected donors. *Proc Natl Acad Sci USA* 1995; **92**: 5773–7

10 Pantaleo G, Demarest JF, Soudeyns H *et al.* Major expansion of CD8+ T cells with a predominant VB usage during the primary immune response to HIV. *Nature* 1994; **370**: 463–7

11 Shankarappa R, Gupta P, Learn Jr G *et al.* Evolution of human immunodeficiency virus type 1 envelope sequences in infected individuals with differing disease progression profiles. *Virology* 1998; **241**: 251–9

12 Levy J, Mackewicz C, Barker E. Controlling HIV pathogenesis: the role of noncytotoxic anti-HIV response of CD8+ T cells. *Immunol Today* 1996; **17**: 217–24

13 Rosenberg E, Altfeld M, Poon S *et al.* Immune control of HIV-1 after early treatment of acute infection. *Nature* 2000; **407**: 523–6

14 Chun TW, Carruth L, Finzi D *et al.* Quantification of latent tissue reservoirs and total body viral load in HIV-1 infection. *Nature* 1997; **387**: 183–8

15 Finzi D, Hermankova M, Pierson T *et al.* Identification of a reservoir for HIV-1 in patients on highly active antiretroviral therapy. *Science* 1997; **278**: 1295–300

16 DeGruttola V, Hughes M, Gilbert P, Phillips A. Trial design in the era of highly effective antiviral drug combinations for HIV infection. *AIDS* 1998; **12 (Suppl A)**: S149–56

17 Autran B, Carcelain G, Li TS *et al.* Positive effects of combined antiretroviral therapy on CD4+ T cell homeostasis and function in advanced HIV disease. *Science* 1997; **277**: 112–6

18 Pakker NG, Kroon EDMB, Roos MTL *et al.* Immune restoration does not invariably occur following long-term HIV-1 suppression during antiretroviral therapy. *AIDS* 1999; **13**: 203–12

19 Furrer H, Egger M, Opravil M *et al.* Discontinuation of primary prophylaxis against *Pneumocystis carinii* pneumonia in HIV-1-infected adults treated with combination antiretroviral therapy. Swiss HIV Cohort Study. *N Engl J Med* 1999; **340**: 1301–6

20 Kelleher AD, Carr A, Zaunders J, Cooper DA. Alterations in the immune response of human immunodeficiency virus (HIV)-infected subjects treated with an HIV-specific protease inhibitor, ritonavir. *J Infect Dis* 1996; **173**: 321–9

21 Pakker NG, Roos MT, van Leeuwen R *et al.* Patterns of T-cell repopulation, virus load reduction, and restoration of T-cell function in HIV-infected persons during therapy with different antiretroviral agents. *J Acquir Immune Defic Syndr Hum Retrovirol* 1997; **16**: 318–26

22 Bouscarat F, Levacher M, Landman R *et al.* Changes in blood CD8+ lymphocyte activation status and plasma HIV RNA levels during antiretroviral therapy. *AIDS* 1998; **12**: 1267–73

23 Rinaldo Jr CR, Liebmann JM, Huang XL *et al.* Prolonged suppression of human immunodeficiency virus type 1 (HIV-1) viremia in persons with advanced disease results in enhancement of CD4 T cell reactivity to microbial antigens but not to HIV-1 antigens. *J Infect Dis* 1999; **179**: 329–36

24 Lederman MM, Connick E, Landay A *et al*. Immunologic responses associated with 12 weeks of combination antiretroviral therapy consisting of zidovudine, lamivudine, and ritonavir: results of AIDS Clinical Trials Group Protocol 315. *J Infect Dis* 1998; **178**: 70–9

25 Li TS, Tubiana R, Katlama C, Calvez V, Ait Mohand H, Autran B. Long-lasting recovery in CD4 T-cell function and viral-load reduction after highly active antiretroviral therapy in advanced HIV-1 disease. *Lancet* 1998; **351**: 1682–6

26 Malhotra U, Berrey M, Huang Y *et al*. Effect of combination antiretroviral therapy on HIV-1 specific cellular immunity in acute HIV-1 infection. *6th Conference on Retroviruses and Opportunistic Infections*. Chicago, IL, USA, 1999; Abstract #23

27 Plana M, Garcia F, Gallart T, Miro JM, Gatell JM. Lack of T-cell proliferative response to HIV-1 antigens after 1 year of highly active antiretroviral treatment in early HIV-1 disease. Immunology Study Group of Spanish EARTH-1 Study. *Lancet* 1998; **352**: 1194–5

28 Ogg GS, Jin X, Bonhoeffer S *et al*. Quantitation of HIV-1-specific cytotoxic T lymphocytes and plasma load of viral RNA. *Science* 1998; **279**: 2103–6

29 Wilkinson J, Zaunders J, Carr A, Cooper D. CD8+ anti-HIV-1 suppressor activity (CASA) in response to antiretroviral therapy: loss of CASA is associated with loss of viremia. *J Infect Dis* 1999; **180**: 68–75

30 Pitcher CJ, Quittner C, Peterson DM *et al*. HIV-1-specific CD4+ T cells are detectable in most individuals with active HIV-1 infection, but decline with prolonged viral suppression. *Nat Med* 1999; **5**: 518–25

31 Stellbrink HJ, Zoller B, Fenner T *et al*. Rapid plasma virus and CD4+ T-cell turnover in HIV-1 infection: evidence for an only transient interruption by treatment. *AIDS* 1996; **10**: 849–57

32 Youle M, Janossy G, Turnbull W *et al*. Changes in CD4 lymphocyte counts after interruption of therapy in patients with viral failure on protease inhibitor-containing regimens. *AIDS* 2000; **14**: 1717–20

33 Orenstein J, Bhat N, Yoder C *et al*. Rapid activation of lymph nodes upon interrupting HAART in HIV-infected patients following prolonged viral suppression. *7th Conference on Retroviruses and Opportunistic Infections*. San Francisco, CA, USA, 2000; Abstract #358

34 Carcelain G, Tubiana R, Mollet L *et al*. Intermittent interruptions of antiretroviral therapy in chronically HIV-infected patients do not induce immune control of HIV. *7th Conference on Retroviruses and Opportunistic Infections*. San Francisco, CA, USA, 2000; Abstract #356

35 Palella FJ, Delaney KM, Moorman AC *et al*. Declining morbidity and mortality among patients with advanced human immunodeficiency virus infection. HIV Outpatient Study Investigators. *N Engl J Med* 1998; **338**: 853–60

36 French M. Antiretroviral therapy immune restoration disease in HIV-infected patients on HAART. *AIDS Reader* 1999; **9**: 548–62

37 Finzi D, Blankson J, Siliciano J *et al*. Latent infection of CD4+ T cells provides a mechanism for lifelong persistence of HIV-1, even in patients on effective combination therapy. *Nat Med* 1999; **5**: 512–7

38 Pantaleo G. How immune-based interventions can change HIV therapy. *Nat Med* 1997; **3**: 483–6

39 Emery S, Lane HC. Immune-based therapies in HIV infection: recent developments. *AIDS* 1996; **10 (Suppl A)**: S159–63

40 Davey R, Chaitt D, Albert J *et al*. A randomised trial of high- versus low-dose subcutaneous interleukin-2 outpatient therapy for early HIV-1 infection. *J Infect Dis* 1999; **179**: 849–58

41 Youle M, Fisher M, Nelson M *et al*. Randomised study of intermittent subcutaneous IL-2 therapy without antiretrovirals versus no treatment. *XIII International AIDS Conference*. Durban, South Africa, 2000; Abstract #LbOr028

42 Chun T, Engel D, Mizell S *et al*. Effect of interleukin-2 on the pool of latently infected, resting CD4+ T cells in HIV-1-infected patients receiving HAART. *Nat Med* 1999; **5**: 651–5

43 Kedzierska K, Mak J, Mijch A *et al*. Granulocyte macrophage colony stimulating factor augments phagocytosis of *Mycobacterium avium* complex by HIV-1 infected monocytes/macrophages *in vitro* and *in vivo*. *J Infect Dis* 2000; **181**: 390–4

44 Imami N, Hardy G, Nelson M *et al*. Induction of HIV-1-specific T cell responses by administration of cytokines in late-stage patients receiving HAART. *Clin Exp Immunol* 1999; **118**: 78–86

45 Tan R, Xu X, Ogg G *et al*. Rapid death of adoptively transferred T cells in acquired immunodeficiency syndrome. *Blood* 1999; **93**: 1506–10

46 Hoff R, McNamara J. Therapeutic vaccines for preventing AIDS: their use with HAART. *Lancet* 1999; **353**: 1723–4

47 Schooley R, Spino C, Kuritzkes D *et al*. Two double-blind, randomised, comparative trials of 4 HIV-1 envelope vaccines in HIV-1-infected individuals across a spectrum of disease severity: AIDS clinical trials groups 209 and 214. *J Infect Dis* 2000; **182**: 1357–64

48 Gotch F, Hardy G, Imami N. Therapeutic vaccines in HIV-1 infection. *Immunol Rev* 1999; **170**: 173–82

49 Moss R, Wallace M, Giermakowska W *et al*. Phenotypic analysis of HIV-1 cell-mediated immune responses after treatment with an HIV-1 Immunogen. *J Infect Dis* 1999; **180**: 641–8

50 Kahn J, Weng Cherng D, Mayer K, Murray H, Lagakos S. Evaluation of HIV-1 Immunogen, an immunologic modifier, administered to patients infected with HIV having 300 to 549 x 106/l CD4 cell counts. *JAMA* 2000; **284**: 2193–202

51 Sandstrom E, Wahren B. Therapeutic immunisation with recombinant gp160 in HIV-1 infection: a randomised double-blind placebo-controlled trial. *Lancet* 1999; **353**: 1735–42

52 Rosenberg ES, Billingsley JM, Caliendo AM *et al*. Vigorous HIV-1-specific CD4[+] T cell responses associated with control of viremia. *Science* 1997; **278**: 1447–50

53 Barker E, Mackewicz C, Reyes-Teran G *et al*. Virological and immunological features of long-term HIV-infected individuals who have remained asymptomatic compared with those who have progressed to AIDS. *Blood* 1998; **92**: 3105–14

54 Gea-Banacloche J, Migueles S, Martino L *et al*. Maintenance of large numbers of virus-specific CD8[+] T cells in HIV-infected progressors and long-term nonprogressors. *J Immunol* 2000; **165**: 1082–92

Prospect of a prophylactic vaccine for HIV

T Hanke

MRC Human Immunology Unit, Institute of Molecular Medicine, John Radcliffe Hospital, Oxford, UK

Human immunodeficiency virus (HIV) continues to infect about 15,000 people every day, 90% of whom live in non-industrialised countries. So far, education programmes have only managed to slow, but not cease, the HIV spread, while powerful drug combinations are too costly and complex for the majority of HIV-infected people and in any case fail to clear HIV from the body. Under these circumstances, the best hope for controlling the HIV pandemic is the development of an effective prophylactic vaccine. With a series of new technologies and increased political and financial commitments, a growing momentum in the field of HIV-vaccine development promises exciting years ahead.

Without going into the details of the devastation that human immunodeficiency virus (HIV) infection and acquired immunodeficiency syndrome (AIDS) cause around the world, particularly in some non-industrialised countries, it is generally agreed that the best hope for halting the spread of HIV is the development of a safe, effective, accessible prophylactic vaccine. Indeed, vaccination remains the most effective method for prevention of infectious diseases since the sanitation of water and milk. Its success has been well illustrated by the world-wide eradication of smallpox and a control of a number of other infectious diseases in industrialised countries.

Despite a considerable effort, no effective vaccine against HIV is yet available. Isolation of HIV in 1983 triggered a phase of optimism and a belief that a vaccine would be available within the next 10 years. Without a real understanding of which immune responses are important for containing the HIV replication, researchers applied the 'good old' strategies. A period of frustration followed when it was realized that traditional immunization approaches of live attenuated or whole inactivated virus vaccines cannot be easily applied for HIV and that antibodies neutralizing primary HIV isolates were nearly impossible to induce. It is only recently that advances in molecular biology and basic HIV research have led to the development of novel promising strategies and renewed optimism among scientists that an effective vaccine against HIV is possible. These together with an increased awareness and commitment of the politicians, drive from organizations such as the International AIDS Vaccine Initiative and major financial injections from national

Correspondence to:
Dr T Hanke, MRC Human
Immunology Unit,
Institute of
Molecular Medicine,
John Radcliffe Hospital,
Oxford OX3 9DS, UK

governments, charities, foundations and generous individuals have created a feeling that the prospects for a development of a successful HIV vaccine have never been greater than now.

The HIV challenge

Scientifically, HIV is a fascinating virus. Unfortunately for the prevention, all the fascinating features of HIV put together make the development of vaccines extremely difficult. First, a successful HIV vaccine may have to induce both neutralizing antibody (nAb) and cell-mediated immunity, which is sometimes expressed more mysteriously as 'a barrier created by the sum of several immune defences'. This is because no clear single immunological correlate of protection has yet been identified. Second, HIV has a tropism for many cell types in the body including the very cells that play essential roles in eliciting and maintaining the immune responses such as CD4+ T-cells, macrophages and dendritic cells[1]. Third, HIV integrates into the host chromosome and can make at least some of the HIV-carrying cells invisible to the immune system. Fourth, HIV has multiple ways of transmission. The most common route is through a heterosexual contact, but it can be also passed from mother-to-child or reach the blood stream directly, thus bypassing all natural protective barriers against environmental micro-organisms. Moreover, HIV can be transmitted as both a cell-free virus and virus-infected cells. Fifth, even if an effective vaccine becomes available, total eradication of HIV will be complicated by an animal reservoir of SIV in feral chimps and African monkeys, from which multiple independent transmissions to humans have been documented[2]. Finally, HIV evades effectively both humoral and cellular immune responses. This is mainly due to a high antigenic variability facilitated by a combination of an error-prone reverse transcriptase (10^{-4} per base), recombination between the diploid HIV genome during reverse transcription, and a high replication rate (10^9 new virions per day in an infected individual) even during the asymptomatic phase of infection. Also, other sophisticated strategies that HIV employs contribute to the immune evasion.

Thus, the structure of the HIV envelope glycoprotein protects effectively HIV from neutralization by antibodies[3]. In viral and cellular membranes, the envelope forms a trimer of gp120–gp41 heterodimers, which is mediated by the interaction between the most conserved surfaces on the heterodimers. This makes these conserved regions on the virus inaccessible, while the exposed areas are highly variable and masked by bulky polysaccharide structures. The CD4-binding site is buried deep in the molecule and can be more easily reached by the extended CD4 loop than the complementarity-determining regions of antibodies. The chemokine co-receptor-binding site is hidden and becomes available only after the gp120 interaction with the CD4 receptor. Both of these sites are guarded by flexible V1, V2 and V3 loops with highly variable amino acid sequences, which obscure the neutralization epitopes and contribute to the inefficiency of affinity maturation of the antibody responses. In summary, the biggest problem of neutralization is reaching the neutralizing epitopes on HIV by antibodies.

There is much more hope in killing of HIV-infected cells by CTL, but it is not without challenges either[4]. A quick accumulation of mutations cause an escape from the CTL by altering epitopes so that they either cannot be recognized or antagonize the index peptide-specific responses. Down-regulation of MHC class I molecules was described, although this may be insufficient to prevent CTL killing. A selective loss of HIV-specific T cell responses may occur through exhaustion, anergy and up-regulation of Fas ligand (CD95L) on HIV infected cells, which may induce apoptosis in approaching CTL.

All these mechanisms come down to a single fact: HIV persists in the face of vigorous anti-HIV immune responses, which do abate the initial viraemia, but in a vast majority of cases fail to clear the virus from the body or provide a life-long protection from progression to AIDS. Therefore, a successful vaccination strategy has to train the immune system to respond faster and/or elicit qualitatively or quantitatively better immune responses than the natural HIV infection does. The immune response has to win the battle very early during the primary infection (Fig. 1; see below).

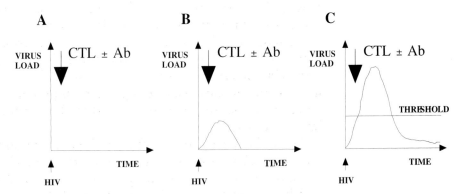

Fig. 1 Protective immune responses have to act very early to minimize HIV replication, generation of HIV variants and the damage which HIV inflicts. As a result of a successful vaccination, HIV is never detected in the body (A), only a transient replication occurs after which HIV is cleared (B), or the level of HIV viraemia is kept below the threshold of transmission and development of AIDS (C).

Light at the end of the HIV tunnel

Despite these multiple defences that HIV employs, observations and experimental data are accumulating which suggest that an immunological protection against the HIV infection is achievable. The identification of exposed seronegative/uninfected individuals with CTL responses against HIV raised the possibility that the CTL responses could have at least contributed to the prevention of infection[5]. The immunological bases of this protection was further supported[6] by the fact that re-exposure to HIV appeared necessary for maintaining the 'resistance'. Furthermore, in the SIV and HIV infections of non-human primates, complete resistance or partial protection has been achieved by an active immunization employing a series of vaccine modalities. Recently, promising subunit vaccine approaches inducing protection are on the increase[7-11].

Aims of a preventive vaccine

Ideally, the goal of an effective prophylactic vaccine is to prevent HIV infection or induce so-called 'sterilizing immunity' so that, after exposure, the virus is never detected in the body. However, most vaccines in use today work by preventing disease symptoms rather than the infection itself. For HIV, sterilizing immunity may not be an achievable objective either. Rather, vaccination may aim at elicitation of such an immunity that allows a limited and transient virus replication, after which the virus is cleared from the body, there are no signs of disease and no transmission to other individuals. Alternatively, a potentially successful vaccine may induce immune responses that decrease the primary viraemia and suppress virus load to levels so low, that both progression to AIDS and transmission are totally prevented (Fig. 1). Anything less would constitute a partial protection, but even a partially protective vaccine may be useful in some parts of the world. While in the industrialised countries, a prophylactic vaccine only delaying disease may not be that advantageous because of the highly active anti-retroviral therapy (HAART), vaccinated individuals infected with HIV in non-industrialised countries, *i.e.* without the possibility of HAART, may benefit enormously just from a substantial delay of the disease.

Importance of HIV clades

The significance of the genetic diversity among individual HIV isolates and its implication for vaccine design have been long debated. The predominant HIV-1 clade in Europe and North America is clade B, which is also the most studied one. In central and Eastern Africa, the predominant circulating HIV-1 strain is clade A, while clade C is dominating Southern Africa, India and China. Generally, a clade-specific vaccine design requires a more careful consideration for the induction of nAb than for CTL. Although there are some important inter-clade differences in CTL epitopes, many epitopes are conserved across-clades partially due to structure/function constraints[12]. However, to facilitate the interpretation of efficacy studies, vaccines should attempt to match the local strains prevalent in the trial population with the view that any successful approaches can be adapted for other clades if cross-protection is not achieved.

Non-human primate models of AIDS

Central to the development and preclinical evaluation of new vaccine strategies is the use of suitable animal models. They allow the assessment in a relatively faster and cheaper way the basic safety, immunogenicity and in some instances efficacy of new vaccines, and provide a platform for a more effective planning of clinical trials. Infection of non-human primates with immunodeficiency viruses offers a spectrum of models in terms of difficulty in preventing virus infection and severity of disease. These models range from the non-pathogenic infection of chimpanzees with HIV-1 SF2, in which a protection is achieved relatively easily, to infection of rhesus macaques with simian immunodeficiency virus (SIV)mac, which usually causes AIDS within the first year after infection and in which protection is much harder to obtain[13]. Infection of humans with HIV-1 lies somewhere in the middle and it still remains to be determined which of the above models are the most useful ones and for what, *i.e.* immunopathology, vaccine immunogenicity, protection against infection or disease, and determination of protection correlates. While a vaccine-induced immunity is enormously encouraging, the interpretation of a failed protection is less clear. First, to establish an infection in all of a small number of control animals, monkey challenge doses are at least 100-fold higher than the estimated HIV doses infecting humans and, second, the challenge viruses are usually more pathogenic. Thus, a vaccine protecting monkeys against an experimental SIV challenge may not have any protective effect in humans, while an immunogenic vaccine failing to protect monkeys may still be beneficial for people. Therefore, a 'fine-tuning' of immunogenicity in, and/or protection of, monkeys may be a useful exercise only as far as providing a starting basis for clinical trials; the final optimization of vaccination parameters for humans will have to be carried out in humans. In essence, certain level of vaccine immunogenicity in non-human primates should be the necessary condition and sufficient drive for testing that approach in humans. For such vaccines, the bridging process between the laboratory and clinic should be facilitated and accelerated. (A near complete list of all monkey challenge experiments is published biennially[14].)

Live attenuated vaccines

Live attenuated vaccines have undergone an extensive evaluation in non-human primates. Studies showed that it was possible to engineer viruses with mutations in several genes, all of which to some degree attenuated the virus and provided a protection against infection greater than other vaccine strategies[15]. However, most attenuated viruses retained pathogenicity and caused AIDS in both adult (after a long incubation period) and new-born monkeys[16]. Also, detection of virulent revertants in monkeys originally immunized with *nef*-deletion mutants may signal that this protection is not always complete[17]. In humans, several subjects in a small group of patients, the Sydney Blood Bank Cohort, experienced a decline in the CD4+ T-cell counts after about 12 years of infection with a *nef*-deleted virus and several developed AIDS[18]. Thus, the development of a safe attenuated HIV vaccine, which replicates sufficiently to confer protection, seems remote. Furthermore, the advent of a number of very safe technologies, which can induce good immune responses, may make the deployment of a potentially lethal preventive vaccine very difficult to justify.

Whole killed vaccines

Whole killed vaccines are non-infectious non-replicating virus particles that have been used successfully as vaccines for other infections such as polio, mumps, influenza and typhoid fever. As AIDS vaccines, inactivated SIV showed some promise in the SIV monkey model. However, while there is no doubt that HIV can be safely inactivated, these vaccines are relatively inefficient in the induction of both neutralizing antibodies and particularly CTL.

Subunit vaccines

Subunit vaccines represent a more rational approach to the vaccine development, which for practical, safety and immunogenicity reasons is almost certain to be favoured for AIDS vaccines to attenuated or whole inactivated HIV preparations[19]. Conceptually, subunit vaccines are

Table 1 Most commonly studied vehicles for genetic vaccines

DNA-based vaccines	Plasmid DNA
Live bacterial vectors	*Mycobacteria*
	Salmonella
	Listeria monocytogenes
	Shigella
Live viral vectors	Retroviruses
	Adeno-associated virus
	Adenoviruses
	Alphaviruses
	Sindbis virus
	Semliki forest virus
	Venezuelan equine encephalitis virus
	Poxviruses
	Modified vaccinia virus Ankara
	NYVAC
	ALVAC
	Fowlpox virus
	Herpes simplex virus

composed of up to three major components: (i) the compulsory **immunogen**, which is an HIV-derived molecule, most frequently and especially for CTL a protein, to which the immune responses are directed; (ii) a **vaccine vehicle**, which is a carrier facilitating the delivery of the immunogen or its gene to the host's body; and (iii) an optional **immunomodulator**, which can be a molecule, signal or adjuvant, often an integral part of the vehicle, modulating the induction of immune responses in terms of type, potency and longevity. While the immunogen defines vaccine specificity and provides a basic level of 'intrinsic' immunogenicity, vaccine vehicles and immunomodulators help to optimize the elicitation of immune responses. Although many processes involved in the induction of immune responses are currently unknown, it is very likely that the immunogenicities of subunit vaccines are in great part determined by the choice of a vaccine vehicle (Table 1) and route of administration.

Furthermore, there is a growing body of data demonstrating that heterologous vaccine vehicles delivering a common immunogen in a sequential prime-boost protocol are more potent inducers of specific immune responses than single vaccine modalities[8,10,20–26]. It is intriguing that some vectors are better for priming and others for boosting. The reasons for the efficiency of the heterologous prime-boost strategies are not clear, but may have to do with: (i) different 'professional' antigen-presenting cells and processing pathways, to which the immunogens are introduced; (ii) focusing of immune responses to the immunogens by priming with simple vectors and boosting with more complex, but at the same time more immunogenic, ones; (iii) allowing for better affinity maturation by initial low level expression of immunogens from a non-complex vehicle; or (iv) inducing the desired Th1/Th2 cytokine milieu during the priming immunization. For the same reasons, certain combinations of vehicles more than others may induce longer-lasting immunological memory.

Antibody responses

As most vaccines currently in use work by inducing virus-neutralizing antibodies, also for the development of HIV vaccines the HIV envelope glycoprotein has been the immunogen of choice. Although some success was reported in inducing nAb against laboratory HIV strains, extreme difficulties with neutralizing primary isolates halted the progress in this area[27]. To date, only a few antibodies neutralizing a broad range of primary HIV isolates have been identified: two bind to the CD4-binding-site and 2G12 epitopes on gp120, and one recognizes the 2F5 epitope on gp41[28].

Nevertheless, approaches focusing on the induction of a strong HIV nAb response continue to be a high priority research area. A vaccine utilizing monomeric HIV gp120 is the only AIDS vaccine so far that has reached phase III efficacy trials in humans. Although the outcome of these trials will not be known for several years, the expectation are low due to the results of phases I and II. In these trials, vaccinees have developed little, if any, antibodies capable of neutralizing field HIV isolates and no differences were observed in breakthrough infections between placebo- and vaccine-immunized subjects[29]. Various other approaches under investigation include the use of gp160 and gp140 oligomers, variable loop deletion mutants, stabilized gp120–gp41 subunits, *env* deglycosylation mutants, envelopes from CD4-independent viruses, gp120–ligand complexes, fusion-competent antigens, gp41 peptides and envelops presented on a carrier which facilitates trimer formation[28]. Many of these strategies are novel and promising, although they may not solve the main problem of accessibility, *i.e.* even if neutralizing antibodies were generated by active immunization, they might not readily reach the neutralizing epitopes on HIV which they recognize. This was reflected in experiments passively transferring antibodies capable of HIV neutralization, in which sterilizing immunity was achieved, but only with very high concentrations which would be hard to achieve and maintain by active vaccination[30]. Moreover, there is a danger of inducing infection-enhancing antibodies. Studies demonstrated that sera neutralizing HIV at high titres (10^{-1} to 10^{-2}) may at lower concentrations (10^{-3} to 10^{-6}) increase its infectivity. Thus, induction of env-specific antibodies by vaccination may not be desirable at all, a possibility that should be resolved by the phase III trial of gp120. In any case, a reliable method for induction of antibodies neutralizing primary HIV isolates by active immunization is still awaited.

Cytotoxic T-lymphocyte responses

CTL are usually CD8[+] cells, which defend an organism against intracellular pathogens such as HIV. They do so through a recognition of 8–10 amino acid-long HIV-derived peptides, which the infected cells process and display on their surface. Upon recognition, CTLs kill virus-infected cells and thus limit the production of new virions, and secrete a variety of soluble factors that directly or indirectly contribute to the suppression of virus replication. Just like for antibodies, these effector functions are adaptive, require a cascade of specific molecular and cellular interactions for their generation, and display a long-term memory[31].

The immunological correlates of protection against HIV remain undefined, but a picture is emerging. While there is still only limited evidence from humans for a protective ability of neutralizing antibodies, compelling data from several laboratories point to the central role of CD8[+] CTL for containing viral replication in both acute and chronic simian and human immunodeficiency virus infections[32].

CTL and prevention of HIV infection

For a successful control of HIV replication, CTLs have to kill virus-infected cells before they shed new virions. The exact timing of the expression of the first viral proteins, *i.e.* susceptibility to CTL killing, and virus release may depend on the cell type and activation status. Thus, although *tat* and *nef* mRNAs were detected in H9 cells as early as 2–3 h postinfection, HIV-infected cells are generally believed to produce rev, tat and nef at about 8–12 h and release new viruses at about 24 h postentry. *In vitro*, this left enough time for CTL to kill HIV-infected cells before these produced new virions and inhibit HIV spread through a release of soluble factors. Therefore, *in vivo*, CTL may be able to clear the initial small number of infected cells before HIV establishes generalized infection. This might explain detection of HIV-specific CTL responses in exposed, but uninfected, commercial sex workers whose cells were fully susceptible to infection with HIV, in uninfected infants born to HIV-infected mothers and seronegative health care workers occupationally exposed to HIV-contaminated body fluids[5].

At the organism level, CTLs have to suppress HIV replication very early after transmission, which in turn can be done most efficiently by targeting the transmitting virus. The more HIV is allowed to replicate, the better chance it has to generate escape mutants and the bigger insult it delivers to the immune system, from which this may never recover completely[33]. In humans, many CTL responses and corresponding epitopes were identified during the asymptomatic phase of infection, *i.e.* weeks to years after the initial CTL response. It is almost by definition that the identified

CTLs were directed against viruses that had been unaffected by or escaped the initial immune responses. And even studies that looked at CTL during the acute HIV infection are likely to have missed the most important events[34]. In addition, analyses of the CTL-HIV interactions usually suffer from not knowing the sequences of the transmitting viruses. Thus, definition of the very first CTL responses induced by natural transmission may pave the way towards an effective prophylactic vaccine. It is in this area that the non-human primate models can become extremely useful as demonstrated by an elegant work, which pointed to the tat protein as being one of the first CTL targets *in vivo* imposing a selective pressure on HIV[35].

Another potential caveat of the current approaches lies in the fact that our knowledge of the CTL responses is based, with a few exceptions[36], on the circulating peripheral blood lymphocytes. However, as the most common route of HIV transmission is through a heterosexual contact, *i.e. via* mucosa, the early battle may not be won in the blood. Although there is a belief in a close correspondence between the blood, lymphoid organs and mucosal CTL, which is supported by limited reports mainly from primate models, a more comprehensive analysis of the mucosal CTL responses in man may have to await further technological advances.

The effectiveness of vaccination is going to be determined by several characteristics of the CTL population. First, the sheer numbers of vaccine-induced memory CTLs influence critically the head-start of the immune system[37], which may require regular boosts to stay above the protection threshold[6]. Second, the homing pattern of memory CTL effectors may affect the HIV control. Third, the specificity of CTL for the transmitting virus[35], proteins expressed early rather than late in the replication cycle[9,23,37], and epitopes derived from structurally constrained regions of proteins, which limits the generation of escape mutants, is likely to be important. Fourth, CTL responses against multiple epitopes may be required for the control of HIV replication[4]. Finally, the CTL success in the time-race with HIV may depend on the CTL killing efficiency, which is determined by, for example, their overall functionality, perforin load, T-cell-receptor affinity for MHC-peptide complexes, and surface density of Fas-ligand and other functional or auxiliary molecules.

Subunit vaccine challenge experiments in non-human primates

Protecting monkeys with semi-rationally designed subunit vaccines has been harder to achieve compared to vaccines based on live attenuated viruses. This is especially true for the early experiments when the knowledge of the HIV pathogenicity was limited. This situation may now be changing due to our increased understanding of the HIV–host interaction and more advanced vaccine vehicle technologies[19]. Thus, protection of macaques may depend of the route of immunization. Subunit DNA vaccines have protected chimpanzees from infection with HIV-1, but provided very limited protection of macaques against pathogenic SIV and non-pathogenic SIV/HIV chimera (SHIV)$_{HXBc2}$ challenges. A control of viraemia and prevention of clinical AIDS was achieved by a vaccine combined from three plasmids expressing gag, env and an IL-2/Ig fusion protein and was mediated by cellular immune responses[11]. Env protein boosting after DNA priming increased antibody, but not CTL responses and protected macaques against a non-pathogenic SHIV$_{HXBc2}$ challenge[20]. Trivalent modified vaccinia virus Ankara (MVA) immunization reduced post-challenge virus burden[38,39], recombinant vaccinia virus-based regimens gave some protection against an SIVmac challenge[37,40] and in a combination with DNA significantly decreased virus loads after infection[41]. Adjuvanted tat protein[9] and recombinant Semliki forest virus priming followed by MVA boosting delivering tat and rev[23] protected macaques against pathogenic challenges with SHIV$_{89.6PD}$ and SIVmacJ5, respectively. A containment of challenge infections by subunit vaccines was also achieved by DNA prime-recombinant fowlpox boost vaccinations, which held non-pathogenic HIV[8] and non-pathogenic SHIV$_{IIIB}$[10] below the level of detection.

Candidate HIV vaccines in clinical trials

There has been about 30 different types of vaccine candidates tested in about 60 clinical trials involving about 5000 HIV-uninfected volunteers (http://www.scharp.org/public/home.htm).

In terms of formulations, the candidate HIV vaccines taken into the phase I studies include peptides mostly corresponding to gp120 V3 loop, but also gag- and nef-derived lipopeptides, yeast transposon-derived Ty virus-like particles carrying p17/p24, DNA-based vaccines, recombinant vaccinia virus, ALVAC (canarypox virus) and *Salmonella typhi* of which the last two vaccines are tested in a combination with monomeric env protein boosts. The majority of these vaccines employed HIV clade B immunogens. New trials are in the pipeline of recombinant MVA leading to a DNA prime-MVA boost protocol, Venezuelan equine encephalitis virus and a novel *Salmonella* vector, all using clade A or C immunogens[26,42]. The vast majority of the above strategies attempt to induce nAb, about half of the studies also include other than env HIV proteins and only a few focus solely on the elicitation of CTL. Recombinant monomeric gp120 protein and ALVAC vectors have reached phase II trials and adjuvanted monomeric gp120 from clades B and E is the only HIV vaccine candidate that has been taken as far as phase III efficacy trials.

So far, the reported immunogenicities in humans of the above vaccines have been unimpressive. Nevertheless, these studies have provided a 'baseline' for new technologies including novel immunogens for induction of neutralizing antibodies, and early proteins, better vaccine vehicles and their combinations for induction of CTL, which showed promise in non-human primate models.

Therapeutic vaccines

Similar immunogenic strategies as employed for a prophylactic vaccine may be used for immunotherapy of HIV-infected individuals. As the replication fitness of HIV within an individual does not correspond directly to the efficiency of transmission, *i.e.* there appears to be a certain transmission 'bottleneck', therapeutic vaccines may require a different set of immunogens and possibly vaccine vehicles for an optimal induction of both humoral and cell-mediated immune responses. Also, therapeutic vaccines may have to be used together with HAART to suppress HIV replication resulting from immune activation.

Perspectives

So what is the prospect of a prophylactic vaccine for HIV? Providing that scientists can outsmart 10,000 nucleotides (the size of the HIV genome), the collection of all the safety, immunogenicity and efficacy data necessary for a deployment of a successful HIV vaccine may still take up to 10 years. The final delivery of an effective vaccine to the people who need it the most and in as short a time as possible will require intense international commitment, collaboration and co-ordination in areas such as preparedness for and management of clinical trials, trial ethics concerning (*e.g.* inclusion of placebo groups and the level of care offered to volunteers infected in the course of the trials), agreements on the intellectual property rights, product manufacture and price. Although vaccine research is an inherently slow process, the recently acquired scientific and political momentum has put the HIV vaccine development back on the road, possibly on a motorway.

References

1   Levy JA. *HIV and the Pathogenesis of AIDS*. Washington, DC: American Society for Microbiology, 1998 or www.amazon.com
2   Hahn BH, Shaw GM, De Cock KM *et al*. AIDS as a zoonosis: scientific and health implications. *Science* 2000; **287**: 607–14
3   Sattentau QJ. HIV gp120: double lock strategy foils host defences. *Structure* 1998; **6**: 945–9

4   McMichael A. T cell responses and viral escape. *Cell* 1998; **93**: 673–6

5   Rowland-Jones SL, McMichael A. Immune responses in HIV-exposed seronegatives: have they repelled the virus? *Curr Opin Immunol* 1995; **7**: 448–55

6   Kaul R, Kimani J, Dong T *et al.* Late seroconversion in HIV 'resistant' Nairobi prostitutes is associated with a preceding decrease in HIV exposure [abstract 489]. In: *Program and Abstracts of the 7th Conference on Retroviruses and Opportunistic Infections.* San Francisco, CA: Foundation for Retrovirology and Human Health, 2000; 168

7   Boyer JD, Ugen KE, Wang B *et al.* Protection of chimpanzees from high-dose heterologous HIV-1 challenge by DNA vaccination. *Nat Med* 1997; **3**: 526–32

8   Kent SJ, Zhao A, Best SJ *et al.* Enhanced T-cell immunogenicity and protective efficacy of a human immunodeficiency virus type 1 vaccine regimen consisting of consecutive priming with DNA and boosting with recombinant fowlpox virus. *J Virol* 1998; **72**: 10180–8

9   Cafaro A, Caputo A, Fracasso C *et al.* Control of SHIV-89.6P infection of cynomologus monkeys by HIV-1 Tat protein vaccine. *Nat Med* 1999; **5**: 643–50

10   Robinson HL, Montefiori DC, Johnson RP *et al.* Neutralizing antibody-independent containment of immunodeficiency virus challenges by DNA priming and recombinant pox virus booster immunizations. *Nat Med* 1999; **5**: 526–34

11   Barouch DH, Santra S, Schmitz JE *et al.* Control of viremia and prevention of clinical AIDS in rhesus monkeys by cytokine-augmented DNA vaccination. *Science* 2000; **290**: 486–92

12   Goulder PJR, Rowland-Jones SL, McMichael AJ *et al.* Anti-HIV cellular immunity: recent advances towards vaccine design. *AIDS* 1999; **13 (Suppl A)**: S121–36

13   Hu SL. Recombinant subunit vaccines against primate lentiviruses. *AIDS Res Hum Retroviruses* 1996; **12**: 451–3

14   Warren JT, Levinson MA. AIDS preclinical vaccine development: biennial survey of HIV, SIV, and SHIV challenge studies in vaccinated nonhuman primates. *J Med Primatol* 1999; **28**: 249–73

15   Mills J, Desrosiers R, Rud E *et al.* Live attenuated HIV vaccines: a proposal for further research and development. *AIDS Res Hum Retroviruses* 2000; **16**: 1453–61

16   Ruprecht RM. Live attenuated AIDS viruses as vaccines: promise or peril? *Immunol Rev* 1999; **170**: 135–49

17   Whatmore AM, Cook N, Hall GA *et al.* Repair and evolution of nef *in vivo* modulates simian immunodeficiency virus virulence. *J Virol* 1995; **69**: 5117–23

18   Learmont JC, Geczy AF, Mills J *et al.* Immunologic and virologic status after 14 and 18 years of infection with an attenuated strain of HIV-1: a report from the Sydney Blood Bank Cohort. *N Engl J Med* 1999; **340**: 1715–22

19   Hanke T. Vehicles for genetic vaccines against human immunodeficiency virus: induction of T cell-mediated immune responses. *Curr Mol Med* 2001; **1**: 123–35

20   Letvin NL, Montefiori DC, Yasutomi Y *et al.* Potent, protective anti-HIV immune responses generated by bimodal HIV envelope DNA plus protein vaccination. *Proc Natl Acad Sci USA* 1997; **94**: 9378–83

21   Hanke T, Blanchard TJ, Schneider J *et al.* Enhancement of MHC class I-restricted peptide-specific T cell induction by a DNA prime/MVA boost vaccination regime. *Vaccine* 1998; **16**: 439–45

22   Schneider J, Gilbert SC, Blanchard TJ *et al.* Enhanced immunogenicity for CD8+ T cell induction and complete protective efficacy of malaria DNA vaccination by boosting with modified vaccinia virus Ankara. *Nat Med* 1998; **4**: 397–402

23   Osterhaus AD, van Baalen CA, Gruters RA *et al.* Vaccination with Rev and Tat against AIDS. *Vaccine* 1999; **17**: 2713–4

24   Hanke T, Samuel RV, Blanchard TJ *et al.* Effective induction of simian immunodeficiency virus-specific cytotoxic T lymphocytes in macaques by using a multiepitope gene and DNA prime-modified vaccinia virus Ankara boost vaccination regimen. *J Virol* 1999; **73**: 7524–32

25   Allen TM, Vogel TU, Fuller DH *et al.* Induction of AIDS virus-specific CTL activity in fresh, unstimulated peripheral blood lymphocytes from rhesus macaques vaccinated with a DNA prime/modified vaccinia virus Ankara boost regimen. *J Immunol* 2000; **164**: 4968–78

26   Hanke T and McMichael AJ. Design and construction of an experimental HIV-1 vaccine for a year-2000 clinical trial in Kenya. *Nat Med* 2000; **6**: 951–5

27   Burton DR, Moore JP. Why do we not have an HIV vaccine and how can we make one? *Nat Med* 1998; **4**: 495–8

28   Sattentau QJ, Moulard M, Brivet B *et al*. Antibody neutralization of HIV-1 and the potential for vaccine design. *Immunol Lett* 1999; **66**: 143–9

29   Connor RI, Korber BT, Graham BS *et al*. Immunological and immunological analyses of persons infected by human immunodeficiency virus type 1 while participating in trials of recombinant gp120 subunit vaccines. *J Virol* 1998; **72**: 1552–76

30   Moore JP, Burton DR. HIV-1 neutralizing antibodies: how full is the bottle? *Nat Med* 1999; **5**: 204–16

31   McMichael AJ, Ogg G, Wilson J *et al*. Memory CD8⁺ T cells in HIV infection. *Philos Trans R Soc Lond B Biol Sci* 2000; **355**: 363–7

32   Hanke T, McMichael AJ. Role for cytotoxic T lymphocytes in protection against HIV infection and AIDS. In: Wong-Staal F, Gallo RC. (eds) *AIDS Vaccine Research in Perspective*. New York: Marcel Dekker, 2001: In press

33   Rosenberg ES, Altfeld M, Poon SH *et al*. Immune control of HIV-1 after early treatment of acute infection. *Nature* 2000; **407**: 523–6

34   Walker BD, Goulder PJ. AIDS. Escape from the immune system. *Nature* 2000; **407**: 313–4

35   Allen TM, O'Connor DH, Jing P *et al*. Tat-specific cytotoxic T lymphocytes select for SIV escape variants during resolution of primary viremia. *Nature* 2000; **407**: 386–90

36   Kaul R, Plummer FA, Kimani J *et al*. HIV-1-specific mucosal CD8⁺ lymphocyte responses in the cervix of HIV-1-resistant prostitutes in Nairobi. *J Immunol* 2000; **164**: 1602–11

37   Gallimore A, Cranage M, Cook N *et al*. Early suppression of SIV replication by CD8⁺ nef-specific cytotoxic T cells in vaccinated animals. *Nat Med* 1995; **1**: 1167–73

38   Hirsch VM, Fuerst TR, Sutter G *et al*. Patterns of viral replication correlate with outcome in simian immunodeficiency virus (SIV)-infected macaques: effect of prior immunization with a trivalent SIV vaccine in modified vaccinia virus Ankara. *J Virol* 1996; **70**: 3741–52

39   Seth A, Ourmanov I, Schmitz JE *et al*. Immunization with a modified vaccinia virus expressing simian immunodeficiency virus (SIV) Gag-Pol primes for an anamnestic Gag-specific cytotoxic T-lymphocyte response and is associated with reduction of viremia after SIV challenge. *J Virol* 2000; **74**: 2502–9

40   Daniel MD, Mazzara GP, Simon MA *et al*. High-titer immune responses elicited by recombinant vaccinia virus priming and particle boosting are ineffective in preventing virulent SIV infection. *AIDS Res Hum Retroviruses* 1994; **10**: 839–51

41   Fuller DH, Simpson L, Cole KS *et al*. Gene gun-based nucleic acid immunization alone or in combination with recombinant vaccinia vectors suppresses virus burden in rhesus macaques challenged with a heterologous SIV. *Immunol Cell Biol* 1997; **75**: 389–96

Index

Ischemic heart disease: therapeutic issues

Scientific Editors: Anthony Gershlick and Simon Davies